STUDY GUIDE *to accompany*

POTTER • PERRY

Fundamentals *of* *Nursing*

CONCEPTS, PROCESS, AND PRACTICE

FOURTH EDITION

GERALYN OCHS, RN, BSN, MSN
Instructor
School of Nursing
Saint Louis University
St. Louis, Missouri

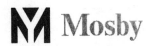 Mosby

St. Louis Baltimore Boston Carlsbad Chicago Naples New York Philadelphia Portland
London Madrid Mexico City Singapore Sydney Tokyo Toronto Wiesbaden

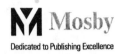

Mosby
Dedicated to Publishing Excellence

A Times Mirror
Company

Vice President and Publisher   Nancy L. Coon
Senior Editor   Susan Epstein
Senior Developmental Editor   Beverly J. Copland
Project Manager   John Rogers
Senior Production Editor   Lavon Wirch Peters
Book Design   Amy Buxton
Manufacturing Manager   Theresa Fuchs

Printed in the United States of America
Composition by Top Graphics
Printing/binding by Plus Communications

Mosby–Year Book, Inc.
11830 Westline Industrial Drive
St. Louis, Missouri 63146

International Standard Book Number 0-8151-4656-6

96 97 98 99 00 / 9 8 7 6 5 4 3 2 1

PREFACE

This Study Guide to accompany the fourth edition of *Fundamentals of Nursing* has been developed to encourage independent learning for beginning nursing students. As you begin to read the text, you may be struck by the difference in style or format from other books you've used in the past; the terms are new, and the focus of content is different. You may be wondering, "How will I possibly learn all the material in this chapter?" The essential objective of this Study Guide is to assist you in this endeavor—to help you learn **what** you need to know and then self-test from more than 500 review questions.

This Study Guide follows the text chapter for chapter. Whatever chapter your instructor assigns, you will use the same chapter number in this Study Guide. The outline format was designed to help you learn to read nursing content more effectively and with greater understanding. Each chapter of this Study Guide has the following sections to assist you to comprehend and recall.

The Preliminary Reading section is designed to teach prereading strategies. You need to become familiar with the chapter by first reading the chapter title, the key concepts and key terms (found at the end of each chapter), and all headings, as well as reviewing all photographs, drawings, tables, and boxes. This can be done rather quickly and will give you an overall idea of the content of the chapter.

The Comprehensive Understanding section is next and is in outline format. This will prove to be a very valuable tool not only as you first read the chapter but also as you review for tests. This outline identifies the topics and main ideas of each chapter as an aid to concentration, comprehension, and retaining textbook information. By completing this outline you will learn to "pull-out" key information in the chapter. As you write the answers in the Study Guide, you will be reinforcing that content. Once completed this outline will serve as a review tool for exams.

The Review Questions in each chapter provide an invaluable means of testing and reinforcing your knowledge of the material read and the answers written in the outline. Each question is multiple-choice and written in the NCLEX format. As a further aid for independent learning, each answer requires a rationale (the reason **why** the option you selected is correct). After you have completed the review questions, you can check the answers in the back of the Study Guide. Page references for rationales are also provided.

For the clinical chapters, Chapters 27-49, a special feature has been added to help you learn to apply your knowledge to clinical practice. The Clinical Situations present real-life scenarios to give you practice in thinking about how to handle clients. Answers are also included at the end of the Study Guide to provide immediate feedback about these situations.

When you finish answering the review questions and clinical situations, take a few minutes for self-evaluation. If you answered a question incorrectly, begin to analyze the thoughts that led you to the wrong answer:

- Did you miss the key word or key phrase?
- Did you read into the question something that wasn't stated?
- Did you not understand the subject matter?
- Did you use an incorrect rationale for selecting your response?

Each incorrect response is an opportunity to learn. Go back to the text and reread any content that is still unclear. In the long run, it will be a time-saving activity and you will complete the semester with a firm understanding of nursing concepts that you can rely on all of your professional career.

To my husband, Jim, for his quiet, reassuring strength and
his generous gift of time.

To my children, Shannon, Patrick, Luke, and Caitlin,
whose love has reshaped my life.
Each day with you is more precious than the one before.

CONTENTS

Chapter 1 | Health-Illness Continuum

Viewing health as an either-or situation ignores the health-illness continuum. In the approaching twenty-first century, health will be viewed from a broader perspective.

PRELIMINARY READING

Chapter 1, pp. 2-20

COMPREHENSIVE UNDERSTANDING

∎ HEALTHY PEOPLE 2000

➤ Healthy People 2000 focuses on three broad public health goals for Americans. List them.

a. _____

b. _____

c. _____

∎ DEFINITION OF HEALTH

➤ Define *health*: _____

_____

➤ The WHO definition of health promotes a positive concept of health. Identify the characteristics.

a. _____

_____

_____

b. _____

_____

_____

c. _____

_____

_____

➤ The individual adapts to changes in internal and external environments to maintain a state of well-being. State examples of each.

a. Internal environmental factors: _____

_____

_____

_____

b. External environmental factors: _____

_____

_____

_____

∎ MODELS OF HEALTH AND ILLNESS

➤ Health and illness are complex concepts. Models are used to understand the relationships between these concepts and the client's attitudes toward health and health practices.

➤ Health beliefs usually cause health behavior. They can positively or negatively affect a client's level of health. Identify practices of each behavior.

a. Positive health behavior: _____

_____

b. Negative health behavior: _____

_____

➤ Models represent different ways of approaching complex issues and understanding a client's attitudes and values about health and illness.

Health-Illness Continuum

➤ Define the health-illness continuum model:

_____

_____

_____

➤ Identify advantages and disadvantages of this model.

a. Advantages: _____

_____

b. Disadvantages: _____

_____

High-Level Wellness Model

➤ This model describes health as an integrated method of functioning and is oriented at maximizing an individual's potential.

➤ Identify the three major components of this model.

a. _____

_____

b. _____

_____

c. _____

_____

➤ Identify the client population(s) for whom this model could be used to ensure effective health care:

_____

_____

_____

▌ NURSE-CLIENT PARTNERSHIP

➤ In this model nurses using the nursing process consider clients the ultimate experts regarding their own

health and _____

_____

_____

_____.

Agent-Host-Environment Model

➤ According to this model, the level of health or illness of an individual or group depends on the dynamic relationship of the agent, host, and environment.
➤ Define the following:

Agent _____

_____

Host _____

_____

Environment _____

_____

Health-Belief Model

➤ The health-belief model demonstrates the relationship between a person's belief and behavior.
➤ Identify the three components of this model.

a. _____

b. _____

c. _____

Health-Promotion Model

➤ The focus of this model is to explain the reasons that individuals engage in health activities.
➤ Identify the three functions on which this model focuses.

a. _____

b. _____

c. _____

▌ VARIABLES INFLUENCING HEALTH BELIEFS AND PRACTICES

➤ Internal and external variables can influence how a person thinks and acts. Understanding the way in which these variables affect a client allows the nurse to plan and deliver individualized care.

Internal Variables

➤ Internal variables include a person's developmental stage, intellectual background, perception of personal functioning, and emotional and spiritual factors. Identify and cite a personal example of how each of the following internal variables affects the client's health belief and practices:

a. Developmental stage _____

_____

_____

b. Intellectual background _____

_____

_____

c. Perception of functioning _____

_____

_____

d. Emotional and spiritual functioning _____

_____

_____

External Variables

➤ External variables influence a person's health beliefs and practices, including family practices, socioeconomic factors, and cultural variables. Identify and cite a personal example of how each of the following external variables affects the client's health belief and practices:

a. Family practices _____

_____

_____

b. Socioeconomic factors _____

_____

_____

c. Cultural background _____

_____

▋ HEALTH PROMOTION AND DISEASE PREVENTION

➤ Activities involving health promotion help clients maintain or enhance their present levels of health.

➤ Activities for illness prevention protect clients from actual or potential threats to health.

➤ The difference between the two involves _____

_____

and _____

_____ .

➤ There are passive and active strategies for health promotion. Give two examples of each.

Passive strategies: _____

_____

_____

Active strategies: _____

_____

_____

➤ The goal of a total health program is to _____

_____

_____

_____ .

➤ Give examples of the following practices or factors that affect health status:

Individual practices _____

_____

Physical stressors _____

_____

Psychological stressors _____

_____

Levels of Preventive Care

➤ Identify the health activities of each of the following levels of preventive care:

Primary _____

_____

_____

_____

_____

Secondary _____

_____

_____

_____

_____

Tertiary _____

_____

_____

_____

_____

▋ RISK FACTORS

➤ Define risk factor: _____

_____

➤ For each of the following categories, identify at least two risk factors:
Genetic and physiological factors _____

_____

_____

_____

Age _____

_____

_____

_____

Environment _____

_____

_____

_____

Life-style _____

_____

_____

_____

▋ ILLNESS AND ILLNESS BEHAVIOR

➤ Define the following:

Illness _____

_____

Illness behavior _____

_____

Variables Influencing Illness Behavior

➤ Give examples of the following:

Internal variables _____

_____

_____

External variables _____

_____

_____

REVIEW QUESTIONS

(The student should select the appropriate answer and cite the rationale for choosing that particular answer.)

1. Internal variables influencing health beliefs and practices include:
   a. Family practices and cultural background
   b. Socioeconomic factors and intellectual background
   c. Spiritual factors and developmental stage
   d. Cultural background and perception of functioning

   Answer ( ) Rationale: _____
   _____
   _____

2. An active health-promotion strategy would include:
   a. Fluoridating drinking water
   b. Fortifying milk with vitamin D
   c. Working in a smoke-free environment
   d. Beginning a weight-reduction program

   Answer ( ) Rationale: _____
   _____
   _____

3. Any variable increasing the vulnerability of an individual or a group to an illness or accident is a (an):
   a. Illness behavior
   b. Risk factor
   c. Negative health behavior
   d. Life-style determinant

   Answer ( ) Rationale: _____
   _____
   _____

4. All of the following characterize illness behavior except:
   a. Calling a physician
   b. Ignoring a physical symptom
   c. Interpreting physical symptoms
   d. Withdrawing from work activities

   Answer ( ) Rationale: _____
   _____
   _____

5. The term *high-level wellness* is best defined as:
   a. Being free of chronic disease
   b. Surviving beyond one's life expectancy
   c. Fluctuating on a wellness-illness continuum within the health spectrum
   d. Functioning at one's best biophysical level

   Answer ( ) Rationale: _____
   _____
   _____

6. A chemical plant had a malfunction. As a result, toxic fumes were emitted over a 10-mile area, causing nausea and vomiting in residents. The agent in this agent-host-environment model is:
   a. The chemical plant
   b. Toxic fumes
   c. Nausea and vomiting
   d. People living in the area

   Answer ( ) Rationale: _____
   _____
   _____

7. Marsha states, "My chubby size runs in our family. It's a glandular condition. Exercise and diet won't change things much." The nurse determines that this is an example of Marsha's:
   a. Acute situation
   b. Active strategy
   c. Positive health behavior
   d. Health beliefs

   Answer ( ) Rationale: _____
   _____
   _____

8. Which of the following nursing activities is an example of primary level preventive caregiving?
   a. Teaching Mrs. Cane to ambulate with her walker
   b. Calculating the correct insulin dosage for Mr. Harper
   c. Informing Mrs. Smith that immunizations for her new infant are available through the health department
   d. Arranging for a hospice nurse to visit with the family of a cancer patient

   Answer ( ) Rationale: _____
   _____
   _____

b. _____

_____

c. _____

_____

➤ Give two examples of illness-prevention activities.

a. _____

_____

b. _____

_____

Primary Care

➤ Primary care services involve the client directly and usually involve the client's first contact with a primary care provider. The focus is _____

_____ and

_____.

➤ Critical to the success of primary care is _____

_____ and

_____.

Diagnosis and Treatment

➤ These services can be delivered in primary care settings. However, once the client's condition becomes

more complicated, _____
care is needed.

➤ Identify the sites for acute secondary care.

a. _____

b. _____

c. _____

Rehabilitation

➤ Define *rehabilitation*: _____

_____.

➤ Services begin the moment a client enters the health care system. The initial focus of rehabilitation is

_____.

As the client's condition stabilizes, the focus is

_____

_____.

➤ Rehabilitation programs take place in:

a. _____

b. _____

c. _____

d. _____

Continuing Care

➤ Continuing care services offer clients ongoing supportive care for chronic, long-term health problems. This includes services for clients with physical disabilities as well as mental illness. Give two examples.

a. _____

b. _____

TYPES OF HEALTH CARE AGENCIES

Health care is provided in a variety of settings. With health care reform, fewer clients are cared for in hospitals.

Outpatient Agencies

➤ Outpatient services are directed at _____

_____ and

_____ care.

➤ Briefly explain the design of the following:

Physician's office _____

_____

_____

_____

Clinics _____

_____

_____

_____

Ambulatory care centers _____

_____

_____

_____

_____

Institutions

➤ Institutional agencies offer health care services to inpatients and outpatients.
➤ Clients who enter hospitals are acutely ill and need comprehensive and specialized tertiary health care. Define the following types of hospitals:

Public _____

_____

_____

Private _____

_____

_____

Military _____

_____

VA _____

_____

_____

➤ Subacute care units were designed for _____

_____

_____

_____.

➤ An extended care facility provides intermediate and long-term medical, nursing, or custodial care for clients recovering from acute and chronic illnesses or disabilities. Briefly explain the following three types of facilities:

Intermediate care _____

_____

_____

_____

Long-term care _____

_____

_____

_____

Residential community _____

_____

_____

_____

➤ Clients may enter psychiatric facilities voluntarily or involuntarily. Identify two emotional or behavioral problems that would require special counseling and treatment.

a. _____

b. _____

➤ Rehabilitation centers are a _____

_____.

Community-Based Agencies

➤ Community-based health care agencies focus on providing health care to clients within their neighborhoods. Explain how each of the following agencies provides health care, and give an example of each.

Adult day-care centers: _____

_____

_____

_____

Home health care agencies: _____

_____

_____

_____

Rural hospitals: _____

_____

_____

_____

Crisis intervention centers: _____

_____

_____

_____

Support Groups

➤ Support groups provide self-help services for clients with select health problems. Participants receive emotional support and information on ways to adjust to personal and health problems. Give two examples.

a. _____

b. _____

Volunteer Agencies

➤ Volunteer agencies are not-for-profit health care agencies established nationally or within a community to meet a specific need. Give two examples.

a. _____

b. _____

Hospices

➤ A hospice is a system of family-centered care designed to allow clients to live and remain at home with _____,

_____,

and _____,
while alleviating the strains caused by terminal illness.

➤ The focus of hospice care is _____

_____.

➤ The client entering a hospice has reached the ____

_____

phase of illness, and the _____,

_____,

and _____
have agreed that no further treatment can reverse
the disease process.

➤ Respite care provides _____

_____.

Government Agencies

➤ Give an example of each of the following agencies:

Local government _____

_____

State _____

_____

National _____

_____

■ HEALTH CARE DELIVERY ISSUES

➤ Health care delivery is changing in response to the
critical issues of health care reform. It is important
to understand the social factors that influence health
care delivery so that appropriate changes can be
made to create better ways of providing nursing care
and to develop new nursing roles.

Competency of Health Care Providers

➤ Identify the six critical competencies needed for
health professions by the year 2005.

a. _____

_____

b. _____

_____

c. _____

_____

d. _____

_____

e. _____

_____

f. _____

_____

Society and the Consumer's Movement

➤ Identify two societal trends that are occurring with
today's health care consumers.

a. _____

b. _____

New Knowledge and Technology

➤ Identify the three disadvantages of the current
knowledge explosion.

a. _____

b. _____

c. _____

Legal Issues and Ethics

➤ _____,_____,

and _____ health care
is an expectation of society. When this expectation is
not met, legal actions can be taken against caregivers.

■ THE CLIENT AND THE HEALTH CARE DELIVERY SYSTEM

➤ Clients entering the health care system have rights.
Identify them.

a. _____

b. _____

Right to Health Care

➤ Rising costs are requiring clients to assume more of the
financial burden for health care. How is this affecting

nursing? _____

_____

_____

_____

Rights within the System

➤ Define *informed consent:* _____

_____.

➤ Identify two committees that evaluate client suggestions and complaints about the delivery of health
care.

a. _____

b. _____

Entry into the System

➤ Identify the three common ways that clients enter
the health care system.

a. _____

b. _____

c. _____

■ FINANCING HEALTH CARE SERVICES

➤ Government agencies and private companies have developed a variety of prepaid health care, insurance, and social service programs to subsidize the cost of health care.

Private Insurance Plans

➤ Define *third-party reimbursements:* _____

_____

_____

_____

Managed Care Plans

➤ Identify the three reasons why managed care plans have been growing.

   a. _____

     _____

     _____

   b. _____

     _____

     _____

   c. _____

     _____

     _____

Long-Term Insurance

➤ Name the two plans that are beginning to identify coverage for long-term care.

   a. _____

   b. _____

U.S. Government Insurance Plans

➤ Briefly explain the following:

   Medicare _____

   _____

   _____

   _____

   Medicaid _____

   _____

   _____

   _____

   _____

Catastrophic health insurance _____

_____

_____

_____

_____

Canadian Government Health Insurance

➤ All citizens of Canada are covered by a mandatory program financed with tax dollars. However, unlike U.S. clients, Canadian clients may experience long waiting periods for elective procedures.

■ INNOVATIONS IN HEALTH CARE DELIVERY

➤ Nursing's Agenda for Health Care Reform (ANA, 1991) presented nursing recommendations for achieving immediate health care reform (see the box on p. 39).

Care Management and Critical Pathways

➤ Briefly identify the following:

   Care management _____

   _____

   _____

   _____

   CareMap _____

   _____

   _____

   _____

Case Management

➤ Define *case management:* _____

_____

_____

_____

Patient-Focused Care

➤ Define *patient-focused care:* _____

_____

_____

_____

Assistive Personnel

➤ Explain the rationale behind the use of assistive personnel in the delivery of care: _____

_____

_____

Advance Practice Nursing

➤ Advance practice nurses consist of

_____,

_____,

_____,

and _____.

➤ Identify some of the responsibilities of an APN:

_____

_____

_____

_____

Quality Improvement

➤ Define the following:

Quality assurance _____

_____

_____

Quality improvement _____

_____

_____

_____

REVIEW QUESTIONS

(The student should select the appropriate answer and cite the rationale for choosing that particular answer.)

1. Third-party payment for financing health care was introduced in the 1920s because:
   a. Affluent people could not afford quality health care
   b. Middle-class people could afford only home care
   c. Hospitals were successfully supported by patient payment
   ✓d. Hospitals were experiencing financial losses

Answer ( ) Rationale: _____

_____

_____

2. The federal law allowing nurse practitioners to deliver primary health care in underserved areas is the:
   ✓a. Rural Health Clinics Act
   ✓b. Hill-Burton Act
   c. National Health Planning and Resources Development Act
   d. Social Security Amendment Act of 1972

Answer ( ) Rationale: _____

_____

_____

3. Health promotion activities are designed to help clients:
   a. Reduce the risk of illness
   b. Maintain maximal function
   c. Promote habits related to health care
   ✓d. All of the above

Answer ( ) Rationale: _____

_____

_____

4. Illness prevention activities are designed to help clients:
   ✓a. Reduce risk factors
   b. Promote habits related to good health
   c. Manage stress
   d. Identify disease symptoms

Answer ( ) Rationale: _____

_____

_____

5. Rehabilitation services begin:
   ✓a. When the client enters the health care system
   b. After the client requests rehabilitation services
   c. After the client's physical condition stabilizes
   d. When the client is discharged from the hospital

Answer ( ) Rationale: _____

_____

_____

6. An example of an extended care facility is a:
   a. Home health agency
   b. Suicide prevention center
   c. State-owned psychiatric hospital
   ✓d. Nursing home

Answer ( ) Rationale: _____

_____

_____

7. An adult day-care center would be best for which of the following clients?
   ✓a. Mrs. Tindale is slightly confused, and her daughter works during the day.
   b. Mr. Valentino lives alone and has frequent shortness of breath requiring intervention.
   c. Baby Ann has frequent periods of seizures.
   d. Francis is severely psychotic and belligerent.

Answer ( ) Rationale: _____

_____

_____

8. A client and his or her family facing the end stages of a terminal illness might best be served by a:
   a. Rehabilitation center
   b. Extended care facility
   ✓c. Hospice
   d. Crisis intervention center

Answer ( ) Rationale: _____

_____

_____

9. The influence of the consumer on health care and its delivery has led to a demand for:
   ✓a. Knowledge and services to promote health and prevent illness
   b. More comfortable facilities
   c. Lower costs for health care
   d. More inpatient services

Answer ( ) Rationale: _____

_____

_____

10. Which feature is unique to the HMO?
    ✓a. The client receives services on a prepaid basis.
    b. Entrance is voluntary and free.
    c. The fee is based on service.
    d. The HMO assumes no risk.

Answer ( ) Rationale: _____

_____

_____

11. One important advantage of managed nursing care is:
    ✓a. Improved coordination of services by health care providers
    b. More emphasis on nursing care tasks
    c. Multiple plans for care are available
    d. The primary caregiver is the staff nurse

Answer ( ) Rationale: _____

_____

_____

Chapter 3 | Health Promotion and Primary Health Care

Health promotion involves behavior that helps prevent disease and protect health. Primary care is a personal health care system that provides for first contact, continuous, comprehensive, and coordinated care.

PRELIMINARY READING

Chapter 3, pp. 47-60

COMPREHENSIVE UNDERSTANDING

■ HEALTH PROMOTION AND DISEASE PREVENTION

➤ Nursing's role in health promotion within primary care settings has three main components. Name them.

a. _____

_____

b. _____

_____

c. _____

_____

Primary Prevention

➤ Primary prevention involves _____

and _____ .

Secondary Prevention

➤ Secondary prevention involves _____

_____

and _____ .

Tertiary Prevention

➤ Tertiary prevention involves _____

_____ .

■ PRIMARY HEALTH CARE

➤ Define *primary health care:* _____

_____

_____ .

➤ Identify some of the settings in which primary care is

delivered: _____

_____

Primary Care Environment

➤ Identify the areas about which the nurse needs to be knowledgeable to deliver care in the primary care en-

vironment: _____

_____

_____

_____

_____

_____

➤ Briefly explain how the following trends impact the primary care environment.

Demographic: _____

_____

_____

_____

Economic: _____

_____

_____

_____

Workforce: _____

_____

_____

_____

Society

➤ Healthy People 2000 includes _____,

_____, _____,

and _____,

and _____ needs.

Primary Care Delivery System

➤ Identify the community-based settings that compose

the primary care delivery system: _____

_____

_____

_____

_____

➤ Briefly explain the managed care model: _____

_____

_____

_____

_____

➤ The focus in the past has been on hospital-based or
private medical care settings (with the emphasis on
controlling overall health care costs). The focus now
is shifting to community-based and primary care settings.

Primary Health Care Providers

➤ Identify the competencies needed of providers in pri-

mary health care services: _____

_____

_____

_____

_____

_____

_____

➤ Primary health care generalists are: _____

_____

_____

_____

_____

_____

_____

➤ Briefly explain the competencies required of the
nurse in primary care.

Professional: _____

_____

_____

_____

Interpersonal: _____

_____

_____

_____

Intraprofessional and interprofessional: _____

_____

_____

_____

Multicultural: _____

_____

_____

_____

Client and Family

➤ The "client" is the person seeking health care and his
or her family or significant other.

➤ Define *health promotion behaviors:* _____

_____

➤ Define *health promotion activities:* _____

_____

_____

➤ Define *disease prevention behaviors:* _____

_____

_____

➤ Identify *disease preventing activities:* _____

_____

_____

➤ Define *health protecting behaviors:* _____

_____

_____

➤ Identify *health protecting activities:* _____

_____

_____

Technological Resources

➤ Explain the impact that technology has on primary health care.

Positive: _____

_____

_____

_____

Negative: _____

_____

_____

_____

■ NURSES' ROLE IN THE DELIVERY OF PRIMARY CARE

➤ The focus of the professional nurse is on maintaining or maximizing health *before* a new problem or a complication of an old problem occurs.

Community-Based Practice

➤ Briefly explain the health care focus on the following groups:

Parish nurse _____

_____

_____

_____

Home health _____

_____

_____

_____

Community-Oriented Primary Care

➤ Define *community-oriented primary care:* _____

_____

_____

_____

The Community as a Partner in Primary Care

➤ Identify the key components in developing a health

care partnership with the community: _____

_____

_____

_____

_____

_____

■ THE NURSING PROCESS AND THE DELIVERY OF PRIMARY CARE SERVICES

➤ In the primary care setting, standard written nursing care plans are not generated. Instead a nurse does a

_____,

_____,

and _____.

➤ The case study method demonstrates how the nursing process is used in a primary care setting. Review the case study.

REVIEW QUESTIONS

(The student should select the appropriate answer and cite the rationale for choosing that particular answer.)

1. The focus of primary care is:
   a. Early detection of illness and its complications
   b. Maintaining optimal health care once the disease has occurred
   c. Health promotion and disease prevention

Answer ( ) Rationale: _____

_____

_____

2. Which of the following is an example of a disease prevention activity?
   a. Keeping one's tetanus immunizations up-to-date
   b. Walking 3 miles a day
   c. Eating a low-fat diet
   d. Fluoridation of municipal drinking water

Answer ( ) Rationale: _____

_____

_____

3. Which of the following is an example of secondary prevention?
   a. Enrolling in a "Eat Healthy" nutritional program
   b. Taking medication daily to control high blood pressure
   c. Learning to walk again after a stroke
   d. Routinely using seat belts when driving

Answer ( ) Rationale: _____

_____

_____

4. Which of the following is an example of a health promotion activity?
   a. Routine exercise program
   b. Cancer screening
   c. Smoking cessation class
   d. Vision screening

Answer ( ) Rationale: _____

_____

5. Which of the following is *not* an example of a primary care setting:
   a. Elementary school
   b. Hospital
   c. Business
   d. Neighborhood health center

Answer ( ) Rationale: _____

_____

_____

6. Which is *not* an example of a health protecting behavior:
   a. Rat and pest control
   b. Bicycle helmets
   c. Immunizations
   d. Fall prevention practices

Answer ( ) Rationale: _____

_____

_____

Chapter
4

Acute Care

When clients experience an abrupt or severe episode of illness, major surgery, or physical injuries resulting from trauma, acute health care becomes necessary.

PRELIMINARY READING

Chapter 4, pp. 61-78

COMPREHENSIVE UNDERSTANDING

■ THE ACUTE CARE ENVIRONMENT

➤ The acute care hospital is in the middle of health care reform, and the changes are influencing nursing staff, clients, physicians, and the services that they provide.

Staff

➤ The nurse who works in an acute care setting is the most critical health care provider.
➤ Many hospitals have reduced the percentage of registered nurses. As a result, the nurse's responsibilities

are more involved with _____,

_____,

and _____.

➤ Define the role of unlicensed assistive personnel:

_____

_____

➤ Appropriate delegation requires critical thinking on the part of the nurse in deciding the needs of each client and making sure appropriate supervision is available as needed. List the five rights of delegation.

a. _____

b. _____

c. _____

d. _____

e. _____

Clients

➤ What clients experience and what they think of that experience will influence how they choose to use a health care system in the future.

➤ Explain the purpose of customer service programs:

_____

_____

➤ Identify and give an example of the seven dimensions of patient-centered care defined by the Picker/Commonwealth Program:

a. _____

_____

b. _____

_____

c. _____

_____

d. _____

_____

e. _____

_____

f. _____

_____

g. _____

_____

Physicians

➤ The medical profession is not held in the same regard as it once was. The reasons for this are

_____,

_____,

_____,

and _____.

➤ Hospitals have demanded that physicians work more efficiently and maintain or improve clinical outcomes.
➤ Physicians want to believe that hospitals are focused on the client's needs and welfare.
➤ A multidisciplinary team is successful in developing sound clinical guidelines only when a physician plays an active role in pathway development.

Services

➤ The changes in health care have brought services into the acute care setting.
➤ Hospitals have added special procedure and recovery units to manage clients on an outpatient basis.
➤ Both procedure and surgical units require nurses to be

highly competent in client _____,

_____,

and _____.

➤ Medical-surgical and intensive care units have become busier since client acuity has risen.

■ THE ACUTE CARE CONTINUUM

➤ Identify the nurse's key role in acute care: _____

_____

_____

_____

Continuum of Care

➤ To ensure a continuum of care, all caregivers must

know _____

_____.

➤ Fragmentation of care occurs when _____

_____

_____.

➤ A well-coordinated, multidisciplinary approach ensures a continuum of care from admission to discharge.

Regulatory Requirements

➤ The purpose of regulatory agency standards for the

acute care setting is to _____

_____.

➤ It is believed that a client receives the best quality care within a shorter time frame if the health care is well coordinated immediately upon admission to the acute care facility.

Admission to an Acute Care Agency

➤ A client can access the health care system in a variety of ways.

Initial Admission Procedures

➤ A client's condition determines the extent of the admitting procedure.

➤ _____

and _____
are the personnel primarily involved with the preliminary procedures for admitting clients into an agency.

➤ Briefly define the following steps within the admission process.

Identifying information: _____

_____

_____

Identification bracelet: _____

_____

_____

Patient's Bill of Rights: _____

_____

_____

Information of available services: _____

_____

_____

Testing: _____

_____

_____

Admission to a Nursing Unit

➤ Briefly identify the procedures a nurse completes

during the admission process: _____

_____

_____

_____

_____

■ MULTIDISCIPLINARY DISCHARGE PLANNING

➤ As soon as a client is admitted to a hospital, all members of health care team begin preparations for discharge.
➤ Successful discharge planning is a _____,

_____, _____
process that ensures that the client has a plan for continuing care after leaving the hospital.
➤ The following outcome levels must be ensured for a client's successful discharge plan:

a. _____

b. _____

c. _____

d. _____

➤ Identify the clients to consider for home care:

_____

_____

_____

_____

▮ NURSING ROLES AND RESPONSIBILITIES

Clinical Practice

➤ Skillful clinical practice in caring for the acutely ill

can minimize _____,

reduce _____,

return _____,

and assist _____.

➤ Briefly summarize the nursing process that ensures

effective discharge planning: _____

_____

_____

_____

_____

_____

_____

➤ Hospitals conduct the discharge planning process differently. Discuss the following roles:

Primary nursing _____

_____

_____

_____

Discharge planning rounds _____

_____

_____

_____

Case manager _____

_____

_____

_____

Referrals for Health Care Services

➤ It is important to remember that other health professionals specialize in skills and knowledge that give a client services that the nurse cannot offer.
➤ It is ideal to have clients participate in referral processes so that they are involved in decision making.
➤ When multiple referrals are made for a client's plan of care, the staff nurse or case manager coordinates referral activities.

Transfers within an Agency

➤ Discharge planning can become more complicated when a client transfers from one nursing unit to another.

➤ Explain the responsibilities of the following nurses in relation to transfers.

Nurses on the sending unit: _____

_____

_____

_____

_____

_____

_____

Nurses on the new unit: _____

_____

_____

_____

_____

_____

Teaching as Part of the Discharge Plan

➤ Identify the responsibilities of the nurse:

_____

_____

_____

_____

_____

_____

_____

_____

➤ Nurses need to be alert for possible learning barriers that affect all clients, and in particular the older adult client.
➤ Identify the goal of educating clients: _____

_____

_____

_____

➤ JCAHO has set minimum standards for information to be provided to clients and their families. Briefly

explain them: _____

_____

_____

_____

_____

_____

_____

_____

Discharge from the Hospital

➤ Summarize the steps to take in the successful discharge

of a client: _____

_____

_____

_____

_____

_____

_____

_____

➤ Explain the responsibilities of the nurse in the event
that a client chooses to leave a hospital against medi-

cal advice (AMA): _____

_____

_____

_____

Home Health Care Planning

➤ Summarize the responsibilities of the home health

nurse: _____

_____

_____

_____

_____

_____

_____

▌ DELIVERY OF ACUTE NURSING CARE

➤ Delivery of care in an acute setting is unique because
of the acuity of clients, the urgency in providing
treatments, and coordinating the contributions of
multiple health care providers.

Assessment

➤ In the acute care setting, assessment becomes more
important because decisions about the data must often be made quickly.

➤ Identify the data that should be included in a comprehensive assessment.

a. _____

b. _____

c. _____

d. _____

e. _____

f. _____

g. _____

h. _____

Nursing Diagnosis

➤ After collecting data about the client, priority nursing diagnoses are developed.
➤ The diagnostic process requires the correct use of assessment skills in revealing defining characteristics
for client problems.

Planning

➤ The plan of care identifies _____

and establishes _____.

➤ In the acute care setting, _____
goals are more realistic to achieve.

➤ Goals and outcomes are established to help the client

achieve _____.

➤ Goals and outcomes for the terminally ill or clients

with serious disabilities are directed at _____

_____.

Implementation

➤ Identify the domain of nursing practice that has particular importance in acute care (Benner): _____

_____

_____

_____

_____

_____

Evaluation

➤ Nurses must critically review and determine if a client is improving and how the client is responding to therapies.

➤ Another important aspect of evaluation is determining the client's continuing needs at the time of discharge.

➤ The nurse evaluates the extent to which

_____,

_____,

and _____

are needed to ensure successful transfer of the client's care to other caregivers.

➤ Outcomes of care must be documented for

_____,

_____,

_____,

and _____.

REVIEW QUESTIONS

(The student should select the appropriate answer and cite the rationale for choosing that particular answer.)

1. All of the following are part of the nurse's role in the admission process *except:*
   a. Teaching the client and family
   b. Providing the client safety and comfort
   c. Maintaining the client's legal rights as a health care recipient
   d. Increasing the client's sense of powerlessness

Answer (　) Rationale: _____

_____

_____

2. The client's signature on the general consent for treatment form gives hospital personnel permission to:
   a. Administer medications
   b. Perform invasive radiological procedures
   c. Perform surgery
   d. Involve the client in experimental protocols

Answer (　) Rationale: _____

_____

_____

3. Discharge planning begins:
   a. When the physician writes the discharge order
   b. The day before the client's anticipated discharge
   c. Toward the end of the client's first week of hospitalization
   d. At the time of the client's admission

Answer (　) Rationale: _____

_____

_____

4. Mr. R is unhappy with the care he has received at the hospital, and he is threatening to leave the hospital against medical advice. The nurse will need to:
   a. Give Mr. R the remainder of the medications he is to receive so he can take them at home.
   b. Discuss with Mr. R the possible outcomes of his decision to leave the hospital.
   c. Tell Mr. R that he cannot leave the hospital without his physician's permission.
   d. Assist Mr. R with dressing and packing his personal belongings.

Answer (　) Rationale: _____

_____

_____

5. At 10 AM, Mr. X arrives on the nursing unit from the admission office. He is in a wheelchair and is complaining of severe pain in his abdomen. His wife and daughter are with him. What would be the most appropriate action for the nurse to take at this time?
   a. Help Mr. X into bed and explain to him how the bed controls are operated.
   b. Help Mr. X into bed and begin a detailed nursing history including family and occupational history.
   c. Explain to Mr. X's family that visiting hours don't start until 11 AM and that they will have to leave now.
   d. Help Mr. X into bed and ask him questions to determine the exact location, duration, and intensity of his pain.

Answer (　) Rationale: _____

_____

_____

6. Mrs. P is an 85-year-old client admitted to your nursing unit with a diagnosis of pneumonia. During your admission assessment you find out that she lives alone and has no relatives or friends to assist her. All of the following would be appropriate initial nursing actions *except:*
   a. Ask Mrs. P questions to determine if she is able to do her own shopping and cooking.
   b. Observe Mrs. P to see if she is able to feed, dress, and bathe herself.
   c. Call social services to begin making arrangements for Mrs. P to be discharged to a nursing home.
   d. Discuss with Mrs. P how she will obtain transportation to her doctor's office for follow-up appointments.

Answer (　) Rationale: _____

_____

_____

Chapter 5

Restorative and Home Health Care

Nurses assist clients to achieve their maximum level of health and functioning by intervening at the primary level to promote health, at the secondary level to maintain health, or at the tertiary level to restore health.

PRELIMINARY READING

Chapter 5, pp. 79-95

COMPREHENSIVE UNDERSTANDING

▌RESTORATIVE CARE

➤ Identify the settings where restorative care services are provided.

a. _____

b. _____

c. _____

d. _____

➤ The services provided in the restorative care settings are those designed to bring the client to the maximum level of health and functioning.

Historical Perspective

➤ The need for restorative care services is directionally proportional to _____
_____.

➤ Restorative care minimizes the impact of morbidity. So as morbidity increases, so does the need for _____.

➤ Briefly explain the Rehabilitation Act of 1973 and the role of nursing: _____
_____
_____
_____

▌FUNCTIONAL STATUS AND RESTORATIVE CARE

➤ Define the following terms:

Functional capacity _____
_____
_____
_____

Residual functional capacity _____
_____
_____

Rehabilitation _____
_____
_____
_____

Restorative _____
_____
_____
_____

➤ Identify the nurse's role in restorative care:
_____
_____
_____

Goal of Restorative Care

➤ Identify the goal of restorative care: _____
_____
_____

➤ Central to restorative care are the client's adaptation to _____

_____

and fulfillment of _____

_____.

Restorative Health Care Team

➤ Identify the core members of the restorative health care team: _____

_____

_____

_____

➤ The function of the team is to: _____

_____

_____

➤ For the restorative health team to function efficiently, the following must occur (explain briefly):

Leadership _____

_____

_____

_____

Communication _____

_____

_____

_____

Collaboration _____

_____

_____

_____

Conflict resolution _____

_____

_____

_____

Restorative Care: Functional Problems and Considerations

➤ Various illnesses or injuries create the need for restorative care to maximize the client's functional

abilities. Give some examples: _____

_____

_____

_____

➤ When working in a restorative care setting, the following must be taken into account: _____

_____

_____

_____

_____

_____

_____

_____

_____

▌ HOME HEALTH IN THE CONTINUUM OF CARE

➤ Define *home health care:* _____

_____

_____

_____

_____

➤ Identify the objectives of home health care: _____

_____

_____

_____

▌ TYPES OF HOME HEALTH CARE SERVICES AND REIMBURSEMENT

➤ Home health care services are reimbursed by

_____,

_____,

and _____.

Home Health Care Agencies

➤ Explain the following aspects of home health care agencies:

Services _____

_____

_____

_____

Reimbursement _____

_____

_____

_____

Private Duty Agencies

➤ Explain the following aspects of private duty agencies:

Services _____

_____

_____

_____

Reimbursement _____

_____

_____

_____

Durable Medical Equipment Companies

➤ Explain the following aspects of medical equipment companies:

Services _____

_____

_____

_____

Reimbursement _____

_____

_____

_____

∎ INCREASED DEMAND FOR HOME HEALTH CARE

➤ Identify the forces causing the demand for home

health care services: _____

_____

_____

_____

_____

_____

_____

∎ NURSING ROLES AND THE RESTORATIVE CARE TEAM

➤ The nurse continuously assists the client in restoration and coordinates the restorative care team.

Clinical Practice

➤ Nursing focus in home health care: _____

_____

_____

_____

➤ Nursing requirements: _____

_____

_____

_____

Home Health Care Management

➤ Nursing focus: _____

_____

_____

_____

➤ Nursing requirements: _____

_____

_____

_____

Teaching and Research Activities

➤ Nursing focus: _____

_____

_____

_____

➤ Nursing requirements: _____

_____

_____

_____

Legal and Ethical Responsibilities

➤ Nursing focus: _____

_____

_____

➤ Identify the three most controversial issues in home health clinical practice.

a. _____

_____

b. _____

_____

c. _____

_____

➤ Identify an ethical dilemma for nurses in home health care: _____

_____

_____

_____

Discharge Planning

➤ Nursing focus: _____

_____

_____

_____

▮ RESTORATIVE CARE AND THE NURSING PROCESS

➤ The nurse uses the nursing process to individualize care so that the client is assisted to regain the maximum level of functioning and independence that is possible.

Assessment

➤ Identify the data that should be included on an assessment form.

a. _____

b. _____

c. _____

d. _____

e. _____

f. _____

g. _____

Nursing Diagnosis

➤ Any nursing diagnosis may apply to a client in the home.
➤ Identify some nursing diagnoses for clients requiring home health care: _____

_____

_____

_____

_____

Planning

➤ The nursing diagnoses and goals should be related to

the _____;

_____;

_____

and _____;

_____;

and _____ problems.

➤ Identify the five factors that must be considered when planning home care.

a. _____

b. _____

c. _____

d. _____

e. _____

Implementation

➤ Identify some of the skilled interventions: _____

_____

_____

_____

➤ Government and private insurers pay for visits only until the client and family have had time to learn the procedures.

Evaluation

➤ Outcomes of care must be documented for

_____,

_____,

_____,

and _____.

▮ CLINICAL ASPECTS OF QUALITY IMPROVEMENT

➤ Explain how the following have an impact on the practice of home health care nurses:

Government agencies _____

_____

_____

_____

JCAHO and CHAP _____

_____

_____

Client's clinical record _____

_____

_____

_____

Case manager _____

_____

_____

_____

Goal of case management _____

_____

_____

_____

■ SPECIALTY NURSING AREAS

➤ Home health care clients increasingly need more specialized and technically advanced services.

Hospice

➤ Define *hospice care,* and identify the role of the nurse in

hospice care: _____

_____

_____

_____

Home Intravenous Therapy

➤ Define *home IV therapies* that are available:

_____

_____

_____

_____

Home Respiratory Care

➤ Identify the role of the nurse in home respiratory care:

_____

_____

_____

_____

■ ISSUES AND CONSIDERATIONS IN RESTORATIVE CARE

➤ Identify the rationale for the increases in restorative

services: _____

_____

_____

_____

_____

_____

_____

REVIEW QUESTIONS

(The student needs to select the appropriate answer and cite the rationale for choosing that particular answer.)

1. Residual functional capacity is referred to as:
   a. Baseline level of functioning
   b. The level of functioning during the illness stage
   c. The level of functioning remaining after the health problem occurred
   d. Limited functioning

   Answer ( ) Rationale: _____

   _____

   _____

2. The core members of the restorative health care team are:
   a. The client
   b. The doctor
   c. The nurse
   d. Every person caring for the client

   Answer ( ) Rationale: _____

   _____

   _____

3. The nurse working in a restorative care setting must take into account:
   a. The client's willingness to participate in care
   b. Family dynamics
   c. Environmental situations
   d. All of the above

   Answer ( ) Rationale: _____

   _____

   _____

4. Sarah's mother will be going home with the services of a home health agency. Sarah is worried about the cost of home health care. The nurse knows that under Medicare and Medicaid regulations, government funds can be used to pay for:
   a. Private duty nursing care
   b. Housekeeping services
   c. Durable medical equipment
   d. Companion services

Answer (   ) Rationale: _____

_____

_____

5. A home health nurse is visiting Ms. W, a 77-year-old client. For Medicare to pay for the home health visits, reports made by the nurse must contain all of the following *except:*
   a. Evidence that the client is able to care for herself
   b. Evidence that skilled care was given
   c. Documentation of the client's homebound status
   d. Statements regarding the client's progress toward discharge

Answer (   ) Rationale: _____

_____

_____

6. The government agency responsible for monitoring compliance with home care regulations and distributing funds for claims is:
   a. Community Health Accreditation Program (CHAP)
   b. Joint Commission on Accreditation of Healthcare Organizations (JCAHO)
   c. Health Care Financing Administration (HCFA)
   d. National Institutes of Health (NIH)

Answer (   ) Rationale: _____

_____

_____

7. The most important action to ensure accreditation and reimbursement for home health care services is:
   a. Provide highly technical, innovative nursing care.
   b. Carefully document nursing assessments, plans, actions, and client response.
   c. Identify all professional and nonprofessional services that the client requests or requires.
   d. Document the agency need for specialty nursing teams and implement continuing education programs for the staff.

Answer (   ) Rationale: _____

_____

_____

Chapter 6

Critical Thinking and Nursing Judgment

When given the responsibility to assist a person in regaining or improving his or her health, a nurse must be able to think critically to problem-solve and find the best solution to a client's needs.

PRELIMINARY READING

Chapter 6, pp. 97-106

COMPREHENSIVE UNDERSTANDING

■ CRITICAL THINKING

➤ How the nurse uses information to reason, make inferences, and form a mental picture of what is happening to a client is critical thinking.

➤ Describe the process of critical thinking in nursing:

_____

_____

_____

_____

➤ To think critically, identify what an individual must be able to do.

a. _____

b. _____

c. _____

d. _____

e. _____

Thinking and Learning

➤ As new knowledge becomes available, professionals must always challenge the old ways of doing things and look at what is most effective, what has been supported by scientific evidence, and what results in better client outcomes.

■ A CRITICAL THINKING MODEL

➤ The critical thinking model defines the outcome of critical thinking as nursing judgment that is relevant to nursing problems in a variety of settings. There are 5 components of critical thinking.

Specific Knowledge Base

➤ Identify what constitutes a nurse's knowledge base:

_____

_____

_____

_____

Experience

➤ Identify the ways that critical thinking is developed

through experience: _____

_____

_____

_____

Competencies

➤ There are three types of critical thinking competencies. Briefly explain and give an example of each one.

General critical thinking: _____

_____

_____

_____

Specific critical thinking (clinical situations): _____

_____

_____

_____

Specific critical thinking (nursing): _____

_____

_____

_____

Attitudes for Critical Thinking

➤ Briefly explain each of the following attributes, which are important for critical thinking:

Accountability _____

_____

_____

_____

Thinking independently _____

_____

_____

_____

Risk-taking _____

_____

_____

_____

Humility _____

_____

_____

_____

Integrity _____

_____

_____

_____

Perseverance _____

_____

_____

_____

Creativity _____

_____

_____

_____

Standards for Critical Thinking

➤ The fifth component of critical thinking includes

_____

and _____.

➤ Professional standards for critical thinking refer to

_____

and _____.

Levels of Critical Thinking in Nursing

➤ There are three levels of critical thinking in nursing that have been identified. Briefly describe each one.

Basic: _____

_____

_____

_____

Complex: _____

_____

_____

_____

Commitment: _____

_____

_____

_____

▌NURSING PROCESS OVERVIEW

➤ The three characteristics of a process are purpose, organization, and creativity. Briefly describe how the nursing process addresses each one of these characteristics.

Purpose: _____

_____

_____

_____

Organization: _____

_____

_____

_____

Creativity: _____

_____

_____

_____

➤ The purpose of the nursing process is to:

a. _____

b. _____

c. _____

d. _____

e. _____

f. _____

Application in Practice

➤ Define *scientific method:* _____

_____

➤ The nursing process is an approach that allows nurses to differentiate their practice from that of physicians and other health care professionals.

The Five-Step Nursing Process

➤ The framework of the nursing process includes the following steps; briefly describe each one.

Assessment: _____

_____

_____

_____

Nursing diagnosis: _____

_____

_____

_____

Planning: _____

_____

_____

_____

Implementation: _____

_____

_____

_____

Evaluation: _____

_____

_____

_____

➤ The entire nursing process is sequential and interrelated. The sequence is _____.

The plan is based on _____.

Nursing care is provided according to _____

_____.

Nursing care is evaluated in terms of achievement of

_____.

REVIEW QUESTIONS

(The student should select the appropriate answer and cite the rationale for choosing that particular answer.)

1. Clinical decision-making requires the nurse to:
   a. Improve a client's health
   b. Establish and weigh criteria in deciding the best choice of therapy for a client
   c. Follow the physician's orders for client care
   d. Standardize care for the client

Answer ( ) Rationale: _____

_____

_____

2. The benefits of the nursing process include all of the following *except:*
   a. The client receives comprehensive and consistent care.
   b. Cost-containment is enhanced because nursing care is based on client needs.
   c. Precise medical diagnoses are more easily defined.
   d. Nurses increase their autonomy and fulfill their legal responsibilities.

Answer ( ) Rationale: _____

_____

_____

3. Which of the following is not one of the five steps of the nursing process?
   a. Planning
   b. Evaluation
   c. Hypothesis testing
   d. Assessment

Answer ( ) Rationale: _____

_____

_____

4. The nurse identifies the client's goals, determines priorities, designs nursing strategies, and determines outcome criteria. This is an example of what component of the nursing process?
   a. Assessment
   b. Planning
   c. Evaluation
   d. Nursing diagnosis
   e. Implementation

Answer ( ) Rationale: _____

_____

_____

5. Gathering, verifying, and communicating data about the client to establish a database is an example of which component of the nursing process?
   a. Assessment
   b. Planning
   c. Evaluation
   d. Nursing diagnosis
   e. Implementation

Answer ( ) Rationale: _____

_____

_____

6. Determining the extent to which goals of care have been achieved is an example of which component of the nursing process?
   a. Assessment
   b. Planning
   c. Evaluation
   d. Nursing diagnosis
   e. Implementation

Answer ( ) Rationale: _____

_____

_____

7. Completing nursing actions necessary for accomplishing a care plan is an example of which component of the nursing process?
   a. Assessment
   b. Planning
   c. Evaluation
   d. Nursing diagnosis
   e. Implementation

Answer ( ) Rationale: _____

_____

_____

8. Identifying the health care needs of the client is an example of which component of the nursing process?
   a. Assessment
   b. Planning
   c. Evaluation
   d. Nursing diagnosis
   e. Implementation

Answer ( ) Rationale: _____

_____

_____

Chapter 7 | Assessment

Assessment begins with the nurse applying knowledge and experience to collect data about a client. Accurate assessment is crucial to ensure that needs are properly identified and the right course of action is implemented by the nurse.

PRELIMINARY READING

Chapter 7, pp. 107-123

COMPREHENSIVE UNDERSTANDING

■ A CRITICAL THINKING APPROACH TO ASSESSMENT

➤ Nursing assessment is the systematic process of _____

_____,

_____,

and _____ data about a client.

➤ This phase of the nursing process includes two steps. Name them.

a. _____

b. _____

➤ Identify the purpose of the assessment: _____

_____

_____

_____

➤ Define *database:* _____

_____

➤ Standardized assessment forms are designed to provide a minimal accountability of the nursing profession to the public.

➤ A comprehensive database includes: _____

_____

_____

➤ Identify and briefly explain two approaches to collecting comprehensive data.

a. _____

_____

_____

b. _____

_____

_____

➤ Whatever approach is used, the nurse must cluster cues of information and identify emerging patterns and potential problems.

Organization of Data Gathering

➤ Accurate assessment makes it possible to devise appropriate goals and strategies.

➤ It is important for the nurse's assessment to first consider the _____.

➤ Identify some nonverbal behavior that a nurse may observe during an assessment: _____

_____.

Data Collection

➤ Define *inferences:* _____

_____

➤ Descriptive data originate in:

a. _____

b. _____

c. _____

d. _____

➤ The collection of inaccurate, incomplete, or inappropriate data leads to incorrect identification of the client's health care needs and subsequent inaccurate, incomplete, or inappropriate nursing diagnoses.

➤ Data are incomplete if the nurse _____,

_____,

or _____.

■ TYPES OF DATA

➤ Define:

Subjective data _____

_____

Objective data _____

_____

■ SOURCES OF DATA

➤ Name the eight sources from which data are obtained.

a. _____

b. _____

c. _____

d. _____

e. _____

f. _____

g. _____

h. _____

➤ Each source provides information about the client's level of wellness, anticipated prognosis, risk factors, health practices and goals, and patterns of health and illness.

Client

➤ Identify the types of information a client can provide.

a. _____

b. _____

c. _____

d. _____

e. _____

Family and Significant Others

➤ Families can be an important source of information about the client's health status. Give an example of each source.

Primary source: _____

_____

_____

_____

Secondary source: _____

_____

_____

_____

Health Care Team Members

➤ Identify the ways that health care team members identify data.

a. _____

b. _____

c. _____

Medical Records

➤ By reviewing medical records, the nurse can

_____,

_____,

and _____.

Other Records

➤ Identify records that may contain pertinent health care information: _____

_____

_____

_____

Literature Review

➤ Reviewing nursing, medical, and pharmacological literature about an illness helps the nurse complete the database.

Nurse's Experience

➤ A nurses's ability to make an assessment will improve

as he or she uses _____,

applies _____,

and focuses _____.

METHODS OF DATA COLLECTION

Interview

➤ The first step in establishing the database is to interview the client.

➤ Identify the major purposes of an interview.

a. _____

b. _____

c. _____

➤ Define *nurse-client relationship:* _____

_____

_____

➤ During an interview the nurse obtains the following information from a client. Explain each dimension.

Physical: _____

_____

Developmental: _____

_____

Emotional: _____

_____

Intellectual: _____

_____

Social: _____

_____

Spiritual: _____

_____

➤ If a positive nurse-client relationship has been established, the client will feel comfortable asking the nurse questions, allowing the client to participate in decision-making regarding goals and the plan of care.

➤ To interview a client successfully the nurse needs

_____,

_____,

and _____.

➤ Define the following types of interview techniques:

Problem-seeking _____

_____

_____

Problem-solving _____

_____

_____

Direct-question _____

_____

_____

_____

Open-ended question _____

_____

_____

➤ There are three phases of the interview. Briefly explain each one.

Orientation phase: _____

_____

_____

Working phase: _____

_____

_____

Termination phase: _____

_____

_____

➤ An important goal for the initial interview is to lay the groundwork for the nurse to understand the client's needs and to begin a relationship that allows the client to become an active partner in decisions about care.

➤ The nurse's _____,

_____,

and _____

encourage a supportive therapeutic relationship with the client.

Nursing Health History

➤ The nursing health history is data collected about:

a. _____

b. _____

c. _____

d. _____

e. _____

➤ Identify the four purposes (objectives) for obtaining a nursing health history.

a. _____

b. _____

c. _____

d. _____

➤ Briefly explain the following components of a health history:

Biological information _____

_____

Reason for seeking health care _____

_____

Client expectations _____

_____

Present illness _____

_____

Past health history _____

_____

Family history _____

_____

Environmental history _____

_____

Psychological history _____

_____

Review of systems _____

_____

Physical Examination

➤ The physical examination and the collection of diagnostic and laboratory data involve the _____

_____.

➤ Define:

Standard _____

Norm _____

➤ The examination is carried out in a systematic manner.

Begin with _____

Followed by _____

_____

Lastly _____

➤ Define the following physical examination techniques:

Inspection _____

Palpation _____

Percussion _____

Auscultation _____

Diagnostic and Laboratory Data

➤ Identify at least two contributions that laboratory data make to the nursing assessment.

a. _____

b. _____

▌ FORMULATING NURSING JUDGMENTS

➤ List the ways to validate information obtained during a nursing history.

a. _____

b. _____

c. _____

d. _____

Data Interpretation

➤ Through a process of inferential reasoning and judgment, the nurse decides what information has meaning in relation to the client's health status.

➤ Define *inferential reasoning:* _____

_____

_____

Data Clustering

➤ After collecting and validating subjective and objective data and interpreting the data, the nurse organizes the information into meaningful clusters. This depends on recognizing _____.

➤ During data clustering, the nurse organizes data and focuses attention on client functions needing support and assistance for recovery.

▌ DATA DOCUMENTATION

➤ Identify the two essential reasons for thoroughness in data documentation.

a. _____

b. _____

REVIEW QUESTIONS

(The student should select the appropriate answer and cite the rationale for choosing that particular answer.)

1. In most circumstances, the best source of information for nursing assessment of the adult client is the:
   a. Nursing literature
   b. Physician
   c. Client
   d. Medical record

Answer ( ) Rationale: _____

_____

_____

2. The interview technique that is most effective in strengthening the nurse-client relationship by demonstrating the nurse's willingness to hear the client's thoughts is:
   a. Open-ended question
   b. Direct question
   c. Problem-solving
   d. Problem-seeking

Answer ( ) Rationale: _____

_____

_____

3. While obtaining a health history, the nurse asks Mr. Jones if he has noted any change in his activity tolerance. This is an example of which interview technique?
   a. Direct question
   b. Problem-seeking
   c. Problem-solving
   d. Open-ended question

Answer ( ) Rationale: _____

_____

_____

4. Mr. Davis tells the nurse that he has been experiencing more frequent episodes of indigestion. The nurse asks if the indigestion is associated with meals or a reclining position and about what relieves the indigestion. This is an example of which interview technique?
   a. Problem-seeking
   b. Problem-solving
   c. Direct question
   d. Open-ended question

Answer (　) Rationale: _____
_____
_____

5. The information obtained in a review of systems (ROS) is:
   a. Objective
   b. Subjective
   c. Based on physical examination findings
   d. Based on the nurse's perspective

Answer (　) Rationale: _____
_____
_____

6. An example of an objective symptom is:
   a. Headache
   b. Itching
   c. Burning
   d. Swelling

Answer (　) Rationale: _____
_____
_____

7. The nurse uses both subjective and objective data in the assessment of a client's pain. Which of the following would be subjective data?
   a. The client stops in the middle of his exercise regimen.
   b. There is a change in the muscle tension on the client's face.
   c. The client states that the pain increases with movement.
   d. The client sleeps for long periods.

Answer (　) Rationale: _____
_____
_____

8. Which of the following statements would be appropriate in the working phase of the admission interview?
   a. "Good morning. I'm Joe Smith, and I'll be your nurse today."
   b. "Why didn't you come to the hospital earlier, Mrs. James?"
   c. "Tell me about the diet you eat at home."
   d. "I've just got one more question, Mrs. James."

Answer (　) Rationale: _____
_____
_____

9. The physical examination technique in which the examiner uses his or her fingers to locate masses and tender areas and to feel pulses is termed:
   a. Auscultation
   b. Palpation
   c. Percussion
   d. Inspection

Answer (　) Rationale: _____
_____
_____

10. When validating data, which question does the nurse seek to answer?
    a. Is information complete and accurate?
    b. Am I ready to plan care?
    c. Has quality care been ensured?
    d. Is the problem statement correct?

Answer (　) Rationale: _____
_____
_____

11. A nurse seeks relationships between factors and symptoms in the database and thus:
    a. Performs a peer review
    b. Formulates a problem statement
    c. Validates data
    d. Clusters data

Answer (　) Rationale: _____
_____
_____

Chapter

8 Nursing Diagnosis

The nursing diagnosis is a clinical judgment about individual, family, or community responses to actual or potential health problems or life processes.

PRELIMINARY READING

Chapter 8, pp. 124-135

COMPREHENSIVE UNDERSTANDING

■ EVOLUTION OF NURSING DIAGNOSIS

➤ Nursing has attempted to define itself professionally and functionally since the writings of Florence Nightingale.

➤ Define:

Client-centered problems _____

_____

_____

_____

The purpose of NANDA _____

_____

_____

_____

■ DEFINITION

➤ *Nursing diagnosis,* as defined by Carpenito (1995):

_____

_____

_____

_____

■ CRITICAL THINKING AND THE NURSING DIAGNOSTIC PROCESS

➤ Define:

Critical thinking _____

_____

_____

_____

Diagnostic process _____

_____

_____

_____

Analysis and Interpretation of Data

➤ Analysis involves recognizing _____,

comparing _____,

and drawing _____.

➤ *Defining characteristics* are _____

_____

_____.

➤ *Clinical criteria* are _____

_____

_____.

➤ Defining characteristics that are beyond healthy norms form the basis for problem-identification.

Identification of Client Problems

➤ An actual health problem is _____

_____

_____.

➤ An at-risk health problem is _____

_____

_____

_____.

■ NURSING DIAGNOSIS STATEMENT
Nursing Diagnosis Format

➤ Nursing diagnoses are stated in a two-part format:

The _____

followed by a _____.

➤ Nursing interventions are directed toward altering or resolving etiologic or related factors.

Formulation of the Nursing Diagnosis

➤ The formulation of the nursing diagnosis is based on identification of client needs.

➤ The diagnostic label is supported by _____

_____

present in the client's _____

_____ database.

➤ The problem is _____;

the related factors are _____.

➤ The etiology, or cause, of the nursing diagnosis must be within the domain of _____

_____

and a condition that responds to _____

_____.

➤ The modification of nursing diagnoses is ongoing. As the level of nursing care and the level of wellness change, these changes are reflected in the statement of nursing diagnosis.

Assessment Data and the Diagnostic Statement

➤ Nursing assessment data must support the diagnostic label, and related factors support the etiology. Review Tables 8-4 and 8-5.

Nursing Diagnosis and Medical Diagnosis

➤ Compare the characteristics of medical and nursing diagnoses in each of the following areas:

	MEDICAL DIAGNOSIS	NURSING DIAGNOSIS
Nature of diagnosis	_____	_____
	_____	_____
	_____	_____
Goal	_____	_____
	_____	_____
	_____	_____
Objective	_____	_____
	_____	_____
	_____	_____

■ SOURCES OF DIAGNOSTIC ERROR

➤ Identify the four areas that are potential sources of diagnostic error.

a. _____

b. _____

c. _____

d. _____

Errors in Data Collection

➤ Identify the four practices that are essential during assessment to avoid data collection errors.

a. _____

b. _____

c. _____

d. _____

Errors in Interpretation and Analysis of Data

➤ Identify ways the nurse determines if data are accurate and complete.

a. _____

b. _____

c. _____

Errors in Data Clustering

➤ Identify ways that incorrect data clustering occurs.

a. _____

b. _____

c. _____

Errors in the Diagnostic Statement

➤ Identify some common guidelines to reduce errors in the diagnostic statement.

a. _____

b. _____

c. _____

d. _____

e. _____

■ NURSING DIAGNOSES: APPLICATION TO CARE PLANNING

➤ The formulated nursing diagnoses provide direction for the planning process and the selection of nursing interventions to achieve the desired outcomes.

Advantages of Nursing Diagnoses

➤ Explain the advantages of using nursing diagnoses in the following:

Communication tool _____

_____

_____

_____

Documentation _____

_____

_____

_____

Discharge teaching _____

_____

_____

_____

Quality assurance and improvement _____

_____

_____

_____

Professionally _____

_____

_____

_____

Limitations of Nursing Diagnoses

➤ List two limitations of nursing diagnoses.

a. _____

_____

b. _____

_____

REVIEW QUESTIONS

(The student should select the appropriate answer and cite the rationale for choosing that particular answer.)

1. A nursing diagnosis:
   a. Is a statement of a client response to a health problem that requires nursing intervention
   b. Identifies nursing problems
   c. Is derived from the physician's history and physical examination
   d. Is not changed during the course of a client's hospitalization

Answer ( ) Rationale: _____

_____

_____

2. Which of the following is *not* a nursing diagnostic category?
   a. Anxiety
   b. Activity intolerance
   c. Respiratory failure
   d. Hopelessness

Answer ( ) Rationale: _____

_____

_____

3. The first part of the nursing diagnosis statement:
   a. Identifies an actual or potential health problem
   b. Identifies the cause of the client problem
   c. May be stated as a medical diagnosis
   d. Identifies appropriate nursing interventions

Answer ( ) Rationale: _____

_____

_____

4. The second part of the nursing diagnosis statement:
   a. Is connected to the first part of the statement with the phrase "due to"
   b. Identifies the probable cause of the client problem
   c. Identifies the expected outcomes of nursing care
   d. Is usually stated as a medical diagnosis

Answer ( ) Rationale: _____

_____

_____

5. Which of the following is the correctly stated nursing diagnosis?
   a. Needs to be fed related to broken right arm
   b. Abnormal breath sounds caused by weak cough reflex
   c. Impaired physical mobility related to rheumatoid arthritis
   d. Impaired skin integrity related to fecal incontinence

Answer (   ) Rationale: _____

_____

_____

6. Mrs. French is a 45-year-old mother of two who is 50 lbs overweight. She has a smoking history of two packs per day for 20 years. She is to have a hysterectomy tomorrow. Which nursing diagnosis should appear on Mrs. French's nursing care plan?
   a. Social isolation
   b. Potential uterine cancer
   c. Risk for ineffective airway clearance related to obesity and smoking
   d. Altered urinary elimination related to incisional pain

Answer (   ) Rationale: _____

_____

_____

7. Mr. Margauz, a 52-year-old business executive, is admitted to the coronary care unit. During his admission interview he denies chest pain or shortness of breath. His pulse and blood pressure are normal. He appears tense and does not want the nurse to leave his bedside. When questioned, he states that he is very nervous. At this moment, which nursing diagnosis is most appropriate?
   a. Alteration in comfort, chest pain
   b. Alteration in bowel elimination related to restricted mobility
   c. High risk for altered cardiac output related to heart attack
   d. Anxiety related to intensive care unit admission

Answer (   ) Rationale: _____

_____

_____

8. If a nurse were to record a client's diagnosis as, "High risk for malnutrition," it would be incorrect because it is:
   a. Stated as a medical diagnosis
   b. Stated as a nursing intervention
   c. An error of omission
   d. An error of commission

Answer (   ) Rationale: _____

_____

_____

9. If a nurse were to record a client's nursing diagnosis as, "Encourage client to verbalize fear," it would be incorrect because it is:
   a. Stated as a medical diagnosis
   b. Stated as a nursing intervention
   c. An error of omission
   d. An error of commission

Answer (   ) Rationale: _____

_____

_____

Chapter 9 | Planning

Planning is the category of nursing in which client-centered goals and expected outcomes are established, and nursing interventions are designed to achieve those goals.

PRELIMINARY READING

Chapter 9, pp. 136-154

COMPREHENSIVE UNDERSTANDING

▌ ESTABLISHING PRIORITIES

➤ Priority selection is the method the nurse and client use to mutually rank the diagnoses in order of importance based on the client's _____,

_____,

and _____.

➤ Maslow's hierarchy of needs arranges basic needs in five levels of priority. Give an example of each.

Physiological: _____

_____

Safety and security: _____

_____

Love and belonging: _____

_____

Self-esteem: _____

_____

Self-actualization: _____

_____

➤ Priorities depend on the urgency of the problem, the nature of the treatment indicated, and the interactions among the nursing diagnoses. Explain each one.

High: _____

_____

Intermediate: _____

_____

Low: _____

_____

▌ CRITICAL THINKING AND ESTABLISHING GOALS AND EXPECTED OUTCOMES

➤ Establishing goals and expected outcomes requires that the nurse critically evaluate the _____

_____,

the _____

_____, and the _____

_____.

➤ Goals and expected outcomes are specific statements of client _____

or _____
that the nurse anticipates from the nursing care.

➤ Identify the two purposes for writing goals and expected outcomes.

a. _____

_____

b. _____

_____

➤ Each goal and expected outcome statement must have a time frame for evaluation.

Goals of Care

➤ Define:

Goals _____

_____

Mutual goal setting _____

_____

Client-centered goal _____

_____

_____

Short-term goal _____

_____

_____

Long-term goal _____
_____
_____

Expected Outcomes

➤ Define *expected outcomes:* _____
_____
_____
_____

➤ Outcomes are desired responses of the client's condition in the _____,
_____,
_____,
_____,

or _____ dimensions.

➤ Identify the functions of an expected outcome.

a. _____

b. _____

c. _____

d. _____

➤ Expected outcomes are derived from _____

and _____ goals and

are based on _____ developed during the second component of the nursing process.

➤ The rationale for several expected outcomes is _____
_____
_____.

Guidelines for Writing Goals and Expected Outcomes

➤ There are seven guidelines to use for writing goals and expected outcomes. Define and give an example of each.

Client-centered factors: _____
_____
_____

Singular factors: _____
_____
_____

Observable factors: _____
_____
_____

Measurable factors: _____
_____
_____

Time-limited factors: _____
_____
_____

Mutual factors: _____
_____
_____

Realistic factors: _____
_____
_____

■ CRITICAL THINKING AND DESIGNING NURSING INTERVENTIONS

➤ Nursing interventions are those actions designed to assist the client in moving from the present level of health to that described in the expected outcome.

➤ Each expected outcome has interventions. The method of intervention selection is always the same,

but the types of interventions are _____

_____ to the client's needs.

Types of Interventions

➤ There are three categories of interventions, and category selection is based on the client's needs. Define and give an example of each.

Nurse-initiated: _____
_____
_____

Physician-initiated: _____
_____
_____

Collaborative: _____
_____
_____

Selection of Interventions

➤ Identify the six factors the nurse uses to select nursing interventions for a specific client.

a. _____

b. _____

c. _____

d. _____

e. _____

f. _____

▌ PLANNING NURSING CARE

➤ Define the following methods for planning nursing care:

Nursing care plan _____

_____

_____

Critical pathways _____

_____

_____

Patient-focused care _____

_____

_____

Purpose of Care Plans

➤ Briefly explain the purpose of a nursing care plan in relation to the following:

Communication _____

_____

_____

Delivery of high-quality care _____

_____

_____

Nurse's shift report _____

_____

_____

Discharge needs _____

_____

_____

Expected outcome criteria _____

_____

_____

➤ The complete care plan is the blueprint for nursing action. It provides direction for implementation of the plan and a framework for evaluation of the client's response to nursing actions.

Care Plans in Various Settings

➤ The structure of the care plan varies, depending on the setting. Its overall purpose is to provide a written guideline for care so that the health care needs of the client and subsequent therapies are communicated among the members of the health care team. Briefly explain the following:

Institutional care plans (Kardex) _____

_____

_____

_____

Computerized care plans (standardized) ___

_____

_____

_____

Student care plans (scientific rationale) ___

_____

_____

_____

Care plans for community-based settings __

_____

_____

_____

Critical Pathways

➤ Critical pathways allow staff from all disciplines to develop integrated care plans for a projected length of stay for clients with a specific case type.
➤ The nurse and other health care team members use the pathway to monitor a client's progress and as a documentation tool.
➤ When using the critical pathways to plan care, forms such as _____,
_____, and
_____ are eliminated.

▌ WRITING THE NURSING CARE PLAN

➤ The nursing diagnosis with the highest priority is the beginning point for the nursing care plan and is followed by other nursing diagnoses in order of assigned priority.
➤ Using the five-column plan, identify the information in each column.

1: _____

_____

_____

2: _____

_____

_____

3: _____

_____

_____

4: _____

_____

_____

5: _____

_____

_____

▌ WRITING CRITICAL PATHWAYS

➤ Critical pathways are a case management tool, which delineates client outcomes within specific time frames.
➤ The pathway designates related nursing diagnoses and interventions.
➤ Expected outcomes are developed during the planning phase, and a specific interval for achieving the outcome is included.
➤ Written so that all members of the health care team can document delivery of care or changes in status.

▌ CONSULTING OTHER HEALTH CARE PROFESSIONALS

➤ Consultation is a process in which _____

_____

_____

_____.

➤ Consultation is based on the problem-solving approach, and the consultant is the stimulus for change.

When to Consult

➤ The need to consult occurs when the nurse has identified a problem that cannot be solved using personal knowledge, skills, and resources.

How to Consult

➤ List the six responsibilities of the nurse when seeking consultation.

a. _____

b. _____

c. _____

d. _____

e. _____

f. _____

REVIEW QUESTIONS

(The student should select the appropriate answer and cite the rationale for choosing that particular answer.)

1. Under what circumstance would the nurse or nursing team independently develop client-centered goals?
   a. When directed to do so by the physician
   b. When the hospital uses standardized care plans
   c. If the client is unable to participate in goal-setting
   d. If the client is unable to read or write

Answer ( ) Rationale: _____

_____

_____

2. Well-formulated, client-centered goals should:
   a. Meet immediate client needs
   b. Include preventive health care
   c. Include rehabilitation needs
   d. All of the above

Answer ( ) Rationale: _____

_____

_____

3. The following statement appears on the nursing care plan for an immunosuppressed client: *The client will remain free from infection throughout hospitalization.* This statement is an example of a (an):
   a. Nursing diagnosis
   b. Short-term goal
   c. Long-term goal
   d. Expected outcome

Answer ( ) Rationale: _____

_____

_____

4. The following statements appear on a nursing care plan for a client after a mastectomy: *Incision site approximated; absence of drainage or prolonged erythema at incision site; and client remains afebrile.* These statements are examples of:
   a. Nursing interventions
   b. Short-term goals
   c. Long-term goals
   d. Expected outcomes

Answer ( ) Rationale: _____

_____

_____

5. An example of a nurse-initiated intervention is:
   a. Administering a prescribed pain medication
   b. Administering a laxative according to protocol
   c. Turning a client every 2 hours to prevent skin breakdown
   d. Ambulating a client according to the therapist's recommendation

Answer ( ) Rationale: _____

_____

_____

6. High-priority nursing diagnoses:
   a. Occur in the physiological dimension only
   b. Are client needs unrelated to a specific illness
   c. Must be treated to prevent harm to the client or others
   d. Must always be determined in conjunction with the client

Answer ( ) Raionale: _____

_____

_____

7. The planning step of the nursing process includes which of the following activities?
   a. Assessing and diagnosing
   b. Evaluating goal achievement
   c. Performing nursing actions and documenting them
   d. Setting goals and selecting interventions

Answer ( ) Rationale: _____

_____

_____

8. Nurse Jones asks the diabetes clinical nurse specialist to consult with her in developing an individualized teaching plan for her client. Which of the following actions by Ms. Jones is not appropriate in the consultation process?
   a. Ms. Jones gives the clinical nurse specialist a brief history of the client's illness.
   b. Ms. Jones tells the clinical nurse specialist that the client is uncooperative and will be hard to teach.
   c. Ms. Jones describes to the clinical nurse specialist the teaching strategies tried thus far.
   d. Ms. Jones incorporates the clinical nurse specialist's recommendations into the care plan.

Answer ( ) Rationale: _____

_____

_____

9. The nursing care plan is:
   a. A written guideline for implementation and evaluation
   b. A documentation of client care
   c. A projection of potential alterations in client behaviors
   d. A tool to set goals and project outcomes

Answer ( ) Rationale: _____

_____

_____

Chapter 10 | Implementation

Chapter

10

Implementation is a category of nursing behavior in which the actions necessary for achieving the goals and expected outcomes of nursing care are initiated and completed.

PRELIMINARY READING

Chapter 10, pp. 155-164

COMPREHENSIVE UNDERSTANDING

■ TYPES OF NURSING INTERVENTIONS

➤ After the plan has been developed according to the client needs and priorities, the nurse performs specific

interventions, which include _____

and _____ treatments.

Protocols and Standing Orders

➤ Nursing interventions can be based on protocols and standings orders. Briefly explain each and where they are commonly used.

Protocols: _____

_____

_____

Standing orders: _____

_____

_____

■ CRITICAL THINKING SKILLS AND IMPLEMENTING NURSING INTERVENTIONS

➤ Identify the factors that make decision-making more difficult when choosing among nurse-initiated interventions.

a. _____

b. _____

➤ Identify the sequence of activities in the information-processing model, which is used for determining nursing interventions:

a. _____

b. _____

c. _____

d. _____

■ IMPLEMENTATION PROCESS

➤ The implementation component of the nursing process has five steps.

Reassessing the Client

➤ When new data are obtained, and a new need is identified, the nurse modifies nursing care. This provides a mechanism for the nurse to determine if the proposed nursing action is appropriate.

Reviewing and Modifying the Existing Nursing Care Plan

➤ If the client's status has changed and the nursing diagnosis and related nursing interventions are no longer appropriate, the nursing care plan needs to be modified.

➤ Modification of the existing care plan includes several steps. Identify them.

a. _____

_____

b. _____

_____

c. _____

_____

d. _____

_____

Identifying Areas of Assistance

➤ Before implementing care, the nurse evaluates the plan to determine the need for assistance and the type required. List the three areas from which a nurse can seek assistance when implementing the nursing care plan.

a. _____

_____

b. _____

_____

c. _____

_____

Implementing Nursing Interventions

➤ Describe the five different methods for implementing nursing interventions.

a. _____

_____

b. _____

_____

c. _____

_____

d. _____

_____

e. _____

_____

➤ Nursing practice is composed of three skills. Define and give an example of each.

Cognitive: _____

_____

_____

Interpersonal: _____

_____

_____

Psychomotor: _____

_____

_____

Communicating Nursing Interventions

➤ Nursing interventions are written (via the nursing care plan and medical record) or communicated orally (one nurse to another or to another health care professional).

▌ IMPLEMENTATION METHODS

➤ For each nursing diagnosis the nurse identifies appropriate interventions, each of which requires specific theoretical knowledge and clinical skills.

Assisting with Activities of Daily Living

➤ Define activities of daily living (ADL): _____

_____

_____

➤ Conditions that result in the need for assistance with ADL can be acute, chronic, temporary, permanent, or rehabilitative.

Counseling

➤ Counseling is an _____

_____

_____.

➤ Identify some areas in which clients or families may need counseling.

a. _____

_____

b. _____

_____

c. _____

_____

Teaching

➤ Define:

Teaching _____

_____

_____

Teaching-learning process _____

_____

_____

Providing Direct Nursing Care

➤ To achieve the therapeutic goals for the client, the nurse initiates interventions to (briefly explain each one):

a. _____

_____

b. _____

_____

c. _____

_____

d. _____

_____

➤ The client's health care goals can be achieved by:

a. _____

_____

b. _____

_____

c. _____

_____

d. _____

_____

Supervising and Evaluating the Work of Other Staff Members

➤ The nurse assigning tasks is responsible for ensuring that each task is assigned appropriately and completed according to the standard of care.

REVIEW QUESTIONS

(The student should select the appropriate answer and cite the rationale for choosing that particular answer.)

1. Which of the following is *not* true of standing orders?
   a. Standing orders are approved and signed by the physician in charge of care before implementation.
   b. With standing orders, the nurse relies on the physician's judgment to determine if the intervention is appropriate.
   c. Standing orders are commonly found in critical care and community health settings.
   d. With standing orders, nurses have the legal protection to intervene appropriately in the client's best interest.

Answer ( ) Rationale: _____

_____

_____

2. Which of the following forms the basis for nursing implementation?
   a. Medical diagnosis
   b. Nursing criteria
   c. Outcome criteria
   d. Nursing care plan

Answer ( ) Rationale: _____

_____

_____

3. Mr. W has a nursing diagnosis of high risk for alteration in nutrition less than body requirements related to poor appetite. The stated expected outcome for Mr. W is "Will maintain weight at admission level of 170 lb by 12/6." The nurse weighs Mr. W on 12/3 and finds that he now weighs 165 lb. The nurse should:
   a. Change the expected outcome to read, "Will maintain weight of 160 lb at time of discharge."
   b. Restate the nursing diagnosis as, "Alteration in nutrition less than body requirements related to poor appetite."
   c. Proceed with care plan as stated
   d. Write "resolved" next to the diagnosis on high risk for altered nutrition

Answer ( ) Rationale: _____

_____

_____

4. The nursing care plan calls for the client, a 300-lb woman, to be turned every 2 hours. The client is unable to assist with turning. The nurse knows that she may hurt her back if she attempts to turn the client by herself. The nurse should:
   a. Rewrite the care plan to eliminate the need for turning
   b. Ignore the intervention related to turning in the care plan
   c. Turn the client by herself
   d. Ask another nurse to help her turn the client

Answer ( ) Rationale: _____

_____

_____

5. Being alert to the possibility of the client becoming nauseated after general anesthesia is an example of which type of nursing skill?
   a. Cognitive
   b. Interpersonal
   c. Technical
   d. Psychosocial

Answer ( ) Rationale: _____

_____

_____

6. Which of the following is true regarding the level of assistance that clients require in the implementation phase of the nursing process?
   a. Two clients with the same medical diagnoses will require the same level of assistance in the provision of nursing care.
   b. Only clients who are unconscious will require total care with respect to their physical needs.
   c. At the assistive level of care, the nurse supplements the client's capabilities when necessary.
   d. It is best for clients who are hospitalized to receive total care from the nursing staff.

Answer (   ) Rationale: _____

_____

_____

7. Mrs. Kay comes to the family clinic for birth control. The nurse obtains a health history and performs a pelvic examination and Pap smear. The nurse is functioning according to:
   a. Protocol
   b. Standing order
   c. Nursing care plan
   d. Intervention strategy

Answer (   ) Rationale: _____

_____

_____

8. Mary Jones is a newly diagnosed diabetic patient. The nurse shows Mary how to administer an injection. This intervention activity is:
   a. Counseling
   b. Communicating
   c. Teaching
   d. Managing

Answer (   ) Rationale: _____

_____

_____

9. Mrs. Williams visited the venereal disease clinic where she was given an injection of penicillin. One hour later, she was covered with a bright rash. This is a(n):
   a. Adverse reaction
   b. Expected outcome
   c. Coexisting condition
   d. Emotional response

Answer (   ) Rationale: _____

_____

_____

10. Five-year-old Julie is in surgery. The nurse sits with the family for a few minutes to determine their fears and concerns about Julie's condition. This is an example of which type of nursing skill?
    a. Cognitive
    b. Interpersonal
    c. Psychomotor
    d. Communication

Answer (   ) Rationale: _____

_____

_____

Chapter 11 | Evaluation

The evaluation step of the nursing process measures the client's response to nursing actions and the client's progress toward achieving goals.

PRELIMINARY READING

Chapter 11, pp. 165-177

COMPREHENSIVE UNDERSTANDING

▮ DYNAMICS OF EVALUATING THE NURSING PROCESS

➤ If outcomes are met, the overall goals for the client are also met.

➤ The nurse compares client behaviors and responses assessed before the nursing interventions are delivered with the behaviors and responses that occur following nursing care.

➤ Explain the two types of evaluations.

Positive: _____

_____

Negative: _____

_____

➤ A client whose health status continuously changes requires frequent evaluation.

Goals

➤ A goal specifies the behavior or response that

_____

_____.

➤ Each nursing diagnosis in the client's care plan has a

_____, and every goal

has a _____ for evaluation.

➤ When preparing a client for discharge, the nurse evaluates the status of each _____

and writes an evaluative statement identifying the

client's progress toward _____

and _____.

Expected Outcomes

➤ Expected outcomes are statements of progressive,

step-by-step _____

or _____

that the client needs to accomplish to achieve the goals of care provided.

➤ When outcomes are achieved, the _____
for a nursing diagnosis have been removed.

➤ To provide truly objective measurements, the out-

comes are _____,

stated in _____ terms, and

have _____ frames for evaluation.

▮ EVALUATION OF GOAL ACHIEVEMENT

➤ The purpose of nursing care is to:

a. _____

b. _____

c. _____

➤ Describe the steps for the objective evaluation of client goal achievement.

a. _____

_____

b. _____

_____

c. _____

_____

d. _____

_____

e. _____

_____

➤ Identify the three degrees of goal attainment.

a. _____

b. _____

c. _____

Evaluative Measures and Sources

➤ Evaluative measures are _____

_____.

➤ The new data collected from evaluation measures are critically analyzed and compared with expected outcomes to determine whether or not changes occurred.

➤ The primary source of data for evaluation is the ___

_____.

➤ Documentation and reporting in the evaluation process are of critical importance. Give some examples.

a. _____

b. _____

c. _____

d. _____

▌ CARE PLAN REVISION AND CRITICAL THINKING

➤ Accurate evaluation leads to the appropriate revision of ineffective care plans and discontinuation of therapy that has been successful.

Discontinuing a Care Plan

➤ After determining that expected outcomes and goals have been achieved, the nurse confirms this evaluation with the client and discontinues that care plan.

Modifying a Care Plan

➤ When goals are not met, the nurse identifies the factors that interfered with goal achievement.

➤ Lack of goal achievement may also result from an error in nursing judgment or failure to follow each step of the nursing process.

➤ When there is failure to achieve a goal, the entire

_____ sequence is repeated to discover

changes that need to be made to _____,

_____, or

_____ the client's health.

➤ A complete reassessment of all client factors relating to the nursing diagnosis and etiology is the first step in reevaluating the nursing process.

➤ After reassessment, the nurse evaluates all _____

and determines if the _____ was accurately formulated for the situation.

➤ Determining that each goal and expected outcome is realistic for the _____,

_____, and

_____ frame is important.

➤ When the goal is still appropriate but has not yet been met, the nurse may change the _____ to allow more time.

➤ The evaluation of interventions examines two factors. Name them.

a. _____

_____

b. _____

➤ The exclusion of evaluation from the nursing process prevents the nurse from evaluating nursing practice and determining if the outcomes of client care are beneficial.

▌ QUALITY IMPROVEMENT

➤ The evaluation of health care is a process used to determine the quality of care and service provided to clients.

➤ JCAHO defines quality improvement (QI) as:

_____

_____

_____

Multidisciplinary Approach

➤ To be successful the members of the health care team must share respect for one another's contributions to client care and be open to new ideas and change.

Unit-Based QI Teams

➤ In a unit-based program, members identify:

a. _____

b. _____

c. _____

d. _____

➤ Unit-based teams are participative, which decentralizes decision-making and accountability for practice and places it at the level of the staff.

Components of the QI Program

➤ Ten steps were developed by the JCAHO to ensure a systematic approach for identifying opportunities to improve quality of care and to take appropriate action to resolve any problems (refer to box 11-2). Briefly explain each step.

1. Responsibility for program: _____

_____

2. Scope of service: _____

_____

3. Key aspects of service: _____

_____

4. Developing quality indicators: _____

_____

5. Establishing thresholds for evaluation: _____

_____

6. Data collection and analysis: _____

_____

7. Evaluation of care: _____

_____

8. Resolution of problems: _____

_____

9. Evaluation of improvement: _____

_____

10. Communication of results: _____

_____

REVIEW QUESTIONS

(The student should select the appropriate answer and cite the rationale for choosing that particular answer.)

1. Measuring the client's response to nursing interventions and the client's progress toward achieving goals is done during which phase of the nursing process?
   a. Planning
   b. Nursing diagnosis
   c. Evaluation
   d. Assessment

Answer ( ) Rationale: _____

_____

2. Evaluation is:
   a. Begun immediately before the client's discharge
   b. Only necessary if the physician orders it
   c. Integrated, ongoing nursing care activity
   d. Done primarily by nurses in the quality assurance department

Answer ( ) Rationale: _____

_____

3. The criteria for determining the effectiveness of nursing action are based on the:
   a. Nursing diagnosis
   b. Expected outcomes
   c. Client's satisfaction
   d. Nursing interventions

Answer ( ) Rationale: _____

_____

4. The primary source of data for evaluation is the:
   a. Physician
   b. Client
   c. Nurse
   d. Medical record

Answer ( ) Rationale: _____

_____

5. When a client-centered goal has not been met in the projected time frame, the most appropriate action by the nurse would be to:
   a. Repeat the entire sequence of the nursing process to discover needed changes
   b. Conclude that the goal was inappropriate or unrealistic and eliminate it from the plan
   c. Continue with the same plan until the goal is met
   d. Rewrite the plan using different interventions

Answer ( ) Rationale: _____

_____

6. When a long-term goal is evaluated as having been achieved, the nurse should:
   a. Revise the short-term goal
   b. Revise the long-term goal
   c. Discontinue the care plan for that nursing diagnosis
   d. Discontinue the entire care plan

Answer ( ) Rationale: _____

_____

7. The overall goal of quality assurance is to:
   a. Find nursing errors
   b. Document excellence of nursing care
   c. Discover ways to improve health care
   d. Ensure excellent health care

Answer ( ) Rationale: _____

_____

8. In a unit-based quality improvement program, the responsibility and authority for monitoring and evaluating quality of nursing practice is placed on the:
   a. Unit medical staff
   b. Professional staff nurses
   c. Hospital administration
   d. Director of nursing

Answer (   ) Rationale: _____

_____

_____

9. "Clients receiving blood transfusions will not experience adverse reactions" is an example of:
   a. A structure indicator
   b. A responsibility indicator
   c. An outcome indicator
   d. A process indicator

Answer (   ) Rationale: _____

_____

_____

10. Which of the following is a correctly stated threshold for evaluation in the quality improvement process?
    a. Incidence of skin breakdown in clients with strokes
    b. Clients are able to discuss home medication regimens.
    c. Ninety percent of clients will express satisfaction with the quality of their meals.
    d. Most of the clients who are on bed rest will maintain intact skin integrity.

Answer (   ) Rationale: _____

_____

_____

Documentation and Reporting

The ideal documentation system should provide comprehensive client information, address client outcomes and standards, facilitate reimbursement from government and insurance company payors, and serve as a legal document.

PRELIMINARY READING

Chapter 12, pp. 179-205

COMPREHENSIVE UNDERSTANDING

■ MULTIDISCIPLINARY COMMUNICATION WITHIN THE HEALTH CARE TEAM

➤ Caregivers use a variety of ways to exchange information about clients. Briefly explain the following:

Reports _____

_____

Record _____

_____

Discussions _____

_____

■ DOCUMENTATION

➤ Documentation is defined as: _____

_____

_____

➤ Good documentation reflects not only quality of care but also evidence of each health care team member's accountability in giving care.

Purposes of Records

➤ Briefly explain the following purposes of a record:

Communication _____

_____

Financial billing _____

_____

Assessment _____

_____

Research _____

_____

Auditing and monitoring _____

_____

➤ Four common communication problem areas in malpractice that are caused by inadequate documentation are:

a. _____

b. _____

c. _____

d. _____

■ GUIDELINES FOR QUALITY DOCUMENTATION AND REPORTING

➤ Six important guidelines must be followed to ensure quality documentation and reporting. Explain each one.

Factual basis _____

_____

_____

Accuracy _____

_____

_____

Completeness _____

_____

_____

Currentness _____

_____

_____

Organization _____

_____

_____

Confidentiality _____

_____

_____

Methods of Recording

➤ The nursing service department of each health care agency selects the method that is used for documentation of client care.

➤ The method should reflect the philosophy of the nursing service and incorporate the standards of care and practice for the department.

➤ The JCAHO requires documentation of nursing diagnosis or problems within the context of the nursing process, as well as evidence of client and family teaching and discharge planning.

➤ Narrative documentation is a storylike format to document information specific to client conditions and nursing care. The disadvantages of this style are:

a. _____

_____

b. _____

_____

c. _____

_____

➤ Problem-oriented medical records (POMR) place emphasis on the client's problems. The method corresponds to the nursing process and facilitates communication of client needs. Explain the following major sections of the POMR:

Database _____

_____

Problem list _____

_____

Care plan _____

_____

Progress notes _____

_____

➤ *SOAP* is an acronym for the POMR method of documentation. Briefly describe the information to be included in each of the sections of the SOAP note.

S: _____

_____

O: _____

_____

A: _____

_____

P: _____

_____

➤ PIE charting has a nursing origin. Briefly describe the information to be included in each of the sections of the PIE note.

P: _____

_____

I: _____

_____

E: _____

_____

➤ Briefly explain the other forms of documentation.

Source records: _____

_____

_____

Charting by exception: _____

_____

_____

Focus charting: _____

_____

_____

Case management and critical pathways: _____

_____

_____

Common Record-Keeping Forms

➤ Briefly explain the following formats used for record-keeping:

Nursing history forms _____

_____

_____

Graphic sheets and flow sheets _____

_____

_____

Nursing Kardex _____

_____

_____

24-Hour client chart records and acuity charting systems _____

_____

Standardized care plans _____

_____

_____

Discharge summary forms _____

_____

_____

Home Health Care Documentation

➤ Documentation in the home health care system has different implications than it does in other areas of nursing. The primary difference is _____

_____.

➤ Documentation is both quality control and justification for reimbursement from Medicare, Medicaid, or private insurance companies.
➤ The nurse is the pivotal person in the documentation of the delivery of home health care.

Long-Term Health Care Documentation

➤ Long-term care documentation supports a multidisciplinary approach in the _____

(referred to as *minimum data set*) and _____

_____

(referred to as *resident assessment protocols*).

Computerized Documentation

➤ Explain the many benefits of computerized documentation. _____

_____

_____

_____

■ REPORTING

➤ Nurses communicate information about clients so that all the health care team members can make the best decisions about them and their care.

Change-of-Shift Reports

➤ Identify the eight major areas to include in a change-of-shift report.

   a. _____

   b. _____

   c. _____

   d. _____

   e. _____

   f. _____

   g. _____

   h. _____

Telephone Reports

➤ It is important that information in a telephone report be clear, accurate, and concise.

Telephone Orders

➤ List the guidelines the nurse should follow when receiving telephone orders from physicians.

   a. _____

   b. _____

   c. _____

   d. _____

   e. _____

   f. _____

Transfer Reports

➤ List the six major information areas in a transfer report.

   a. _____

   b. _____

   c. _____

   d. _____

   e. _____

   f. _____

Incident Reports

➤ Define the purpose of an incident report: _____

_____

_____

_____

_____

REVIEW QUESTIONS

(The student should select the appropriate answer and cite the rationale for choosing that particular answer.)

1. The primary purpose of a client's medical record is to:
   a. Satisfy requirements of accreditation agencies
   b. Communicate accurate, timely information about clients
   c. Provide validation for hospital charges
   d. Provide the nurse with a defense against malpractice

   Answer ( ) Rationale: _____
   _____
   _____

2. Which of the following is correctly charted according to the six guidelines for quality recording?
   a. "Respirations rapid; lung sounds clear."
   b. "Was depressed today."
   c. "Crying. States she doesn't want visitors to see her like this."
   d. "Had a good day. Up and about in room."

   Answer ( ) Rationale: _____
   _____
   _____

3. Your neighbor asks you for information regarding a hospitalized friend's condition. Your reply should be influenced by:
   a. The client's right to confidentiality
   b. Your lack of knowledge of the treatment plan
   c. The neighbor's genuine interest in her friend
   d. Your fear of legal involvement in the case

   Answer ( ) Rationale: _____
   _____
   _____

4. During a change-of-shift report:
   a. Two or more nurses always visit all clients to review their plan of care.
   b. Nurses should exchange judgments they have made about client attitudes.
   c. The nurse should identify nursing diagnoses and clarify client priorities.
   d. Client information is communicated from a nurse on a sending unit to a nurse on a receiving unit.

   Answer ( ) Rationale: _____
   _____
   _____

5. An incident report is:
   a. A legal claim against a nurse for negligent nursing care
   b. A summary report of all falls occurring on a nursing unit
   c. A report of an event inconsistent with the routine care of a client
   d. A report of a nurse's behavior submitted to the hospital administration

   Answer ( ) Rationale: _____
   _____
   _____

6. If an error is made while recording, the nurse should:
   a. Erase it or scratch it out.
   b. Obtain a new nurse's note and rewrite the entries.
   c. Leave a blank space in the note.
   d. Draw a single line through the error and initial it.

   Answer ( ) Rationale: _____
   _____
   _____

7. In the source record, the traditional form of the medical record:
   a. Each discipline has a separate section to record data.
   b. Information is well organized according to the client's problems.
   c. Entries are made in random order throughout the chart.
   d. There is a decrease in the fragmentation of data.

   Answer ( ) Rationale: _____
   _____
   _____

8. When charting in a POMR format:
   a. Enter narrative notes according to the client's specific problem.
   b. Continue charting on all problems, even after they are resolved.
   c. Use a different number or label for a problem each time an entry is made.
   d. Use the "A" section of SOAP notes for charting information that is observed.

   Answer ( ) Rationale: _____
   _____
   _____

9. The assessment portion of a SOAP note includes:
   a. A restatement of the diagnosis
   b. Information gathered from the client
   c. Measurable clinical findings
   d. Interpretation of the client's findings

Answer ( ) Rationale: _____

_____

_____

10. All of the following are true of standardized care plans *except:*
   a. Standardized plans attempt to make documentation easier for nurses.
   b. Standardized plans can educate nurses about the nursing care of clients with particular nursing diagnoses.
   c. The plans are based on the institution's standards for nursing practice.
   d. Standardized plans eliminate the need for the nurse's professional judgment and decision-making.

Answer ( ) Rationale: _____

_____

_____

11. All of the following are true of a discharge summary form *except* that it:
   a. Includes information on activity orders or restrictions
   b. Should never be copied for the client or family
   c. Should include guidelines for calling a physician when problems arise
   d. Includes a description of the client's status in relation to planned outcomes

Answer ( ) Rationale: _____

_____

_____

Chapter

13

Profession of Nursing

The profession of nursing evolves as society, health care needs, and policies change. Nursing responds and adapts to changes, meeting new challenges as they arise.

PRELIMINARY READING

Chapter 13, pp. 207-231

COMPREHENSIVE UNDERSTANDING

▌ HISTORICAL PERSPECTIVE

➤ Nursing was distinguished in its early history as a form of community service and was originally related to a strong instinct to preserve and protect the family.

➤ Throughout history, nursing and medicine have been interdependent.

➤ Briefly explain how Christianity influenced nursing.

_____

_____

_____

➤ Nightingale's view on nursing was: _____

_____

_____

➤ Briefly explain how the following influenced nursing:

Benedictine Order _____

_____

_____

Middle Ages _____

_____

_____

Crusades _____

_____

_____

Sisters/Daughters of Charity _____

_____

_____

Eighteenth century _____

_____

_____

Nineteenth century _____

_____

_____

Civil War _____

_____

_____

Lillian Ward and Mary Brewster _____

_____

_____

ANA Code of Ethics 1926 _____

_____

_____

Present _____

_____

_____

▌ CONCEPTUAL AND THEORETICAL MODELS OF NURSING RESEARCH

➤ A conceptual model refers to: _____

_____

_____

➤ Conceptual and theoretical models are used to:

a. _____

b. _____

c. _____

➤ Nursing theories provide the nurse with:

a. _____

b. _____

c. _____

d. _____

e. _____

Nightingale's Theory

➤ Identify the concepts basic to Nightingale's theory.

_____

_____

_____

_____

Peplau's Theory

➤ Identify the concepts basic to Peplau's theory.

_____

_____

_____

_____

Henderson's Theory

➤ Identify the concepts basic to Henderson's theory.

_____

_____

_____

_____

Abdellah's Theory

➤ Identify the concepts basic to Abdellah's theory.

_____

_____

_____

_____

Orlando's Theory

➤ Identify the concepts basic to Orlando's theory.

_____

_____

_____

_____

Levine's Theory

➤ Identify the concepts basic to Levine's theory.

_____

_____

_____

_____

Johnson's Theory

➤ Identify the concepts basic to Johnson's theory.

_____

_____

_____

_____

Roger's Theory

➤ Identify the concepts basic to Roger's theory.

_____

_____

_____

_____

Orem's Theory

➤ Identify the concepts basic to Orem's theory.

_____

_____

_____

_____

King's Theory

➤ Identify the concepts basic to King's theory.

_____

_____

_____

_____

Neuman's Theory

➤ Identify the concepts basic to Neuman's theory.

_____

_____

_____

_____

Roy's Theory

➤ Identify the concepts basic to Roy's theory.

_____

_____

_____

_____

Watson's Theory

➤ Identify the concepts basic to Watson's theory.

_____

_____

_____

_____

▋ AMERICAN NURSES ASSOCIATION (ANA) DEFINITION OF NURSING PRACTICE

➤ Briefly describe the focus of the ANA definition of nursing practice for the following dates:

1955 _____

_____

1965 _____

_____

1979 _____

_____

1980 _____

_____

▋ CANADIAN NURSES ASSOCIATION (CNA) DEFINITION OF NURSING PRACTICE

➤ Briefly explain the CNA definition of nursing and

standards of practice. _____

_____

_____

_____

▋ EDUCATIONAL PREPARATION

Registered Nurse Education

➤ As the profession of nursing grew, various educational routes for becoming an RN were developed. Briefly explain the following:

Associate degree education _____

_____

Diploma education _____

_____

_____

Baccalaureate education _____

_____

Accreditation and Licensure

➤ To be accredited, nursing programs must meet certain criteria established by the National League for Nursing (NLN).

➤ In the United States, RN candidates must pass the National Council Licensure Examination for Registered Nurses (NCLEX-RN).

Graduate Nursing Education

➤ The purpose of graduate education is to: _____

_____

_____

Continuing Education

➤ The goals of continuing education are to: _____

_____

_____

_____

In-Service Education

➤ An in-service program is designed to: _____

_____

_____

_____

Licensed Practical Nurse Education

➤ An LPN or LVN is trained in _____

and _____
and practices under the supervision of a registered nurse in a hospital or community health practice setting.

Career Mobility and Clinical Ladder

➤ The clinical ladder unifies _____,

fosters _____, and

is a professional _____.

➤ The clinical ladder contains:

a. _____

b. _____

c. _____

d. _____

■ NURSING PRACTICE

➤ The practice of nursing is guided only in part by administrators in hospitals and other health care agencies and institutions.

➤ State and provincial nurse practice acts establish

_____

_____, and professional

organizations establish _____

_____.

Standards of Nursing Practice

➤ Standards of practice are important for the following reasons:

a. _____

b. _____

c. _____

d. _____

e. _____

Nurse Practice Acts

➤ Nurse practice acts regulate the licensure and practice of nursing. Each state or province defines for itself the scope of nursing practice, but most have similar practice acts.

Practice Settings

➤ Nursing practice settings are expanding because of the changes in the health care delivery system.

➤ There is greater emphasis on community-based practice and the knowledge base for this practice developed from traditional and nontraditional methods.

➤ The largest group of practicing nurses is those working in hospitals or other health care agencies.

➤ Nursing practice in hospital and skilled nursing facilities is becoming more complex partly because of the increased older adult population and rising acuity rates.

➤ The rapid rise in the number of older adults, clients with chronic illnesses, and clients with functional impairments has resulted in the growth of long-term care facilities.

➤ The rising costs of institutional care create the need for community-based nursing services aimed at ___

_____,

_____, and

_____ care.

➤ Institutional health care focuses on _____

_____.

➤ Community-based nursing is directed toward the

_____ and

_____ within that community.

➤ Community-based nurses are employed in a variety of practice settings. Briefly explain each one.

Community health centers: _____

_____

_____

Schools: _____

_____

_____

Occupational health settings: _____

_____

_____

Home health care agencies: _____

_____

_____

■ ROLES AND FUNCTIONS OF THE NURSE

➤ The contemporary nurse functions in the following roles. Briefly explain each one.

Care giver_____

_____

Clinical decision maker _____

_____

Protector and client advocate_____

_____

Case manager _____

_____

Rehabilitator_____

_____

Comforter _____

_____

Communicator_____

_____

Teacher _____

_____

Career Roles

➤ Explain the following career roles and functions:

Nurse educator _____

_____

_____

Advanced practice nurse _____

_____

_____

Clinical nurse specialist _____

_____

_____

Nurse practitioner _____

_____

_____

Certified nurse-midwife _____

_____

_____

Nurse anesthetist _____

_____

_____

Nurse administrator _____

_____

_____

Nurse researcher _____

_____

_____

Health Care Team

➤ The health care team comprises four general types of professionals. Briefly explain each role.

Physician _____

_____

_____

Physician assistant _____

_____

_____

Therapist _____

_____

_____

Pharmacist _____

_____

_____

Social worker _____

_____

_____

Spiritual advisor _____

_____

_____

▌ NURSING AS A PROFESSION
Professionalism

➤ Professions possess the following primary characteristics. Explain each one.

Education _____

_____

_____

Theory _____

_____

_____

Service _____

_____

_____

Autonomy _____

_____

_____

Code of ethics _____

_____

_____

Professional Organizations

➤ Briefly identify the issues with which the following organizations deal:

ANA and CNA _____

_____

ICN _____

_____

NLN _____

_____

NSNA _____

_____

AORN _____

_____

AWHONN _____

_____

NAPNAP _____

_____

AACN _____

_____

■ SOCIETY'S INFLUENCE ON NURSING

➤ Explain how the following issues have affected nursing practice:

Technological advances _____

_____

_____

Demographic changes _____

_____

_____

Consumer's movement _____

_____

_____

Health promotion _____

_____

_____

Women's movement _____

_____

_____

Human rights movement _____

_____

_____

■ TRENDS IN NURSING

➤ Nursing is continuously growing and evolving as changes occur in society, in health care emphases and methods, in life-styles, and among nurses, themselves.

Political Influence of Professional Nursing

➤ Nurses' involvement in politics is receiving greater emphasis in nursing curricula, professional organizations, and health care settings.

➤ The ANA employs RNs as lobbyists at the federal level, and state nursing organizations also hire lobbyists and legislative specialists to work on state nursing issues and to assist with federal efforts.

Nursing's Influence on Health Care Policy and Practice

➤ Nursing's Agenda for Health Care Reform supports the creation of a health care system that ensures

_____,

_____,

and _____.

➤ The plan for reform focuses on _____

and the _____,

_____, and

_____ of health.

REVIEW QUESTIONS

(The student should select the appropriate answer and cite the rationale for choosing that particular answer.)

1. The factor that best advanced the practice of nursing in the first century was:
   ✓a. Teachings of Christianity
   b. Growth of cities
   c. Better education of nurses
   d. Improved conditions for women

Answer (   ) Rationale: _____

_____

_____

2. Contemporary nursing practice is based on knowledge generated through nursing theories. Nightingale's theory introduced the concept that nursing care focuses on:
   ✓a. Manipulating the client's environment
   b. Promoting the client's self-care needs
   c. Maintaining a maximum level of wellness
   d. Developing interpersonal interactions with the client

Answer (   ) Rationale: _____

_____

_____

3. Which of the following best summarizes the 1980 American Nurses Association definition of nursing?
   a. Nursing is a goal-directed service.
   b. Nursing focuses on health care of the ill client.
   ✓c. Nursing is the diagnosis and treatment of the impact of illness on the client.
   d. Nursing is the extension of medical treatment.

Answer (   ) Rationale: _____

_____

_____

4. Nursing education programs may seek voluntary accreditation by the appropriate council of the:
   a. American Nurses Association
   b. International Council of Nurses
   c. Congress for Nursing Practice
   ✓d. National League for Nursing

Answer ( ) Rationale: _____

_____

_____

5. The graduate nurse must pass a licensure examination administered by the:
   a. Accredited school of nursing
   b. American Nurses Association
   ✓c. State boards of nursing
   d. National League for Nursing

Answer ( ) Rationale: _____

_____

_____

6. In-service education programs are:
   a. Accredited by the ANA or state boards of nursing
   b. Required for state license renewal
   ✓c. Designed to increase the competency of nurses employed by the institution
   d. Goal-directed toward promoting leadership in health care delivery

Answer ( ) Rationale: _____

_____

_____

7. The nurse's roles are interrelated. The role prominently expressed when protecting the client's human rights is:
   a. Caregiver
   b. Manager
   ✓c. Client advocate
   d. Rehabilitator

Answer ( ) Rationale: _____

_____

_____

8. When Mr. Jones had his leg amputated, the nurse assisted him as he learned to cope with the artificial limb and new routine. The nurse's primary role at this time was:
   ✓a. Rehabilitator
   b. Manager
   c. Friend
   d. Advisor

Answer ( ) Rationale: _____

_____

_____

9. An expanded role of the nurse is:
   a. Primary nurse
   b. Team leader
   c. Staff nurse
   ✓d. Nurse practitioner

Answer ( ) Rationale: _____

_____

_____

10. A group that lobbies at the state and federal levels for advancement of the nurse's role, economic interest, and health care is the:
   ✓a. American Nurses Association
   b. State boards of nursing
   c. National Student Nurses' Association
   d. American Hospital Association

Answer ( ) Rationale: _____

_____

_____

Chapter 14

Communication

Communication is the basic element of human interactions that allows people to establish, maintain, and improve contacts with others.

COMPREHENSIVE UNDERSTANDING

▌ LEVELS OF COMMUNICATION

➤ Summarize the following communication interactions:

Intrapersonal _____

_____

Interpersonal _____

_____

Public _____

_____

▌ ELEMENTS OF THE COMMUNICATION PROCESS

➤ Communication is complex, involving _____

_____ and _____
symbols and messages exchanged between persons.

➤ Communication is a process. This process allows

_____

_____.

➤ Communication is a response between two or more persons as they send and receive stimuli and messages.

➤ Communication occurs on a social level, with participants engaged in intrapersonal and interpersonal contact.

➤ Briefly summarize the elements of communication.

Referent _____

_____

Sender _____

_____

Message _____

_____

Channels _____

_____

Receiver _____

_____

Feedback _____

_____

▌ MODES OF COMMUNICATION

➤ People send messages in verbal and nonverbal modes, which are closely bound together during interpersonal interaction.

Verbal Communication

➤ Verbal communication involves spoken or written words. To make a message clear the nurse uses effective verbal communication techniques. Briefly explain each one.

Clarity and brevity: _____

_____

Vocabulary: _____

_____

Denotative and connotative meaning: _____

_____

Pacing: _____

_____

Timing and relevance: _____

_____

Humor: _____

_____

Nonverbal Communication

➤ Nonverbal communication is transmission of messages without the use of words.

➤ Nonverbal cues add meaning to the verbal message.
➤ Nonverbal communication is much more powerful than verbal communication.
➤ Becoming a good observer of nonverbal behavior requires time and practice. Briefly explain the following nonverbal behaviors:

Metacommunication _____

_____

_____

Personal appearance _____

_____

_____

Intonation _____

_____

_____

Facial expression _____

_____

_____

Posture and gait _____

_____

_____

Gestures _____

_____

Touch _____

_____

■ FACTORS INFLUENCING COMMUNICATION

➤ Many factors influence the content of a message and the manner in which it is shared. Briefly explain the following:

Development _____

_____

_____

Perceptions _____

_____

_____

Values _____

_____

_____

Emotions _____

_____

_____

Sociocultural background _____

_____

_____

Gender _____

_____

Knowledge _____

_____

Roles and relationships _____

_____

_____

Environment _____

_____

_____

Space and territoriality _____

_____

_____

■ THERAPEUTIC COMMUNICATION

➤ Therapeutic communication is the process _____

_____

_____.

➤ Therapeutic communication develops an interpersonal relationship between the client and nurse.
➤ Therapeutic communication is based on patient disclosure and confidentiality.
➤ Therapeutic communication ultimately enables the nurse to establish a working relationship with the client.

Social Interaction

➤ The first attempt at communicating with a client usually consists of a brief social interaction.
➤ Superficial interaction makes participants feel safe because the discussion has no hidden intent for personal disclosures.

➤ The goal of social interaction is to _____

_____.

Caring and Methods of Effective Communication

➤ Briefly summarize the following techniques used to foster communication:

Listen attentively _____

_____

_____

Conveying acceptance _____

_____

_____

Asking related questions _____

_____

_____

Paraphrasing _____

_____

_____

Clarifying _____

_____

_____

Focusing _____

_____

_____

Stating observations _____

_____

_____

Offering information _____

_____

_____

Maintaining silence _____

_____

_____

Using assertiveness _____

_____

_____

Summarizing _____

_____

_____

Barriers to Effective Communication

➤ Explain the barriers that are nontherapeutic.

Giving an opinion: _____

_____

_____

Offering false reassurance: _____

_____

_____

Being defensive: _____

_____

_____

Showing approval or disapproval: _____

_____

_____

Stereotyping: _____

_____

_____

Asking Why: _____

_____

_____

Changing the subject inappropriately: _____

_____

_____

❚ HELPING RELATIONSHIPS

➤ The nurse-client relationship is a dynamic process involving a collaborative effort of the nurse and client to resolve a problem and promote the client's health and adaptation abilities.

➤ Creation of a therapeutic environment rests on the nurse's ability to provide physical and psychosocial comfort to the client.

Dimensions of Helping Relationships

➤ The following are the common features of a helping relationship. Briefly explain each one.

Trust: _____

_____

_____

Empathy and sympathy: _____

_____

_____

Caring: _____

_____

_____

Autonomy and mutuality: _____

_____

_____

Phases of a Helping Relationship

➤ A helping relationship is a bond that allows the nurse to be more effective in carrying out the nursing process.

- The nurse is responsible for directing the client through the helping relationship to ensure that the client's needs are met.
- The helping relationship consists of the following phases. Briefly explain each one.

Preinteraction: _____

_____

_____

Orientation: _____

_____

_____

_____

Working: _____

_____

_____

_____

Termination: _____

_____

_____

_____

■ COMMUNICATION AND THE NURSING PROCESS

- Through communication a nurse and client come to an agreement about how to meet the goals of care successfully. These functions are part of the ongoing nursing process.
- The nurse uses the nursing process to ensure that clients communicate in a meaningful and effective way.

Assessment

- List the factors that influence communication.

a. _____

b. _____

c. _____

d. _____

- Review of medical history and physical assessment provides clues to the client's physical ability to communicate. List four mechanisms that allow a client to communicate.

a. _____

b. _____

c. _____

d. _____

- Physical barriers cause _____,

_____,

or _____.

Nursing Diagnosis

- List three nursing diagnoses appropriate for a client with alterations in communication.

a. _____

b. _____

c. _____

Planning

- List three goals for effective interpersonal communication.

a. _____

b. _____

c. _____

Implementation

- List the nursing interventions for helping clients with ineffective coping or impaired social interaction.

a. _____

b. _____

c. _____

d. _____

e. _____

f. _____

- List five methods to control the environment so that it is conducive to interpersonal interactions.

a. _____

b. _____

c. _____

d. _____

e. _____

- Briefly identify the individual approaches used to communicate with the following types of clients:

Those with physical communication barriers _____

_____

_____

A child _____

_____

_____

An older adult _____

_____

_____

An unconscious client _____

_____

_____

Evaluation

➤ List four expected outcomes for the client with impaired communication.

a. _____

b. _____

c. _____

d. _____

REVIEW QUESTIONS

(The student should select the appropriate answer and cite the rationale for choosing that particular answer.)

1. In demonstrating the method for deep breathing exercises, the nurse places his or her hands on the client's abdomen to explain diaphragmatic movement. This technique involves the use of which communication element?
   a. Feedback
   ✓b. Tactile channel
   c. Referent
   d. Message

Answer ( ) Rationale: _____

_____

_____

2. Which statement about nonverbal communication is correct?
   a. It is easy for a nurse to judge the meaning of a client's facial expression.
   ✓b. The nurse's verbal messages should be reinforced by nonverbal cues.
   c. The physical appearance of the nurse rarely influences nurse-client interaction.
   d. Words convey meanings that are usually more significant than nonverbal communication.

Answer ( ) Rationale: _____

_____

_____

3. The term referring to the sender's attitude toward the self, the message, and the listener is:
   a. Nonverbal communication
   ⓑ. Meta communication
   c. Connotative meaning
   d. Denotative meaning

Answer ( ) Rationale: _____

_____

_____

4. Which communication technique would be most effective in eliciting information about a client?
   a. Maintaining silence
   ✓b. Open-ended questions
   c. Stating observations
   d. Summarizing

Answer ( ) Rationale: _____

_____

_____

5. Which of the following statements by the nurse could be considered false reassurance to the client?
   ✓a. "I understand your concern about surgery, but at your age there's nothing to worry about."
   b. "I know that it must be frightening to be in the hospital, but you'll receive the care you need."
   c. "It's a difficult time for you, but be assured that I'm willing to listen to anything you have to say."
   d. "No, I've never lost a close relative to cancer, but I understand how difficult it must be for you."

Answer ( ) Rationale: _____

_____

_____

6. All of the following are important factors when communicating with clients. Which is the most important in establishing effective communication with a child?
   a. Meeting the child at eye level
   b. Providing a quiet, comfortable environment
   c. Informing the child about any discomfort associated with a procedure
   ✓d. Understanding the influence of development on language and thought processes

Answer ( ) Rationale: _____

_____

_____

7. The referent in the communication process is:
   a. That which motivates the communication
   b. The means of conveying messages
   c. Information shared by the sender
   d. The person who initiates the communication

Answer ( ) Rationale: _____

_____

_____

8. The nurse is conducting an admission interview with the client. To maintain the client's territoriality and maximize communication, the nurse should sit:
   a. 0 to 18 inches from the client
   b. 18 inches to 4 feet from the client
   c. 4 to 12 feet from the client
   d. 12 feet or more from the client

Answer ( ) Rationale: _____

_____

_____

9. Mr. Sherwood's care necessitates that an intimate distance be maintained between him and his caregiver. To prevent this from hindering the establishment of a helping relationship, the caregivers must:
   a. Apologize each time and explain the need for close contact
   b. Rotate assignments for his care
   c. Convey confidence and gentleness
   d. Restrict time of close contact to that which is necessary to complete procedures

Answer ( ) Rationale: _____

_____

_____

10. The focus of a working phase of a therapeutic helping relationship is:
    a. Setting the tone
    b. Identifying problems and goals
    c. Evaluating goal achievement
    d. Meeting goals already determined

Answer ( ) Rationale: _____

_____

_____

11. Which of the following is a correctly stated nursing diagnosis for a client with a communication problem?
    a. Impaired verbal communication related to right-side cerebral vascular accident
    b. Inability to communicate related to lack of knowledge of proper English
    c. Impaired verbal communication related to bilateral hearing loss
    d. Poor communication skills related to lack of formal education

Answer ( ) Rationale: _____

_____

_____

Chapter 15 | Teaching-Learning Process

A well-designed, comprehensive teaching plan that fits a client's learning needs can reduce health costs, improve the quality of care, and help clients gain optimum wellness and increased independence.

PRELIMINARY READING

Chapter 15, pp. 259-284

COMPREHENSIVE UNDERSTANDING

∎ STANDARDS FOR CLIENT EDUCATION

➤ Briefly summarize the standards for client and family education (JCAHO, 1994).

a. _____

_____

b. _____

_____

c. _____

_____

d. _____

_____

e. _____

_____

f. _____

_____

➤ The successful accomplishment of these standards is based on nursing assessments, nursing diagnoses, implementation, and evaluation.
➤ Evidence of successful client education must be noted in the client's medical record.

∎ PURPOSES FOR CLIENT EDUCATION

➤ Comprehensive client education includes three important purposes, each involving a separate phase of health care (see the box on text p. 261).

Maintenance and Promotion of Health and Illness Prevention

➤ The nurse is a visible, competent resource for clients intent on improving physical and psychological well-being. In the school, home, clinic, or workplace, the nurse provides information and skills that will allow clients to practice healthier behaviors.

➤ Promoting healthy behaviors through education increases self-esteem by allowing clients to assume more responsibility for their health.
➤ Greater knowledge can result in better health maintenance habits.

Restoration of Health

➤ Injured or ill clients need information and skills that will help them regain or maintain their levels of health.
➤ The family is a vital part of a client's return to health and may need to know as much as the client.
➤ The nurse should not assume that the family should be involved and must first assess the client-family relationship.

Coping with Impaired Functioning

➤ In the case of serious disability, the client's family role may change, making understanding and acceptance by family members necessary.
➤ The family's ability to provide support can result from education, which begins as soon as the client's needs are identified and the family displays a willingness to help.

∎ TEACHING AND LEARNING

➤ Define:

Teaching _____

_____

Learning _____

_____

➤ Teaching is most effective when it responds to a learner's needs.
➤ Interpersonal communication is essential for successful teaching.

Role of the Nurse in Teaching and Learning

➤ The nurse should try to anticipate clients' needs for information (see text p. 262) based on their physical conditions or treatment.
➤ The nurse clarifies information provided by physicians and may become the primary source of information for adjusting to health problems.

➤ Kruger (1991) noted three areas for nurse responsibilities in patient education. List them.

a. _____

_____

b. _____

_____

c. _____

_____

Teaching as Communication

➤ The teaching process closely parallels the communication process.
➤ A teacher applies each element of the _____ process while imparting information to learners.
➤ Define the following terms via the teaching process:

Referent _____

_____

Sender _____

_____

Message _____

_____

Channels _____

_____

Receiver _____

_____

Feedback _____

_____

▮ DOMAINS OF LEARNING

➤ Learning occurs in _____

(understandings), _____ (attitudes),

and _____ (motor skills) domains.
➤ The characteristics of learning within each domain affect the teaching and evaluation methods used.

Cognitive Learning

➤ Bloom (1956) classifies cognitive behaviors in an ordered hierarchy. Summarize each one.

Knowledge: _____

_____

_____

Comprehension: _____

_____

_____

Application: _____

_____

_____

Analysis: _____

_____

_____

Synthesis: _____

_____

_____

Evaluation: _____

_____

_____

Affective Learning

➤ Affective learning deals with expression of feelings and acceptance of attitudes, opinions, and values.
➤ Summarize the following hierarchy behaviors:

Receiving _____

_____

_____

Responding _____

_____

_____

Valuing _____

_____

_____

Organizing _____

_____

_____

Characterizing _____

_____

_____

Psychomotor Learning

➤ Psychomotor learning involves acquiring skills that require the integration of mental and muscular activity.
➤ Summarize the following hierarchy behaviors:

Perception _____

_____

_____

Set _____

_____

_____

Guided response _____

_____

_____

Mechanism _____

_____

_____

Complex overt response _____

_____

_____

Adaptation _____

_____

_____

Origination _____

_____

_____

■ BASIC LEARNING PRINCIPLES

➤ Learning depends on the motivation to learn, the ability to learn, and the learning environment.

Motivation to Learn

➤ An attentional set is _____

_____.

➤ Briefly explain how the following distractions influence the ability to learn:

Physical discomfort _____

_____

_____

Anxiety _____

_____

_____

Environmental _____

_____

_____

➤ Motivation is an _____

_____

_____.

➤ Briefly explain how the following can affect motivation:

Social mastery _____

_____

_____

Task mastery _____

_____

_____

Physical mastery _____

_____

_____

➤ Compliance is _____

_____

_____.

➤ Summarize the major concepts of the health-belief model: _____

_____

_____

➤ The process of grieving gives clients time to adapt psychologically to the emotional and physical implications of illness.
➤ Readiness to learn is significantly related to the stage of grieving.
➤ When the client enters the stage of acceptance, which is compatible with learning, the nurse introduces a teaching plan.
➤ Teaching continues as long as the client remains in a stage conducive to learning.
➤ The client is not seen as a passive recipient or consumer of health care and education but as an active partner in the provision of care.

Ability to Learn

➤ Summarize how the following influence the ability to learn:

Developmental capability _____

_____

_____

Physical capability _____

_____

_____

Learning Environment

➤ Factors in the physical environment where teaching takes place make learning either a pleasant or a difficult experience. List five factors to consider when selecting the learning setting.

a. _____

b. _____

c. _____

d. _____

e. _____

INTEGRATING THE NURSING AND TEACHING PROCESSES

➤ The teaching process requires assessment to _____
_____. A diagnostic statement
specifies _____.

➤ The nurse sets specific learning objectives and implements the teaching plan using teaching and learning
principles to ensure _____
_____.

➤ The teaching process requires an evaluation of learning based on _____.

➤ The nursing and teaching processes are not the same.
The nursing process requires _____
_____
_____.

The teaching process focuses on _____
_____
_____.

Assessment

➤ The client requires the nurse to assess the following
factors. Summarize each one.
Learning needs:

a. _____
_____
_____

b. _____
_____
_____

c. _____
_____
_____

d. _____
_____
_____

e. _____
_____
_____

Motivation to learn:

a. _____
_____
_____

b. _____
_____
_____

c. _____
_____
_____

d. _____
_____
_____

e. _____
_____
_____

f. _____
_____
_____

g. _____
_____
_____

Ability to learn:

a. _____
_____

b. _____
_____

Teaching environment:

a. _____
_____

b. _____
_____

c. _____
_____

Resources for learning:

a. _____

_____

_____

b. _____

_____

_____

c. _____

_____

_____

d. _____

_____

_____

e. _____

_____

_____

Nursing Diagnosis

➤ Classifying diagnoses by the three learning domains helps the nurse focus specifically on subject matter and teaching methods.

Planning

➤ After determining the nursing diagnoses that identify a client's learning needs, the nurse develops a teaching plan, determines goals and expected outcomes, and involves the client in selecting learning experiences. Expected outcomes guide the _____

_____

_____.

➤ A learning objective identifies the _____ of a planned learning experience and helps_____

_____ for learning.

➤ A learning objective includes the same criteria as goals or outcomes in a nursing care plan, which are:

a. _____

b. _____

c. _____

d. _____

➤ The principles of teaching are techniques that incorporate the principles of learning. Explain the following principles:

Setting priorities _____

_____

_____

Timing _____

_____

_____

Organizing teaching material _____

_____

_____

Maintaining learning attention and participation ___

_____

_____

_____

Building on existing knowledge _____

_____

_____

Selection of teaching methods _____

_____

_____

Implementation

➤ Describe 7 principles to apply in any teaching plan.

a. _____

b. _____

c. _____

d. _____

e. _____

f. _____

g. _____

➤ Briefly explain the following teaching approaches:

Telling _____

_____

_____

Selling _____

_____

_____

Participating _____

_____

_____

Entrusting _____

_____

_____

Reinforcing _____

_____

_____

➤ Summarize the following instructional methods:

One-to-one discussion _____

_____

_____

Group instruction _____

_____

_____

Preparatory instruction _____

_____

_____

Demonstrations _____

_____

_____

Analogies _____

_____

_____

Role playing _____

_____

_____

Discovery _____

_____

_____

➤ Identify some teaching tools to be used with the following:

Illiteracy _____

_____

_____

Cultural diversity _____

_____

_____

Children's needs _____

_____

_____

Older adults _____

_____

_____

Evaluation

➤ Evaluation reinforces learners' correct behavior, helps learners realize how they should change incorrect behavior, and helps the teacher determine the adequacy of teaching.

➤ Identify some evaluation measures: _____

_____

_____

_____

_____

➤ List the three areas to be included when documenting client teaching.

a. _____

b. _____

c. _____

REVIEW QUESTIONS

(The student should select the appropriate answer and cite the rationale for choosing that particular answer.)

1. The process of teaching relies on the principles of:
   a. Interpersonal communication
   b. Psychosocial adaptation
   c. Developmental studies
   d. Conceptual development

Answer ( ) Rationale: _____

_____

_____

2. When developing a teaching plan for a client coping with impaired functioning, the nurse should focus on:
   a. Anatomy and physiology of the affected body system
   b. The expected duration of care
   c. The prevention of complications
   d. The cause and origin of symptoms

Answer ( ) Rationale: _____

_____

_____

3. An internal impulse that causes a person to take action is:
   a. Anxiety
   b. Motivation
   c. Compliance
   d. Adaptation

Answer ( ) Rationale: _____

_____

_____

4. Demonstration of the principles of body mechanics used when transferring clients from bed to chair would be classified under which domain of learning?
   a. Cognitive
   b. Social
   c. Psychomotor
   d. Affective

Answer ( ) Rationale: _____

_____

_____

5. Which of the following clients is most ready to begin a patient-teaching session?
   a. Ms. Hernandez, who is unwilling to accept that her back injury may result in permanent paralysis.
   b. Mr. Frank, a newly diagnosed diabetic, who is complaining that he was awake all night because of his noisy roommate.
   c. Mrs. Brown, a client with irritable bowel syndrome, who has just returned from a morning of testing in the GI lab.
   d. Mr. Jones, a client who had a heart attack 4 days ago and now seems somewhat anxious about how this will affect his future.

Answer ( ) Rationale: _____

_____

_____

6. The nurse works with pediatric clients who have diabetes. Which is the youngest age-group to which the nurse can effectively teach psychomotor skills such as insulin administration?
   a. Toddler
   b. Adolescent
   c. School-age
   d. Preschool

Answer ( ) Rationale: _____

_____

_____

7. An appropriately stated nursing diagnosis for a client with a health teaching need would be:
   a. Knowledge deficit related to diabetes
   b. Inability to learn medication administration related to lack of proper motivation
   c. Altered health maintenance related to lack of knowledge about skin care
   d. Knowledge deficit (psychomotor) related to old age

Answer ( ) Rationale: _____

_____

_____

8. Which of the following is an appropriately stated learning objective for Mr. Ryan, a newly diagnosed diabetic?
   a. Mr. Ryan will be taught self-insulin administration by 5/2.
   b. Mr. Ryan will perform blood glucose monitoring with the EZ-Check Monitor by the time of discharge.
   c. Mr. Ryan will know the signs and symptoms of low blood sugar by 5/5.
   d. Mr. Ryan will understand diabetes.

Answer ( ) Rationale: _____

_____

_____

9. The nurse explains the procedure for obtaining a clean catch urine specimen to the client. Which teaching approach will the nurse use?
   a. Telling
   b. Selling
   c. Participating
   d. Entrusting

Answer ( ) Rationale: _____

_____

_____

10. When documenting client teaching, the nurse should include all of the following *except:*
    a. Method of teaching
    b. Evaluation of learning
    c. General information about content taught
    d. Attainment of learning objectives

Answer ( ) Rationale: _____

_____

_____

Chapter
16

Research

Nursing leaders and organizations have made considerable efforts to increase nurses' awareness of the importance of nursing research as a foundation for practice.

PRELIMINARY READING

Chapter 16, pp. 285-297

COMPREHENSIVE UNDERSTANDING

■ HISTORICAL PERSPECTIVE
➤ Briefly explain the significance of the following:

Florence Nightingale _____

_____

_____

_____

Goldmark report _____

_____

_____

_____

1940 _____

_____

1950 _____

_____

1960 _____

_____

1970 _____

_____

1980 _____

_____

1990 _____

_____

■ SCIENTIFIC RESEARCH IN NURSING
Knowledge Acquisition
➤ Knowledge is acquired in many ways. Scientific research is the most reliable and objective of all methods of gaining knowledge.

➤ The following are ways an individual learns. Briefly explain each one:

Tradition _____

_____

_____

_____

Experts _____

_____

_____

_____

Experience _____

_____

_____

Other disciplines _____

_____

_____

_____

Trial and error _____

_____

_____

_____

Logical reasoning and critical thinking _____

_____

_____

Scientific method _____

_____

_____

➤ List the five characteristics of a scientific investigation.

a. _____

b. _____

c. _____

d. _____

e. _____

Nursing and the Scientific Approach

➤ The purpose of the scientific approach is to _____

_____

_____.

➤ Research provides a way for nursing questions and problems to be studied in greater depth within the context of nursing.

Definitions of Scientific and Nursing Research

➤ Define:

Scientific method _____

_____

_____

Scientific approach _____

_____

_____

_____

Phenomena _____

_____

Hypothesis _____

_____

_____

Biomedical research _____

_____

_____

Nursing research _____

_____

_____

_____

Experiment _____

_____

_____

_____

Quantitative research _____

_____

_____

_____

Comparison group _____

_____

_____

Experimental group _____

_____

_____

Subjects _____

_____

_____

Qualitative research _____

_____

_____

_____

Nursing Research and the Nursing Process

➤ The research process consists of phases or steps that can be compared and contrasted with those of the nursing process. Briefly compare the two.

Nursing process: _____

_____

_____

_____

_____

Research process: _____

_____

_____

_____

_____

Nurse Researchers

➤ In 1981 the ANA noted that all levels of nursing preparation have an active role in the process of developing nursing knowledge and implementing this knowledge into practice.

➤ List 5 of the 11 ANA priorities for nursing research.

a. _____

b. _____

c. _____

d. _____

e. _____

➤ Studies that investigate client outcomes and the effectiveness of nursing care are called _____.

➤ Briefly explain the expectations of the following levels of nursing preparation with clinical nursing research:

Doctorally prepared _____

_____

_____

_____

Master's degree _____

_____

_____

_____

Baccalaureate _____

_____

_____

Associate degree _____

_____

_____

▌ ETHICAL ISSUES IN RESEARCH
Rights of Human Subjects

➤ Informed consent means that research subjects:

a. _____

_____

b. _____

_____

c. _____

_____

➤ Confidentiality is _____

_____

_____

_____.

➤ Anonymity is _____

_____

_____.

Rights of Other Research Participants

➤ All participants, including health care professionals caring for clients, have the right to be fully informed about the study, its procedures, and any physical or emotional injury that clients could experience as a result of participation.

➤ Any nurse or student nurse has the right to refuse to carry out any research procedures if he or she is concerned about their ethical aspects.

➤ Withholding proper care or implying that care will be withheld from clients who refuse to participate is unethical.

▌ NURSING RESEARCH IN NURSING PRACTICE
Identifying Research Studies

➤ The typical research report has the following parts. Briefly explain each section:

Abstract _____

_____

_____

Introduction _____

_____

_____

Methods _____

_____

_____

Results _____

_____

_____

Discussion _____

_____

_____

_____

Reference list _____

_____

_____

_____

➤ Explain the difference between primary and secondary

source: _____

_____

_____

_____

Locating Research Studies

➤ Identify some common sources of research studies:

_____

_____

_____

_____

_____

_____

_____

_____

Organizing Information from a Research Study

➤ Define *citations:* _____

_____

_____

_____

Identifying Clinical Nursing Problems

➤ List three characteristics of a clinical nursing problem with the potential to be researched.

a. _____

b. _____

c. _____

Using Findings in Nursing Practice

➤ To use findings in clinical practice, the nurse must be aware of the problems already studied.

➤ List four criteria used to determine if research findings should be applied to nursing practice.

a. _____

b. _____

c. _____

d. _____

➤ Define *research utilization:* _____

_____

_____

_____.

REVIEW QUESTIONS

(The student should select the appropriate answer and cite the rationale for choosing that particular answer.)

1. The purpose of the ANA's priorities for nursing research is to:
   a. Review nurse researchers' ethical standards
   √b. Identify areas of nursing practice needing further knowledge to improve client care
   c. Assess the quality of nursing research proposals
   d. Identify the educational preparation required of nurse researchers

Answer (   ) Rationale: _____

_____

_____

2. The researcher's refusal to disclose the names of subjects is:
   a. Confidentiality
   √b. Anonymity
   c. Informed consent
   d. Protection of clients

Answer (   ) Rationale: _____

_____

_____

3. The purpose of an institutional review board is to:
   a. Ensure that federal funds are equitably appropriated
   b. Conduct research benefiting the public
   c. Determine the risk status of clients in research projects
   √d. Ensure that ethical principles are observed in human-subject research.

Answer (   ) Rationale: _____

_____

_____

4. Research studies can most easily be identified by:
   a. Looking for the word "research" in the title of the report
   b. Looking for the study only in research journals
   √ c. Examining the contents of the report
   d. Reading the abstract and conclusion of the report

Answer ( ) Rationale: _____

_____

5. Which statement concerning research reports is accurate?
   a. Nursing textbooks are primary sources of information.
   √ b. Primary sources are those written by one of the researchers in the study.
   c. The fact that a report is a primary source guarantees its accuracy.
   d. Secondary sources are the best source of information about the research study.

Answer ( ) Rationale: _____

_____

6. To find articles on a particular subject, the nurse first checks:
   a. The citation list at the end of the article
   b. Through pages of related journals
   c. Other articles written by the same authors
   √ d. The subject headings in a cumulative index

Answer ( ) Rationale: _____

_____

7. A research report includes all of the following *except:*
   a. A summary of literature used to identify the research problem
   b. The researcher's interpretation of the study results
   √ c. A summary of other research studies with the same results
   d. A description of methods used to conduct the study

Answer ( ) Rationale: _____

_____

8. When findings were published, the author stated, "Empirical data revealed no difference in pain relief when two approaches were compared." Empirical data refer to:
   a. Interpretations given by leading authorities
   √ b. Testing in the real world, the results of which can be literally observed
   c. Abstract concepts
   d. Data gathered in previous generations

Answer ( ) Rationale: _____

_____

9. A good clinical study is characterized by all the following *except:*
   a. The problem occurs frequently in a definable population.
   b. A way for measuring the problem is available.
   c. The possible solution alters client care.
   √ d. The problem has been satisfactorily dealt with before the study.

Answer ( ) Rationale: _____

_____

Leadership and Management

In today's health care environment all professional nurses must rely on their own leadership and management skills if they are to be successful.

PRELIMINARY READING

Chapter 17, pp. 298-305

COMPREHENSIVE UNDERSTANDING

■ DEFINITIONS OF LEADERSHIP AND MANAGEMENT

➤ Leadership is _____
_____
_____
_____ .

➤ Management is _____
_____
_____
_____ .

■ LEADERSHIP AND MANAGEMENT THEORIES

➤ The development of leadership theory has proceeded along two lines, research on leadership traits and the development of management thought. Briefly explain the following terms:

Trait theory _____
_____
_____
_____

Theory X and theory Y _____
_____
_____
_____

Scientific Management Theory

➤ Briefly summarize the focus of scientific management theory: _____
_____
_____
_____
_____
_____

Management Process

➤ The management process consists of eight tasks. List them.

P _____

O _____

S _____

D _____

C _____

O _____

R _____

B _____

Human Relations Movement

➤ At the core of the human relations movement is the belief that _____
_____
_____ .

➤ Briefly explain the Hawthorne Studies: _____
_____
_____

Systems Theory

➤ The systems theory approach views organizations as
_____
_____ .

LEADERSHIP AND MANAGEMENT STYLE

➤ *Style* refers to _____
_____
_____
_____.

➤ Leadership styles relate to the amount of control or freedom the group is allowed by the manager.

Autocratic Style

➤ The autocratic leader _____
_____
_____
_____.

➤ Identify appropriate situations for the autocratic leadership style: _____
_____.

Democratic Style

➤ The democratic style is _____
_____
_____.

➤ Identify appropriate situations for this leadership style: _____
_____
_____.

Laissez-Faire Style

➤ The laissez-faire style refers to _____
_____
_____.

➤ Identify appropriate situations for the laissez-faire leadership style: _____
_____
_____.

Situational Leadership

➤ The situational leadership style is _____
_____
_____.

➤ The situational leadership style contends that there is no single best leadership style but rather that the style used by the manager should be _____
_____ or _____.

➤ Describe the four styles of leadership behavior in situational management.

a. _____
b. _____
c. _____
d. _____

LEADING AND MANAGING IN A TYPICAL WORK SETTING

➤ The nursing staff involved in providing care to clients or families uses leadership and management skills at a clinical level, while those in management positions use these same skills at a group or unit-wide level to accomplish the goals of the unit.

Typical Work Flow

➤ Summarize the focus, leadership, and management skills on a typical day for the following:

Staff nurse _____
_____
_____
_____

Manager _____
_____
_____
_____

Role of the Nurse Manager

➤ Summarize the responsibilities and the role of the nurse manager: _____
_____
_____
_____
_____
_____

■ LEADERSHIP SKILLS FOR NURSING STUDENTS

➤ Briefly explain how to develop the following leadership skills in the new graduate:

Organization _____

_____

_____

_____

Delegation _____

_____

_____

_____

Team player attitude _____

_____

_____

REVIEW QUESTIONS

(The student should select the appropriate answer and cite the rationale for choosing that particular answer.)

1. One difference between a leader and a manager is that a manager:
   ✓a. Is responsible for day-to-day operations and stability
   b. Has a vision or a goal for the group
   c. Influences others to follow his or her direction
   d. Focuses on innovation and change

Answer ( ) Rationale: _____

_____

_____

2. Which statement best describes the outcome of the research by trait theorists?
   a. Leaders are born not made.
   b. Intelligence has been found to be the predominant trait of effective leaders.
   c. Motivation and persistence are the most important traits of effective leaders.
   ✓d. No one personality type is associated with leadership.

Answer ( ) Rationale: _____

_____

_____

3. Which situation best describes an application of the scientific management theory on a nursing unit?
   a. Group members discuss the loss of two long-term clients.
   ✓b. The supervisor tells the charge nurse that most employees require close supervision to be productive.
   c. The personnel manager and charge nurse agree that people who are committed to goals will have job satisfaction.
   d. Specialists in time and motion studies observe staff members' productivity.

Answer ( ) Rationale: _____

_____

_____

4. A nurse manager who decides to use a staff action committee to resolve a problem related to unit policies is basing her actions on which of the following?
   a. The management process
   b. Theory X and the scientific management approach
   c. Situational leadership and theory X
   ✓d. Theory Y and human relations theory

Answer ( ) Rationale: _____

_____

_____

5. A student nurse practicing primary leadership skills would demonstrate all of the following except:
   a. Being sensitive to the group's feelings
   b. Recognizing others for their contribution
   ✓c. Assuming primary responsibility for planning, implementation, follow-up, and evaluation
   d. Developing listening skills and being aware of personal motivation

Answer ( ) Rationale: _____

_____

_____

6. Mr. Massie is the team leader on a busy surgical floor. The team members are upset with the evening client assignments. Mr. Massie tells the team members to work things out for themselves and that whatever they decide will be satisfactory. Mr. Massie's leadership style could best be described as:
   a. Authoritarian
   b. Democratic
   c. Laissez-faire
   d. Situational

Answer (   ) Rationale: _____

_____

_____

7. The effective nurse manager is able to use different styles and leadership skills depending on the specific situation and the maturity of the employees. This is an example of which leadership style?
   a. Authoritarian
   b. Democratic
   c. Laissez-faire
   d. Situational

Answer (   ) Rationale: _____

_____

_____

8. The authoritarian leader:
   a. Promotes individual initiative and creativity
   b. Is concerned primarily about tasks and goals
   c. Establishes a two-way group communication pattern
   d. Delegates authority and responsibility to others

Answer (   ) Rationale: _____

_____

_____

9. During a cardiac arrest, which leadership style would be most effective?
   a. Authoritarian
   b. Democratic
   c. Laissez-faire
   d. Situational

Answer (   ) Rationale: _____

_____

_____

Chapter 18 | Values

A skillful nurse learns to recognize and work with the power of values while caring for clients. Values give life and identity to individuals, professions, and societies.

PRELIMINARY READING

Chapter 18, pp. 306-318

COMPREHENSIVE UNDERSTANDING

▮ VALUES DEFINED

➤ A value is a _____ _____ _____.

➤ Valuing has _____, _____, _____, and _____ components.

➤ The values an individual holds reflect personal needs, cultural and societal influences, and relationships with significant others.

➤ Values relate to one another to form a _____ _____.

➤ The nurse helps clients clarify or reprioritize personal values, minimize conflict, and achieve consistency among values and behaviors related to health.

▮ NATURE AND FUNCTION OF VALUES

➤ The values that influence behavior may be conscious or unconscious.
➤ A person's values about health determine the choices made about health promotion and the use of health care resources during a time of illness.
➤ Having realistic goals allows the person to be flexible

and to attain greater satisfaction from the _____ _____, _____, and _____ influenced by personal values.

➤ Perceptions of other individuals and our responses toward them are influenced by values.
➤ Values function as a _____ _____ _____.

➤ Values do not determine the worth of any person nor should one's assessment of others' values determine how they are treated in a professional relationship.

▮ FORMATION OF VALUES

➤ Values can be learned through _____, _____, and _____.

➤ Briefly explain how a professional group (e.g., student nurses) learn values.

Observation: _____ _____ _____

Reasoning: _____ _____ _____

Experience: _____ _____ _____

➤ People form values by interacting with others. Give an example of each of the following:

Conscious transmission of values: _____ _____ _____

Unconscious transmission of values: _____ _____ _____

Modes of Value Transmission

➤ Values are learned and evolve over a lifetime.
➤ Many values are not consciously chosen as the values people wish to have.
➤ The process of transmitting values can be deliberate.

➤ There are five traditional modes of value transmission. Briefly explain each one.

Modeling: _____

_____

_____

Moralizing: _____

_____

_____

Laissez-faire: _____

_____

_____

Responsible choice: _____

_____

_____

Reward and punishment: _____

_____

_____

➤ Value formation, modification, and reaffirmation occur throughout a person's life.

Sociocultural Influences

➤ Values are formed in social settings where the _____

_____, _____,

_____, and _____
backgrounds of people may vary.

➤ People take on many values of the dominant culture in which they live.
➤ To give effective care, a nurse strives to understand the

_____,

_____,

_____,

and _____.

■ VALUES IN PROFESSIONAL NURSING

➤ Values give _____,

_____, and _____.
Professions are as strong as the values on which they are based.

➤ All professions exist in relationship to society and are needed only as long as the underlying values of the profession are shared by the persons they serve.
➤ For purposes of identity and education, professions state what they believe to be their organizing and sustaining values.
➤ Nursing's most fundamental value is _____

_____.

➤ Client advocacy has also developed as a primary nursing value.

The Value of Caring

➤ A consensus has emerged within nursing that caring serves as nursing's central value, providing an organizing framework for professional research, education, and theory development.
➤ Name the five perspectives on the nature of caring.

a. _____

_____

b. _____

_____

c. _____

_____

d. _____

_____

e. _____

➤ Nurtured in people by their own experiences of being cared for, care exists as a learned behavior.
➤ Care happens interpersonally and takes on the unique characteristics of each human relationship.
➤ Care always happens within a context, implying that it is not simply an abstract or theoretical value but rather takes its shape and definition by what is needed in each situation.
➤ Certain changes within the health care delivery system threaten nurses' ability to exercise the caring they value.

Give some examples: _____

_____

_____

_____

American Association of Colleges of Nursing Values

➤ There are seven values essential for the professional nurse. Identify each one, and give an example of professional behavior.

a. _____

_____

b. _____

_____

c. _____

_____

d. _____

_____

e. _____

_____

f. _____

_____

g. _____

_____

The Value of Advocacy

➤ Define *client advocacy:* _____

_____

_____

➤ Identify some situations in which client advocacy is

needed: _____

_____

_____

_____

_____

■ VALUES AND HEALTH PROMOTION

➤ Nursing's goal is to help clients establish _____

_____.

➤ The nurse who learns about clients' values devises a more successful teaching program.
➤ Helping persons identify, prize, and act on their values provides a foundation for nursing interventions that promote health.
➤ Values serve an integrating function for _____,

_____, _____, and

_____ dimensions of human life and impact each dimension and the person's overall well-being in many ways.

➤ Changes brought on by injury and illness can result

in values _____, _____,

_____, _____,

_____, and uncertainty, all of which can have a negative impact on a person's health status.

Values Clarification

➤ To promote a healthy awareness of personal values and behaviors in the change process, individuals can use the cognitive processes of values clarification.

➤ Values clarification can be a useful tool in:_____

_____

_____

_____

_____

➤ Values clarification helps clients gain: _____

_____

_____

_____

_____

_____

➤ Values clarification, or valuing, is a process of self-discovery that helps people gain insights into their own values.
➤ The nurse's role is to shape responses to the client's questions or statements to motivate that client to examine personal thoughts and actions.
➤ There are three steps to appraise values. Explain each one.

Choosing: _____

_____

_____

Prizing: _____

_____

_____

Acting: _____

_____

_____

Values Clarification in Various Settings

➤ Values clarification is often more successful when the nurse has repeated contacts with clients.
➤ Explain briefly how nurses explore a client's value system in the following settings:

Acute care _____

_____

_____

Rehabilitation _____

_____

_____

VALUES CHALLENGES IN NURSING

➤ Because values give people meaning and are held very deeply, it is easy to see how conflict arises internally or between people when values are challenged.

➤ As nursing matures, critical shifts in professional values have occurred, sparking controversies and creating new ideals.

➤ Values also impact health at a social level.

Personal Challenges

➤ To make intelligent and thoughtful decisions about care, nurses must be aware of the influence personal values have in caregiving.

➤ Embarrassment can occur both personally and professionally when nurses struggle with negative feelings and behavior when their values are challenged.

➤ A nurse can negotiate a conflict he or she feels inside

first by _____

_____

_____,

second by _____

_____

_____,

and third by _____

_____

_____.

Professional Challenges

➤ In addition to the nursing profession's challenge to uphold its caring ideals through education, research, and expert practice, the nursing profession faces an increasing responsibility to respond collectively to societal health issues.

➤ Assuming an even greater role as health advocates would challenge nursing to examine societal health care values carefully.

➤ Priester (1992) named six values underlying the United States health care system. List them.

a. _____

b. _____

c. _____

d. _____

e. _____

f. _____

REVIEW QUESTIONS

(The student should select the appropriate answer and cite the rationale for choosing that particular answer.)

1. A value is:
   a. A pattern or way of life
   b. The philosophical investigation or study of a particular issue
   c. The actual behavior, customs, and beliefs of groups of people
   ✓d. A personal belief about the worth of a given idea that sets standards and influences behavior

   Answer (   ) Rationale: _____

   _____

   _____

2. You are working with a 15-year-old diabetic girl and her parents. You often overhear the parents telling her that "We were meant to take good care of our bodies," or "Going off your diet is irresponsible and childish. You should be ashamed of yourself." By what mode is this girl's parents attempting to transmit values to her?
   a. Modeling
   ✓b. Moralizing
   c. Laissez-faire
   d. Responsible choice

   Answer (   ) Rationale: _____

   _____

   _____

3. Values clarification is:
   ✓ a. A process of discovery that helps a person gain insight into values
   b. A set of rules designed to interfere with conscientious decision-making
   c. The development of a specific set of values that should be accepted by all persons
   d. A method of indoctrination to religious, moral, or cultural standards

   Answer (   ) Rationale: _____

   _____

   _____

4. Mrs. G, an 88-year-old woman, believes that life should not be prolonged when hope is gone. She has decided that she does not want extraordinary measures taken when her life is at its end. Because she feels this way, she has talked with her daughter about her desires, completed a living will, and left directions with her physician. This is an example of:
   a. Affirming a value
   b. Choosing a value
   ✓ c. Prizing a value
   d. Reflecting a value

   Answer (   ) Rationale: _____

   _____

   _____

5. Which statement about values is correct?
   a. Most individuals possess many personal values.
   ✓ b. A person's values about health will determine decisions about health promotion activities.
   c. Extrinsic values are associated with the maintenance of life.
   d. Personal values rarely influence an individual's perception of others.

   Answer (   ) Rationale: _____

   _____

   _____

6. A nursing instructor is comforting a grieving parent. By actions, the instructor may be transmitting a value of caring through which mode?
   ✓ a. Modeling
   b. Moralizing
   c. Laissez-faire
   d. Responsible behavior

   Answer (   ) Rationale: _____

   _____

   _____

7. In the first step of the values clarification process, which of the following behaviors would reflect appropriate client support?
   a. Encouraging the client to state personal values
   ✓ b. Assisting the client in examining alternative values
   c. Helping the client plan ways to translate values into behaviors
   d. Offering a set of values from which the client may choose those he or she prefers

   Answer (   ) Rationale: _____

   _____

   _____

8. What are the three basic choices inherent in the values clarification steps?
   a. Choosing, acting, evaluating
   b. Assessing, planning, prizing
   c. Assessing, implementing, evaluating
   ✓ d. Choosing, acting, prizing

   Answer (   ) Rationale: _____

   _____

   _____

9. Which of the following correctly states the reason for the values clarification process?
   a. It implies a specific set of values
   b. It is a means for standards indoctrination
   c. It is a set of decision-making rules
   ✓ d. It enhances self-awareness and insight

   Answer (   ) Rationale: _____

   _____

   _____

Chapter 19 | Ethics

Technological advances have pushed to new limits questions about the beginning and end of human life, the quality of life, and professional ethics and virtue.

PRELIMINARY READING

Chapter 19, pp. 319-331

COMPREHENSIVE UNDERSTANDING

■ DEFINITION OF ETHICS

➤ Define *ethics:* _____
_____
_____
_____

➤ Morals describe the _____,
_____, and _____
of people groups.

➤ Health care ethics concerns itself with _____
_____
_____
_____.

➤ Ethics reflects the personal virtues, principles, and standards that govern professional behaviors.
➤ Values influence one's ethical decision-making, relationships, and conduct.
➤ Ethics is a study of _____,
_____, and _____
and is concerned with determining what is good or valuable for all people.

■ ETHICS IN NURSING

➤ A professional code of ethics, mandates for nursing accountability and responsibility, and institutional ethics committees offer support and guidance for ethical practice.

An Ethic of Care

➤ An ethic of care is concerned with _____
_____
_____
_____.

➤ To be able to care is part of human survival.
➤ The professional caregiver is able to go from a self-centered to an other-centered position and is willing to take action on behalf of other persons.
➤ Practitioners who function from an ethic of care are sensitive to unequal relationships, which can lead to an abuse of power, whether it is intentional or not.
➤ An ethic of care leads a nurse to be sensitive to each

situation and to respond with _____

knowledge, _____, _____,

and _____.

Nurses' Codes of Ethics

➤ Nursing has developed codes of ethics that describe ideals for professional conduct.
➤ They give guidelines to assist nurses in their own moral reasoning.
➤ The codes differ slightly, but all reflect a commitment

to the primary principles of: _____
_____
_____
_____
_____
_____
_____

➤ Secondary principles of: _____
_____
_____
_____
_____
_____
_____
_____

■ ACCOUNTABILITY AND RESPONSIBILITY

➤ *Responsibility* refers to: _____

_____

_____

_____

➤ *Accountability* refers to: _____

_____

_____

_____

➤ Professional accountability serves the following purposes:

a. _____

b. _____

c. _____

d. _____

➤ The JCAHO has recommended the establishment of standards for the delivery of nursing care. These standards provide a basic structure against which nursing care is objectively measured.

Foundations for Ethical Deliberations

➤ "Doing ethics" involves participating in a critical thought process about right and wrong or thinking about situations in which one has more than one "right" possible course of action.

➤ Developing an understanding of the complex thought process (_____) involved in processing ethical situations helps nurses participate more fully in the discussion.

➤ Ethical principles guide one's _____.

➤ Principles offer "universal" norms or standards for guidance in reasoning.

Moral Reasoning

➤ Briefly describe the factors that influence a person's thinking.

Emotions: _____

_____

_____

_____

Law: _____

_____

_____

_____

Religious faith: _____

_____

_____

_____

Culture: _____

_____

_____

_____

Moral Theories

➤ There are two basic moral theories that play important roles in the reasoning process. Briefly describe each one.

Deontology: _____

_____

_____

_____

_____

Teleology: _____

_____

_____

_____

_____

Ethical Principles

➤ The moral responsibilities of professionals are guided by primary and secondary principles. Briefly describe each one.

Respect for persons: _____

_____

_____

_____

_____

Respect for autonomy: _____

_____

_____

_____

_____

Nonmaleficence and beneficence: _____

_____

_____

_____

Justice: _____

_____

_____

_____

Veracity, confidentiality, and fidelity: _____

_____

_____

_____

_____

➤ Informed consent: _____

_____

_____

_____

➤ Advance directives: _____

_____

_____

_____

METHODOLOGY FOR ETHICAL DECISION MAKING
➤ The nurse uses the following guidelines for ethical processing and decision-making: Briefly describe each one:

Presume good will _____

_____

_____

_____

Identify all important persons _____

_____

_____

_____

Gather the relevant information _____

_____

_____

_____

Identify important ethical principles _____

_____

_____

_____

Propose alternative courses of action _____

_____

_____

_____

Take action _____

_____

_____

_____

INSTITUTIONAL ETHICS COMMITTEES
➤ To help facilitate ethical dialogue and provide the educational and policy resources necessary to create a climate sensitive to ethical challenges, health care institutions have developed ethics committees.
➤ Identify the functions of institutional ethics committees: _____

_____

_____

_____

Nurses' Relationship to Ethics Committees
➤ The composition of an ethics committee should be multidisciplinary. Having representation from various disciplines helps ensure that the moral interests of all relevant parties are considered.
➤ Nurses hold valuable moral information on client and family values, health status, and coping.

■ ETHICAL HEALTH PROMOTION

➤ Many ethical situations that end in crisis or dilemma happen because good prevention has not been practiced.
➤ The best way to prevent an ethical crisis is to work at establishing relationships of trust and understanding.

REVIEW QUESTIONS

(The student should select the appropriate answer and cite the rationale for choosing that particular answer.)

1. A health care issue often becomes an ethical dilemma because:
   a. A client's legal rights coexist with a health professional's obligations.
   b. Decisions must be made quickly, often under stressful conditions.
   c. Decisions must be made based on value systems.
   √d. The choices involved do not appear to be clearly right or wrong.

   Answer ( ) Rationale: _____
   _____
   _____

2. The personal conviction that something is absolutely right or wrong in all situations is a (an):
   a. Legal obligation
   b. Personal value
   √c. Moral belief
   d. Ethical issue

   Answer ( ) Rationale: _____
   _____
   _____

3. A basic structure against which competent care is objectively measured is a:
   a. Law
   b. Principle
   √c. Standard
   d. Code

   Answer ( ) Rationale: _____
   _____
   _____

4. A document that lists the medical treatment a person chooses to refuse if unable to make decisions is the:
   a. Durable power of attorney
   b. Informed consent
   c. Medical record
   √d. Advance directives

   Answer ( ) Rationale: _____
   _____
   _____

5. Which statement about an institutional ethics committee is correct?
   √a. The ethics committee is an additional resource for clients and health care professionals.
   b. The ethics committee relieves health care professionals from dealing with ethical issues.
   c. The ethics committee would be the first option in addressing an ethical dilemma.
   d. The ethics committee replaces decision-making by the client and health care providers.

   Answer ( ) Rationale: _____
   _____
   _____

6. The nurse is working with parents of a seriously ill newborn. Surgery has been proposed for the infant, but the chances of success are unclear. In helping the parents resolve this ethical conflict, the nurse knows that the first step is:
   a. Exploring reasonable courses of action
   √b. Collecting all available information about the situation
   c. Clarifying values related to the cause of the dilemma.
   d. Identifying people who can solve the difficulty

   Answer ( ) Rationale: _____
   _____
   _____

7. Nonmaleficence refers to:
   a. Showing respect for all persons
   b. Supporting the client's right to informed consent
   √c. Preventing or removing harm to the client when possible
   d. Considering how the client can best be helped

   Answer ( ) Rationale: _____
   _____
   _____

8. The nursing profession has codes of ethics to ensure that:
   a. Nursing programs have the same basic curriculum.
   b. The practice of nursing meets legal requirements.
   c. Nurses administer client care based on scientific knowledge.
   √d. There are accepted principles that serve to guide nursing practice.

   Answer ( ) Rationale: _____
   _____
   _____

Chapter 20 | Legal Issues

Nurses must understand the law not only to protect themselves from liability but also to protect their client's rights.

PRELIMINARY READING

Chapter 20, pp. 332-349

COMPREHENSIVE UNDERSTANDING

▌LEGAL LIMITS OF NURSING
➤ Professional nurses must understand the legal limits influencing their daily practice.

Sources of Law
➤ The legal guidelines that nurses must follow are derived

from _____ law,

_____ law, and _____ law.

➤ Define the following:

Nurse practice acts _____

_____

_____

_____

Civil laws _____

_____

_____

_____

Defamation _____

_____

_____

_____

Slander _____

_____

_____

_____

Criminal law _____

_____

_____

_____

A crime _____

_____

_____

_____

_____

Felony _____

_____

_____

_____

Misdemeanor _____

_____

_____

_____

Regulatory law _____

_____

_____

_____

Common law _____

_____

_____

_____

Licensure
➤ Licensure permits persons to offer special skills to the public, but it also provides legal guidelines for protection of the public.
➤ A license can be suspended or revoked by the Board of Nursing if a nurse's conduct violates provisions in the licensing statute.

➤ If a client is harmed as a direct result of a nursing student's actions, or lack of action, the liability for the incorrect action is generally shared by the student, instructor, hospital or health care facility, and university or educational institution.

➤ If the student nurse is employed as a nurse's aide, he or she should perform tasks that appear in the job description for a nurse's aide.

■ LEGAL LIABILITY IN NURSING

Torts

➤ A tort is _____
_____.

➤ Malpractice is _____
_____.

➤ Negligence is _____
_____
_____.

➤ Nurses have been involved in several common negligent acts or professional malpractice, such as:
_____
_____
_____
_____
_____
_____
_____

➤ Nurses must use professional judgment as they carry out physicians' orders and independent nursing therapies.

➤ Identify the criteria that must be established in a malpractice suit against a nurse.

   a. _____

   b. _____

   c. _____

   d. _____

➤ A nurse's duty of care to a client is defined by the
_____
_____.

➤ The duty of care can be breached through either
_____ or _____.

Minimizing Liability Through Effective Documentation and Client Relationships

➤ Nurses can reduce their chances of being named in lawsuits by following: _____
_____
_____
_____
_____
_____
_____

➤ Identify the importance of good documentation:
_____
_____
_____
_____
_____
_____

Malpractice Insurance

➤ Personal liability insurance protects nurses in all aspects of professional practice.

➤ Employer's insurance only covers nurses while they are working within the scope of their employment.

➤ Good Samaritan laws protect _____
_____
_____.

➤ Since nurses have professional knowledge, they are held to a higher standard than an ordinary untrained good Samaritan.

➤ Gross negligence involves unreasonable recklessness on the part of the good Samaritan, whether that person is a professional or a layperson.

Standards of Care

➤ Standards of care are the guidelines for nursing practice.

➤ In a malpractice lawsuit, these standards are used to determine: _____
_____
_____
_____

➤ All state legislatures have passed nurse practice acts that define the scope of nursing practice, or the framework within which nurses must practice.

➤ Nurse practice acts set: _____

_____

_____

_____

_____

➤ Professional organizations are another source for defining standards of care. Briefly explain each one.

ANA: _____

_____

NLN: _____

_____

AORN: _____

_____

AACN: _____

_____

➤ The written policies and procedures of the employing institution detail how nurses are to perform their duties and be found in _____.

➤ The fact that your institution may require you to perform a procedure will not protect you as an individual if this practice is found to be outside the scope of nursing as defined by your state's nurse practice act.

➤ Nurses need to know the standards of care they are expected to meet within their specific work setting.

➤ An expert nurse may be called to define and explain to the court what a reasonably prudent nurse would have been expected to do in a particular situation.

Confidentiality

➤ Nursing standards for what is confidential information are based upon professional ethics.

➤ Confidential information gained while caring for a client may be privileged and therefore immune from disclosure under the law.

Informed Consent

➤ Identify the factors that must be verified for a consent to be valid.

a. _____

b. _____

c. _____

d. _____

➤ Informed consent is _____.

➤ A person is able to give consent if he or she is of

_____, _____, or has been

legally identified as the _____.

➤ Consent must be received from a person who can understand explanations for them to truly understand the decision they are making.

➤ It is important to clarify clients' understanding of the information they have been given to ensure that the consent being given is truly informed.

➤ A client refusing surgery or other medical treatment must be informed about any harmful consequences.

➤ Many procedures that nurses perform do not require formal written consent, yet clients still deserve the protection of their right to give or refuse consent to treatment.

➤ Implied consent for treatment is involved in nursing procedures.

➤ To force treatment on a client could result in a charge of assault or battery. Briefly explain each one.

Assault: _____

_____

Battery: _____

_____

➤ In some instances, the law presumes the client would wish to be treated. Identify such cases: _____

_____

_____

_____

_____

➤ If a client participates in an experimental treatment program or submits to the use of experimental drugs or treatments, detailed and stringently regulated informed consent is used.

➤ Institutional review boards (IRBs) are responsible for

_____

_____.

➤ Obtaining client consent for medical procedures is not appropriate for the nurse.

Physician Interactions

➤ Nurses may share liability for errors made by physicians and other health care personnel or for inadequate care provided by the employing institution.

➤ Nurses are obligated to follow physician's orders unless

_____

_____.

➤ A nurse should not perform a physician's order if it is foreseeable that harm will come to the client.
➤ If a verbal order is necessary, it should be written out and signed by the physician within 24 hours.
➤ A "no code" order needs to be written, not given verbally.

Short Staffing

➤ The JCAHO requires institutions to have guidelines for determining the number (staffing ratios) of nurses required to give care to a specific number of clients.
➤ Nursing supervisors should be informed when a nurse is assigned to care for more clients than is reasonable, and a written protest should be filed to document such an assignment.
➤ When staffing is inadequate, nurses should not walk out because charges of abandonment can be made.

Floating

➤ Nurses who float should inform the supervisor of any lack of experience they may have caring for the type of clients on the nursing unit.
➤ A supervisor can be held liable if a staff nurse is given an assignment she cannot safely handle.

Contracts and Employment Agreements

➤ A contract is a _____

_____.

➤ A breach of contract occurs _____

_____.

➤ By accepting a job, a nurse enters into an agreement with an employer and will perform _____

and adhere to the _____.

➤ _____, _____, and

_____ may be interpreted as the written terms of a nurse's employment contract.

➤ Nurses also enter into contractual agreements with

clients. Give some examples: _____

_____

_____

_____

_____

∎ LEGAL ISSUES IN NURSING PRACTICE

➤ Legal issues reflect changing trends in the life-styles of people in our society.

Surrogate Pregnancy Contracts and Adoption

➤ Identify the statutes in relation to the following:

Surrogate parenting _____

_____

Baby selling _____

_____

Adoption _____

_____

Abortion Issues

➤ A nurse may work with a client seeking an abortion or one who has had an abortion.
➤ Summarize the legal rights of women relative to abortion.

Roe vs. Wade: _____

_____

_____

_____

_____

Spousal consent: _____

_____

_____

_____

Parental consent: _____

_____

_____

_____

Informed consent: _____

_____

_____

_____

Controlled Substances

➤ Summarize the Comprehensive Drug Abuse Prevention and Control Act: _____

_____

_____

_____

_____

_____

Acquired Immunodeficiency Syndrome (AIDS)

➤ In 1985 the CDC recognized universal precautions as a

necessary protection for both _____

and _____.

➤ Briefly summarize the position of the following with regard to mandatory testing of health care personnel:

CDC _____

_____

_____

_____

ANA _____

_____

_____

_____

➤ Briefly identify the recommendations put forth by

The Americans with Disabilities Act (ADA): _____

_____

_____

_____

_____

_____

_____

➤ Nurses who refuse to care for HIV-infected clients may be reprimanded or fired for insubordination.

Death and Dying

➤ The law specifies that death occurs _____

_____

_____

_____.

➤ Active euthanasia involves _____

_____

_____

_____.

➤ Passive euthanasia involves _____

_____

_____

_____.

➤ Autopsies are required in circumstances such as death resulting from an accident or suspected abuse or other criminal activity.

Living Wills and Health Care Surrogates

➤ The Patient's Self-Determination Act requires _____

_____

_____

_____.

➤ Living wills are _____

_____

_____.

➤ Health care surrogate statutes are sometimes referred

to as _____

_____

_____.

Organ Donations

➤ Summarize the policies and procedures of the institution or the laws of a state regarding the nurse's role

with organ donations: _____

_____

_____

_____

_____

_____

_____

▌ NURSING ROLES RELATED TO LEGAL PRACTICE

➤ Nurses are professionals who are accountable for the autonomous judgments they make while working in a community setting.

➤ Summarize the public health laws pertaining to com-

munity health nurses: _____

_____

_____

_____

_____

_____

The Nurse as an Advocate

➤ Nurses serve as client advocates by _____
_____
_____
_____ .

The Nurse as a Risk Manager

➤ Through minimizing the risk in providing care for clients, the nurse reduces the possibility that clients will be financially and emotionally devastated through being injured by inappropriate care.

➤ Risk management is _____
_____ .

➤ Risk management steps include: _____
_____
_____
_____
_____
_____
_____

➤ Tools used by risk managers are _____
_____ .

➤ The rationale for quality assurance is _____
_____ .

➤ A nurse's documentation is his or her _____
_____
_____
_____ .

➤ If the nurse's credibility becomes questionable as a result of these documents, the risk of greater liability exists for the nurse.

➤ Explain the following:

Professional liability insurance _____
_____
_____
_____

Occurrence policy _____
_____
_____
_____

Statutes of limitation _____
_____
_____
_____

Professional Involvement

➤ The viewpoint of nurses becomes more powerful, and nurses become more effective as a profession when they are organized and cohesive.

REVIEW QUESTIONS

(The student should select the appropriate answer and cite the rationale for choosing that particular answer.)
 1. The scope of nursing practice is legally defined by:
    ✓a. State nurse practice acts
    b. Professional nursing organizations
    c. Hospital policy and procedure manuals
    d. Physicians in the employing institutions

Answer ( ) Rationale: _____
_____
_____

 2. A student nurse who is employed as a nursing assistant may perform any functions that:
    a. Have been learned in school
    b. Are expected of a nurse at that level
    ✓c. Are identified in the position's job description
    d. Require technical rather than professional skill

Answer ( ) Rationale: _____
_____
_____

 3. A confused client who fell out of bed because side rails were not used is an example of which type of liability?
    a. Felony
    b. Assault
    c. Battery
    ✓d. Negligence

Answer ( ) Rationale: _____
_____
_____

4. The best way a nurse can avoid being named in a malpractice lawsuit is to:
   a. Keep documentation vague so that claims are difficult to prove
   ✓b. Develop an empathetic rapport with the client
   c. Use traditional methods in the practice of nursing because old ways are best
   d. Rely on the advice of more experienced nurses rather than the policy and procedure manuals of the institution

Answer ( ) Rationale: _____
_____
_____

5. The nurse puts a restraint jacket on a client without the client's permission and without a physician's order. The nurse may be guilty of:
   a. Assault
   ✓b. Battery
   c. Invasion of privacy
   d. Neglect

Answer ( ) Rationale: _____
_____
_____

6. When obtaining a client's consent for surgery, the nurse determines that the client does not understand what is involved. The nurse's responsibility is to:
   ✓a. Notify the physician
   b. Explain the procedure in layman's terms
   c. Obtain the consent regardless of limitations
   d. Cancel the surgery until the problem is solved

Answer ( ) Rationale: _____
_____
_____

7. In a situation in which there is insufficient staff to implement competent care, a nurse should:
   a. Organize a strike
   b. Inform the clients of the situation
   c. Refuse the assignment
   ✓d. Accept the assignment but make a protest in writing to the administration

Answer ( ) Rationale: _____
_____
_____

8. The nurse receives an order for a medication, and the dosage ordered seems to be too high. The nurse discusses the order with the physician who confirms that the dose ordered is too high. The nurse should:
   a. Give the medication as ordered
   b. Change the ordered dosage to make it more appropriate
   c. Ignore the order
   ✓d. Discuss the medication order with the nursing supervisor

Answer ( ) Rationale: _____
_____
_____

9. When an error occurs, the nurse completes an incident report so that:
   a. The appropriate legal authority might be notified
   ✓b. Hospital liability and possible future claims may be assessed
   c. The client has a written record to submit to the insurance company
   d. A permanent record of the event can be attached to the client's chart

Answer ( ) Rationale: _____
_____
_____

10. Which of the following is the generally accepted definition of death in most states?
   a. Cessation of heartbeat
   ✓b. Absence of brain function
   c. Unattainable blood pressure
   d. Loss of deep tendon reflexes

Answer ( ) Rationale: _____
_____
_____

Chapter 21 | Cultural Diversity

Transcultural rapport and communication occur when someone attempts to understand another's point of view from that person's cultural frame of reference.

PRELIMINARY READING

Chapter 21, pp. 351-369

COMPREHENSIVE UNDERSTANDING

▌ IMMIGRATION AND DEMOGRAPHY
➤ The demographics of the United States population is changing.
➤ Identify the five major cultural groups.

a. _____

b. _____

c. _____

d. _____

e. _____

➤ Each immigrant group has its own cultural attitudes about health and illness.

➤ _____, _____, and _____ changes play a role in observed health care beliefs and practices as well as the use of health services by an individual, a family, or a community.

▌ HERITAGE CONSISTENCY
➤ Define:

Acculturation _____

_____

Heritage consistency _____

_____

Culture
➤ Culture represents _____

_____

_____

_____

_____.

Ethnicity
➤ Ethnicity is a sense of _____

_____

_____

_____.

Religion
➤ Religion is _____

_____

_____

_____.

➤ Ethical values and religious beliefs and practices serve to further clarify ethnicity.
➤ The degree of heritage consistency is evaluated by determining the importance of _____,

_____, and _____ to a person.

➤ Heritage consistency is a way of understanding if a person interprets health or illness in a modern or a traditional way.

▌ CULTURAL PHENOMENA
➤ There are six cultural phenomena that have been identified as varying among cultural groups.

Environmental Control
➤ *Environmental control* refers to _____

_____

_____

_____.

Biological Variations

➤ Identify some examples of how people from one cultural group differ biologically from members of other cultural groups: _____

_____

_____

_____

_____

_____

_____

_____

Social Organization

➤ *Social organization* refers to _____

_____

_____

_____.

➤ Identify some examples of social barriers to health

care: _____

_____

_____

_____

Communication

➤ Language differences are the most important factor in providing transcultural nursing care because they affect all stages of the nursing process.
➤ Identify some common ways that nurses might com-

municate with clients of a different culture: _____

_____

_____

_____

_____

_____

➤ If special attention is given to the communication process, then nurses can work to overcome language differences with clients who do not speak their language.

Space

➤ Personal space involves _____

_____.

➤ Territoriality is _____

_____.

➤ Identify the common behaviors found in the following zones:

Intimate zone _____

Personal distance _____

Social distance _____

Public distance _____

Time

➤ Summarize the concept *future oriented:* _____

_____

_____

_____

▌ TRADITIONAL HEALTH AND ILLNESS BELIEFS
➤ The range of health and illness definitions, beliefs, and practices is infinite, and there are differences within and among groups.

Traditional Beliefs
➤ Traditional health beliefs about the cause of illness may differ vastly from the Western model of epidemiology. Therefore it is important to understand traditional epidemiology, or the causes of illness within a belief system.

Traditional Practices
➤ Summarize the varieties of folk medicine, and give an example of each one.

Natural: _____

_____

_____

_____

Magicoreligious: _____

_____

_____

_____

Use of protective objects: _____

_____

_____

_____

Use of food: _____

_____

_____

_____

Religious practices: _____

_____

_____

_____

Traditional Remedies

➤ When people use the medicines that are from within

their ethnocultural heritage, it is viewed as _____

_____.

➤ Alternative medicine is _____

_____

_____.

Healers

➤ The person sees the healer as one who understands the problem within the cultural context, speaks the same language, and shares a similar world view. Explain the following:

Medicine man _____

Señora _____

Espiritista _____

Curandero _____

Partera _____

Root-worker _____

Chinese doctor _____

■ CULTURAL ASPECTS OF HEALTH AND ILLNESS

➤ Many cultures exist in the United States, and nurses must be aware of these groups and be familiar with the basic characteristics of each.

➤ Clients must be assessed as individuals. Characteristic beliefs of a cultural group are not necessarily shared by each individual in that group. (See table below.)

■ CULTURAL FACTORS AND THE NURSING PROCESS

➤ Nurses should be aware of and sensitive to their own unique heritage and health traditions as well as to the client's sociocultural background.

➤ The nursing process enables the nurse to provide individualized care and can be adapted to provide culturally sensitive care.

➤ Begin assessment by determining the client's _____

_____, _____,

and _____.

➤ When establishing the goals of care and planning specific interventions, the nurse considers _____

_____

_____.

➤ Discussing cultural variables with clients and families during planning helps the nurse implement client's personal health beliefs and practices so that interventions can be individualized.

➤ Nurses should evaluate their attitudes toward providing transcultural nursing care.

	Cultural Background	Causes of Illness	Methods of Prevention	Remedies
Asian Americans				
Black or African Origin Americans				
American Indians				
Hispanic Origin Americans				
European Americans				

REVIEW QUESTIONS

(The student should select the appropriate answer and cite the rationale for choosing that particular answer.)

1. Which of the following is *not* included in evaluating the degree of heritage consistency in a client?
   - ✓a. Gender
   - b. Culture
   - c. Ethnicity
   - d. Religion

Answer (   ) Rationale: _____

_____

_____

2. Which of the following interventions is helpful in communicating with a client who speaks a language other than yours?
   - a. Reassure the client that you have friends of his ethnic or racial background.
   - b. Speak to the client using his ethnic dialect.
   - ✓c. Ask the client for clarification if you don't understand what he is saying.
   - d. At the initial meeting, address the client by his first name.

Answer (   ) Rationale: _____

_____

_____

3. When providing care to clients with varied cultural backgrounds, it is imperative for the nurse to recognize that:
   - a. Cultural considerations must be put aside if basic needs are in jeopardy.
   - ✓b. Generalizations about the behavior of a particular group may be inaccurate.
   - c. Current health standards should determine the acceptability of cultural practices.
   - d. Similar reactions to stress will occur when individuals have the same cultural background.

Answer (   ) Rationale: _____

_____

_____

4. To respect a client's personal space and territoriality, the nurse:
   - a. Avoids the use of touch
   - ✓b. Explains nursing care and procedures
   - c. Keeps the curtains pulled around the client's bed
   - d. Stands 8 feet away from the bed, if possible

Answer (   ) Rationale: _____

_____

_____

5. To be effective in meeting various ethnic needs, the nurse should:
   - a. Treat all clients alike
   - ✓b. Be aware of client's cultural differences
   - c. Act as if he or she is comfortable with the client's behavior
   - d. Avoid asking questions about the client's cultural background

Answer (   ) Rationale: _____

_____

_____

6. In the next century, "average" American residents will no longer include:
   - ✓a. European Americans
   - b. African Americans
   - c. Asian Americans
   - d. Native Americans

Answer (   ) Rationale: _____

_____

_____

7. The most important factor in providing nursing care to clients in a specific ethnic group is:
   - ✓a. Communication
   - b. Time orientation
   - c. Biological variation
   - d. Environmental control

Answer (   ) Rationale: _____

_____

_____

8. Before effectively caring for a client from an ethnic group, the nurse must first:
   - a. Study the ethnic culture
   - ✓b. Determine personal cultural beliefs and values
   - c. Work with an ethnic folk healer
   - d. Minimize transcultural communication

Answer (   ) Rationale: _____

_____

_____

Chapter 22

Stress and Adaptation

Stress is a phenomenon that affects the social, psychological, developmental, spiritual, and physiological dimensions.

PRELIMINARY READING

Chapter 22, pp. 370-387

COMPREHENSIVE UNDERSTANDING

■ CONCEPTS OF STRESS
Stress and Stressors

➤ Stress is _____
_____
_____.

➤ Identify the psychological and physiological responses to stress: _____
_____
_____
_____
_____

➤ Stressors can be classified as *internal* or *external*. Give an example of each.

Internal _____
_____

External _____
_____

Physiological Adaptation

➤ Define *homeostasis:* _____
_____
_____.

➤ Explain the three major mechanisms used in adapting to a stressor.

Medulla oblongata: _____
_____
_____

Reticular formation: _____
_____
_____

Pituitary gland: _____
_____
_____

➤ Physiological mechanisms of adaptation can provide only short-term control over the body's equilibrium.

Models of Stress

➤ Stress models are used to identify the stressors for a particular individual and predict that person's responses to them. Summarize the following models:

Response-based _____
_____
_____

Adaptation model _____
_____
_____

Stimulus-based _____
_____
_____

Transaction-based _____
_____
_____

Factors Influencing Response to Stressors

➤ List the four characteristics of a stressor that influence a person's response.

a. _____

b. _____

c. _____

d. _____

➤ The greater the scope of a stressor, the greater the response of the client to it.

108

ADAPTATION TO STRESSORS

➤ Adaptation is _____

_____

_____

_____ .

➤ There are many forms of adaptation. Give some

examples: _____

_____

_____

_____

_____

➤ List the four requirements for successful family adaptation.

a. _____

b. _____

c. _____

d. _____

Dimensions of Adaptation

➤ Stress can affect the _____,

_____ , _____ ,

_____ , and _____ dimensions.

RESPONSE TO STRESS

➤ When stress occurs, a person uses physiological and psychological energy to respond and adapt.
➤ The stress response is adaptive and protective, and the characteristics of this response are the result of integrated neuroendocrine responses.

Physiological Response

➤ Describe the four common characteristics of the local adaptation response (LAS).

a. _____

b. _____

c. _____

d. _____

➤ List (in sequence) and briefly describe the three stages of the general adaptation syndrome (GAS):

a. _____

b. _____

c. _____

Psychological Response

➤ Exposure to a stressor, whether actual or perceived, produces frustration, anxiety, and tension.
➤ Psychological adaptive behaviors can be constructive or destructive. Give an example of each behavior.

Constructive: _____

_____

_____

Destructive: _____

_____

_____

➤ Physiological adaptive behaviors are referred to as

_____ .

➤ Define:

Task-oriented behaviors _____

_____

_____

Ego-defense mechanisms _____

_____

_____

NURSING PROCESS AND ADAPTATION TO STRESS

Assessment

➤ A person's perception of a stressor is based on _____

_____ , _____ , _____ ,

_____ , _____ , _____ ,

and _____ .

➤ Physiological indicators of stress are objective, more readily identified, and can be commonly observed or measured.
➤ Identify six physical indicators of stress.

a. _____

b. _____

c. _____

d. _____

e. _____

f. _____

➤.Define the following stress situations:

Mild _____

_____

Moderate _____

_____

Severe _____

_____

➤ Prolonged stress can affect the ability to complete developmental tasks. Identify one indicator for each developmental stage.

Infancy: _____

School-age: _____

Adolescence: _____

Young adult: _____

Middle-age: _____

Older adult: _____

➤ Identify three emotional indicators of stress: _____

_____

_____

_____

➤ Identify four intellectual indicators of stress: _____

_____

_____

_____

_____

➤ Identify a social indicator of stress: _____

_____

➤ Identify two spiritual indicators of stress: _____

_____

_____

Nursing Diagnosis

➤ Stress can result in multiple diagnostic statements.

Identify at least 5: _____

_____

_____

_____

_____

_____

_____

Planning

➤ The care plan is individualized to the client's perception of the stressor and response to stress.
➤ Stress-management techniques are designed to match the client's actual and potential stressors.

General goals are: _____

_____

_____

Implementation

➤ Stress management may be seen as a health promotion activity or an intervention that modifies a response to illness.
➤ Identify stress-reduction methods for each stress management goal (see table below).

Evaluation

➤ Clients' perceptions of stress differ; their perceptions of stress reduction do also.
➤ Achievement of care goals can indicate the degree of stress reduction.

Reducing Stressful Situations	Decreasing Psychological Responses	Improving Responses to Stress

REVIEW QUESTIONS

(The student should select the appropriate answer and cite the rationale for choosing that particular answer.)

1. Which definition does *not* characterize stress?
   a. Any situation in which a nonspecific demand requires an individual to respond or take action
   b. A phenomenon affecting social, psychological, developmental, spiritual, and physiological dimensions
   c. A condition eliciting an intellectual, behavioral, or metabolic response
   d. Efforts to maintain relative constancy within the internal environment

Answer ( ) Rationale: _____

_____

_____

2. Which statement about homeostasis is inaccurate?
   a. Homeostatic mechanisms provide long-term and short-term control over the body's equilibrium.
   b. Homeostatic mechanisms are self-regulatory.
   c. Homestatic mechanisms function through negative feedback.
   d. Illness may inhibit normal homeostatic mechanisms.

Answer ( ) Rationale: _____

_____

_____

3. Which nursing intervention is best used when applying the adaptation model of stress?
   a. Interventions to improve or stabilize blood pressure
   b. Interventions to reduce anxiety
   c. Interventions to maintain fluid balance
   d. Interventions to promote reality orientation

Answer ( ) Rationale: _____

_____

_____

4. The body's response to localized stress could include all of the following *except:*
   a. Blood clotting
   b. Wound healing
   c. Inflammatory response
   d. Fever

Answer ( ) Rationale: _____

_____

_____

5. Major homeostatic mechanisms are controlled by all of the following *except:*
   a. Thymus gland
   b. Medulla oblongata
   c. Reticular formation
   d. Pituitary gland

Answer ( ) Rationale: _____

_____

_____

6. Which of the following is an example of the local adaptation syndrome?
   a. Alarm reaction
   b. Flight-or-fight response
   c. Ego-defense mechanisms
   d. Inflammatory response

Answer ( ) Rationale: _____

_____

_____

7. The general adaptation syndrome consists of three stages. During which stage does the body stabilize and hormone levels return to normal?
   a. Exhaustion
   b. Regeneration
   c. Resistance
   d. Compensation

Answer ( ) Rationale: _____

_____

_____

8. Marsha had her first child 3 weeks ago. As she adapts to her new role as mother, which of the following would be an example of a task-oriented behavior?
   a. Marsha tells herself that she may not be a great mother yet, but she is able to keep her house straight and get dinner ready on time.
   b. Marsha joins the New Moms Network at the hospital where she gave birth.
   c. Marsha tells everyone that the reason mothering is a little hard for her is that her own mother was not openly affectionate with her.
   d. Marsha complains of frequent headaches and asks others to come in and care for the baby.

Answer ( ) Rationale: _____

_____

_____

9. Cathy is a 55-year-old woman who is seeking help for complaints of chronic fatigue and migraine headaches. The nurse begins talking with Cathy about the demands of her home, work, and social life. The nurse does this because he knows that middle-age adults often experience stress as a result of:
   a. Conflicts between expectations and desires
   b. Conflicts between trust and mistrust
   c. Feeling that too many responsibilities have been placed on them
   d. Feeling that they need to develop a sense of adequacy

   Answer ( ) Rationale: _____

   _____

   _____

10. Truman has asked his nurse to describe health-enhancing habits that can reduce the impact of stress in his life. Which of the following would be an appropriate response by the nurse?
    a. "Avoid vigorous exercise because it will decrease your energy reserve."
    b. "Eat a diet high in meat and sugar to provide for body fuel reserves."
    c. "Reduce your social and personal contacts to save time for more important things."
    d. "Try developing a list of tasks to be performed in order of priority."

    Answer ( ) Rationale: _____

    _____

    _____

11. Crisis intervention is a specific measure used for helping a client resolve a particular, immediate, stress problem. This approach is based on:
    a. The ability of the nurse to solve the client's problems
    b. An in-depth analysis of a client's situation
    c. Teaching the client how to use ego-defense mechanisms
    d. Effective communication between the nurse and client

    Answer ( ) Rationale: _____

    _____

    _____

23 Self-Concept

Self-concept is a subjective image of the self and a complex mixture of unconscious and conscious feelings, attitudes, and perceptions.

PRELIMINARY READING

Chapter 23, pp. 388-408

COMPREHENSIVE UNDERSTANDING

▮ OVERVIEW OF SELF-CONCEPT

➤ The four components of self-concept are _____ _____, _____, _____, and _____.

➤ Self-concept is a dynamic combination. List five sources from which self-concept is derived.

    a. _____

    b. _____

    c. _____

    d. _____

    e. _____

➤ A healthy self-concept has a high degree of stability and generates positive or negative feelings toward the self.

➤ Self-esteem is _____

_____.

▮ COMPONENTS OF SELF-CONCEPT

➤ Self-concept can be described in terms of a continuum from strong to weak or positive to negative, depending on the individual strengths of the four components.

Identity

➤ Summarize the concept of identity and its development: _____

_____

_____

_____

Body Image

➤ Summarize the concept of body image and its development: _____

_____

_____

_____

Self-Esteem

➤ Summarize the concept of self-esteem and its development: _____

_____

_____

_____

Roles

➤ Summarize the concept of roles and its development:

_____

_____

_____

_____

▮ STRESSORS AFFECTING SELF-CONCEPT

➤ A self-concept stressor is any _____

_____

_____.

➤ A physical change in the body leads to an altered body image. Identity and self-esteem can also be affected.

➤ A crisis occurs when a person cannot overcome obstacles with the usual methods of problem-solving and adapting.

Identity Stressors

➤ Identity is affected by stressors throughout life. Give an example of a stressor for each developmental stage.

Adolescence: _____

_____

Adulthood: _____

_____

Retirement: _____

_____

Body Image Stressors

➤ Identify at least five stressors affecting body image:

_____

_____

_____

_____

_____

Self-Esteem Stressors

➤ Identify at least three stressors that affect self-esteem:

_____

_____

_____

Role Stressors

➤ Identify at least three stressors that affect roles:

_____

_____

_____

➤ Define the following:

Role conflicts _____

_____

_____

Role ambiguity _____

_____

_____

Role strain _____

_____

_____

Development of Self-Concept

➤ Each stage of development has specific activities that assist the client in developing a positive self-concept. Name some for each stage.

Infancy: _____

_____

_____

_____

Toddler: _____

_____

_____

_____

Preschool: _____

_____

_____

_____

School-age: _____

_____

_____

_____

Adolescence: _____

_____

_____

_____

Young adult: _____

_____

_____

_____

Middle adult: _____

_____

_____

_____

Older adult: _____

_____

_____

_____

Family Effect on Self-Concept Development

➤ The family plays a key role in creating and maintaining its members' self-concepts.

➤ Children learn from their parents and siblings a basic sense of who they are and how they are expected to live.

NURSE'S EFFECT ON CLIENT'S SELF-CONCEPT

➤ A nurse's acceptance of a client with an altered self-concept helps stimulate positive rehabilitation.

➤ List five behaviors involved in establishing rapport with a client.

a. _____

b. _____

c. _____

d. _____

e. _____

SELF-CONCEPT AND THE NURSING PROCESS

Assessment

➤ In assessing self-concept, the nurse obtains objective and subjective data that focus on actual and potential self-concept stressors and on behaviors associated with an altered self-concept.

➤ The nursing assessment should include consideration

of previous _____

behaviors; _____ of the stressors;

and the client's _____ resources.

Nursing Diagnosis

➤ Clients with defining characteristics for self-concept disturbances suggest nursing diagnoses pertinent to

deficiencies in _____,

_____, _____,

or _____.

Planning

➤ The nurse, client, and family need to plan care directed at helping the client regain or maintain a healthy self-concept.

➤ Interventions focus on helping the client _____

_____ and on

_____ coping methods.

Implementation

Creating a Therapeutic Environment

➤ Identify at least three ways to create a therapeutic

environment: _____

_____

_____

_____

_____

Establishing a Therapeutic Environment

➤ Identify at least four behaviors that are involved in establishing a therapeutic relationship:

_____

_____

_____

_____

_____

Supporting Self-exploration

➤ Identify seven nursing interventions for the client to engage in self-exploration:

_____

_____

_____

_____

_____

_____

_____

➤ Identify the five points that are essential in addressing a client whose self-concept appears to be in distress:

_____

_____

_____

_____

_____

Evaluation

➤ Desired outcomes for a client with a self-concept disturbance may include statements of self-acceptance and acceptance of change in appearance or function.

REVIEW QUESTIONS

(The student needs to select the appropriate answer and cite the rationale for choosing that particular answer.)

1. Which developmental stage is particularly crucial for identity development?
   a. Infancy
   b. Preschool age
   c. Adolescence
   d. Young adult

Answer (   ) Rationale: _____

_____

_____

2. Which of the following statements about body image is correct?
   a. Physical changes are quickly incorporated into a person's body image.
   b. Body image refers only to the external appearance of a person's body.
   c. Body image is a combination of a person's actual and perceived (ideal) body.
   d. Perceptions by other persons have no influence on a person's body image.

Answer (   ) Rationale: _____

_____

_____

3. Robert, who is 2 years old, is praised for using his potty instead of wetting his pants. This is an example of learning a behavior by:
   a. Identification
   b. Imitation
   c. Substitution
   d. Reinforcement-extinction

Answer (   ) Rationale: _____

_____

_____

4. In which developmental stage is role ambiguity most common?
   a. Older adult
   b. Middle adult
   c. Young adult
   d. Adolescence

Answer (   ) Rationale: _____

_____

_____

5. Mr. Davis tells the nurse he will need to have a private room after surgery. He explains that he is the president of a small business and that the company's success depends on him being available around the clock to make important business decisions. Mr. Davis is showing the nurse his:
   a. Sense of identity
   b. Ego integrity
   c. Self-ideal
   d. Role ambiguity

Answer (   ) Rationale: _____

_____

_____

6. Mrs. Watson has just undergone a radical mastectomy. The nurse is aware that Mrs. Watson will probably have considerable anxiety over:
   a. Role performance
   b. Self-identity
   c. Body image
   d. Self-esteem

Answer (   ) Rationale: _____

_____

_____

7. Johnny Martin was praised by his nurse after correctly self-administering insulin injections four times. Johnny enthusiastically relates his success to all visitors. Which of the following is Johnny demonstrating?
   a. Positive body image
   b. Self-esteem
   c. Positive personal identity
   d. Positive role behavior

Answer (   ) Rationale: _____

_____

_____

8. Which of the following statements demonstrates that the nurse's self-concept is positively affecting the client?
   a. "You've got to take a more active part in caring for your ostomy."
   b. "I know your ostomy is difficult to look at, but you will get used to it in time."
   c. (While grimacing) "Ostomy care isn't so bad."
   d. "Let me show you how to place the bag on your stoma."

Answer (   ) Rationale: _____

_____

_____

9. A college student wishes to study all weekend, but his parents expect him to participate in a family reunion. What type of role conflict is this situation describing?
   a. Interpersonal
   b. Interrole
   c. Person-role
   d. Role overload

Answer (   ) Rationale: _____

_____

_____

Sexuality

Acknowledging values and biases and gaining knowledge about sexual issues may broaden understanding of the vast range of normal sexual behaviors.

PRELIMINARY READING

Chapter 24, pp. 409-439

COMPREHENSIVE UNDERSTANDING

■ CONCEPTS OF SEXUALITY

➤ Define the following:

Sexual health _____

_____

_____

_____

Sexuality _____

_____

_____

_____

Sex _____

_____

_____

_____

➤ The key ingredients of knowing oneself as female or male is being born with female or male genitalia and learned social roles.

Dimensions of Sexuality

➤ Sexuality is influenced by cultural rules and norms that determine what is acceptable behavior within the culture.
➤ Identify some cultural sexual traditions: _____

_____

_____

_____

_____

_____

➤ Sexuality is linked to religious and ethical standards of conduct. Give some examples: _____

_____

_____

_____

_____

➤ Many of the beliefs and attitudes regarding female and male psychological, moral, and psychosexual development are based on theories.

Sexual Identity

➤ Gender identity is _____.
➤ Gender role _____.
➤ Cultural and environmental factors play a key role in defining sex roles.

Sexual Orientation

➤ Sexual orientation is _____.
➤ A continuum exists between heterosexuality and homosexuality, which provides a conceptual model for understanding the variance of sexual orientation in society and the complexity of human behavior.

➤ Homophobia is _____.
➤ Most homosexual men and women define themselves as satisfied with their gender and social role, they simply have a persistent desire to be with members of their own sex.

Variations in Sexual Expression

➤ Transsexuals are _____.

➤ Gender dysphoria is _____.

➤ Transvestites are _____.

■ ATTITUDES TOWARD SEXUAL HEALTH

➤ Attitudes toward sexual feelings and behavior change as people develop and as they grow older.

➤ Identify the areas in which nurses reflect their attitudes toward sexuality: _____

_____

_____

_____

_____

_____

_____

Clients' Sexual Attitudes

➤ All people have sexual value systems _____ concerning sexuality.
➤ Clients may be confused about their own sexual value

systems and thus experience _____ when dealing with their sexuality.

➤ The most common concern of clients is _____

_____.

Nurses' Attitudes Toward Sexuality

➤ Nurses deal with personal attitudes by accepting their existence, exploring their sources, and finding ways to work with them.
➤ Promotion of sex education and honest examination of sexual values and beliefs can help in reducing sexual bias.

▮ SEXUAL ANATOMY AND PHYSIOLOGY

Female Sex Organs

➤ Complete the following table, which outlines the physiology of the female reproductive system:

STRUCTURE/ORGAN	FUNCTION(S)
EXTERNAL SEX ORGANS	
Mons veneris	
Labia	
Clitoris	
Vestibule	

STRUCTURE/ORGAN	FUNCTION(S)
INTERNAL SEX ORGANS	
Vagina	
Uterus	
Fallopian tubes	
Ovaries	
Breast	

➤ Summarize the menstrual cycle in relation to the feedback loop involving hormones of the _____

_____, _____, and _____:

_____

_____

_____

_____

_____

_____

_____

➤ Signs and symptoms experienced by women with

premenstrual syndrome (PMS) are _____

_____

_____.

➤ There is no physiological reason for a woman to abstain from sexual activity during menstruation.

➤ Menopause is _____

_____

_____

_____.

Male Sex Organs

➤ Complete the following table, which outlines the physiology of the male reproductive system:

STRUCTURE/ORGAN	FUNCTION(S)
EXTERNAL SEX ORGANS	
Penis	
Scrotum	
INTERNAL SEX ORGANS	
Testicles	
Epididymis	
Vas deferens	
Urethra	
Seminal vesicles	
Prostate gland	
Cowper's glands	

➤ Men do experience changes in sexual response, or the climacteric. Some examples are: _____

_____

_____

_____

_____

■ SEXUAL DEVELOPMENT

Infancy

➤ Female and male infants are born with the capacity for sexual pleasure and response.
➤ Parents need to be encouraged to accept the infant's exploratory behavior as a positive step toward the

development of a _____.

Toddlerhood and Preschool

➤ Summarize the normal behaviors related to sexual development for toddlers and preschoolers: _____

_____

_____

_____

_____

_____

School-Age Years

➤ Summarize the normal behaviors related to sexual development for school-age children: _____

_____

_____

_____

_____

Puberty and Adolescence

➤ Summarize the normal behaviors related to sexual development during puberty and adolescence:

_____

_____

_____

_____

_____

_____

Adulthood

➤ Summarize the normal behaviors related to sexual development in adulthood: _____

_____

_____

_____

_____

_____

Older Adulthood

➤ List the four areas of concern that affect sexual function in the older adult:

a. _____

b. _____

c. _____

d. _____

▌ SEXUAL RESPONSE
Sexual Response Cycle

➤ The sexual response cycle is defined as _____

_____, _____,

_____, and _____ phases.

➤ The following phases are basic physiological responses to sexual arousal. Explain each one.

Vasoconstriction: _____

_____

Tumescence: _____

_____

Myotonia: _____

_____

▌ PREGNANCY AND SEXUALITY

➤ Identify sexual desires in relation to trimesters of pregnancy.

First: _____

_____

Second: _____

_____

Third: _____

_____

➤ Give some examples of a relationship between coital

activity and premature labor: _____

_____

_____

_____

_____

➤ Briefly explain the changes that occur to a woman

postpartum: _____

_____

_____

_____

▌ ISSUES RELATED TO SEXUALITY

➤ Identify some common issues related to sexuality:

_____

_____

_____

_____

_____

Contraception

➤ The ability to prevent a pregnancy or plan the time between pregnancies should be part of a client's health care plan.

➤ Identify the three major factors influencing the use of contraception.

a. _____

_____

b. _____

_____

c. _____

_____

➤ Identify examples of the following contraception methods, and cite the advantages and disadvantages of each method:
Biological

a. _____

b. _____

c. _____

d. _____
Chemical

a. _____

b. _____

c. _____

d. _____
Mechanical

a. _____

b. _____

c. _____
Surgical

a. _____

b. _____

Infertility

➤ Identify some of the causes of infertility: _____

_____

_____

_____

_____

Abortion

➤ Summarize the issue of abortion in relation to ration-

ales, emotions, and personal values: _____

_____

_____

_____

Sexually Transmitted Diseases

➤ STDs are transmitted from _____

_____.

➤ Persons most likely to be infected share one key char-

acteristic. Name it: _____.

➤ Explain the four bacterial sexually transmitted diseases.

Gonorrhea: _____

_____

Chlamydia: _____

_____

Pelvic inflammatory disease: _____

_____

_____

Syphilis: _____

_____

➤ Explain the two viral sexually transmitted diseases.

Herpes simplex: _____

_____

_____

_____

Genital warts: _____

_____

_____

_____

➤ The primary routes of HIV transmission are: _____

_____

_____

_____

_____

_____

_____

_____

_____

_____

➤ List five measures to improve safe sex.

a. _____

b. _____

c. _____

d. _____

e. _____

Sexual Abuse

➤ Incidents of sexual abuse have a traumatic effect on
the victim and may cause physical and psychological
problems and later sexual dysfunction.

➤ Providers must understand the importance of their
responses to the victim's reactions and adaptations
and refrain from applying personal values and
stereotypes to the victims and their families.

Effects of Illness on Sexuality

➤ Summarize the physiological and psychological

changes that may affect sexuality: _____

_____

_____

_____

_____

_____

_____

_____

➤ Medications can interfere with sexual desire and all
the phases of the sexual response cycle.

➤ Clients leave the security and privacy of their homes
and enter a more public and intrusive environment
when they are admitted to the hospital.

Sexual Dysfunction

➤ List four psychological conditions that contribute to sexual dysfunction.

a. _____

b. _____

c. _____

d. _____

➤ List four physiological factors that may contribute to sexual dysfunction.

a. _____

b. _____

c. _____

d. _____

■ SEXUALITY AND THE NURSING PROCESS

Assessment

➤ Nurses can expect to encounter clients who have problems with one or more of the stages of sexual behavior, including the feeling of wanting sex, the physiology and emotions of having sex, and the feelings experienced after sex.

➤ Briefly explain the following factors that affect sexuality:

Physical _____

_____

_____

_____

Relationship _____

_____

_____

_____

Life-style _____

_____

_____

_____

Self-esteem _____

_____

_____

_____

➤ List five questions a nurse may use to elicit a brief sexual history from an adult: _____

_____

_____

_____

_____

_____

_____

_____

_____

_____

➤ Briefly explain the techniques used in a physical examination for a male and a female:

Male _____

_____

Female _____

_____

Nursing Diagnosis

➤ Diagnosing sexual dysfunction or altered sexuality patterns depends on whether the client _____

_____ or _____.

Planning

➤ List the five general goals for clients experiencing actual or potential alterations in sexual functioning.

a. _____

b. _____

c. _____

d. _____

e. _____

➤ Goals will not be achieved if recommended interventions fail to match the client's sexuality.

Implementation

■ HEALTH PROMOTION

➤ Topics of education vary, depending on the defining characteristics and related factors. Describe some situations: _____

_____

_____

_____

_____

■ ACUTE CARE

➤ The client should be encouraged to investigate and acknowledge social and ethical values and analyze the role of sexuality in his or her self-concept.
➤ Identify situational and developmental crises that

prompt education: _____

_____

_____

_____

_____

■ RESTORATIVE CARE

➤ Clients may still require support to follow through with a referral and reinforcement of explanations of procedures, treatments, or exercises.

Evaluation

➤ Client or spouse verbalizations determine if goals and outcomes have been achieved.
➤ Sexuality is felt more than observed, and sexual expression requires an intimacy not amenable to observation.
➤ All people involved may need to be reminded of the individual nature of sexual expression and the multiple factors that affect perceptions and responses.

REVIEW QUESTIONS

(The student should select the appropriate answer and cite the rationale for choosing that particular answer.)
 1. An individual whose inner sense of sexual identity does not match the biological body is known as a:
    a. Lesbian
    b. Homosexual
    c. Transsexual
    d. Transvestite

Answer ( ) Rationale: _____

_____

_____

 2. The follicular phase of the menstrual cycle is characterized by:
    a. Increasing levels of progesterone
    b. Reduction in ovarian production of estrogen
    c. Inhibition of follicle-stimulating hormone
    d. Rupture of the graafian follicle

Answer ( ) Rationale: _____

_____

_____

 3. Which statement about the uterine secretory phase of the menstrual cycle is accurate?
    a. The secretory phase is the time before ovulation.
    b. The uterus is under the influence of high levels of estrogen.
    c. Cervical mucus becomes more clear, slippery, and stretchable.
    d. In the absence of pregnancy, the endometrium begins to slough.

Answer ( ) Rationale: _____

_____

_____

 4. At what developmental stage is it particularly important for children reared in single-parent families to be exposed to same-sex adults?
    a. Infancy
    b. Toddlerhood and preschool years
    c. School-age
    d. Adolescence

Answer ( ) Rationale: _____

_____

_____

5. In the school-age child, learning and reinforcement of gender-appropriate behaviors are most commonly derived from:
   a. Parents
   b. Teachers
   c. Siblings
   d. Peers

Answer (   ) Rationale: _____

_____

_____

6. Which statement about sexual response in the older adult is correct?
   a. The resolution phase is slower.
   b. The orgasm phase is prolonged.
   c. The plateau phase is prolonged.
   d. The refractory phase is more rapid.

Answer (   ) Rationale: _____

_____

_____

7. Which of the following statements about sexuality during the postpartum period is incorrect?
   a. Couples should refrain from sexual intercourse until vaginal bleeding has stopped and discomfort subsides.
   b. In the early postpartum period, breast-feeding couples need not be concerned about using contraceptives.
   c. The demands of the baby may negatively influence sexual desire in both partners.
   d. Hormonal changes will decrease the amount of vaginal lubrication, necessitating the use of water-soluble lubricants during intercourse.

Answer (   ) Rationale: _____

_____

_____

8. The least effective means of preventing pregnancy is:
   a. Coitus interruptus
   b. Calendar (rhythm) method
   c. Body temperature method
   d. Mucus method

Answer (   ) Rationale: _____

_____

_____

9. Which statement about abortion is correct?
   a. Women who decide to abort an unwanted fetus will not experience any guilt.
   b. Nurses are obliged to participate in an abortion procedure, even if it conflicts with their personal values.
   c. The male partner of a woman who has an abortion may experience loss and grief, requiring professional support.
   d. Women who abort a deformed fetus will not experience any loss or grief.

Answer (   ) Rationale: _____

_____

_____

10. The only 100% effective method to avoid contracting a disease through sex is:
    a. Using condoms
    b. Avoiding sex with partners at risk
    c. Knowing the sexual partner's health history
    d. Abstinence

Answer (   ) Rationale: _____

_____

_____

11. Which sexual dysfunction in females is most often associated with physiological factors?
    a. Primary orgasmic dysfunction
    b. Secondary orgasmic dysfunction
    c. Dyspareunia
    d. Vaginismus

Answer (   ) Rationale: _____

_____

_____

25 | Spiritual Health

Spirituality gives a broad dimension to the holistic view of humanity.

PRELIMINARY READING

Chapter 25, pp. 440-455

COMPREHENSIVE UNDERSTANDING

▌ SPIRITUALITY AND RELIGION

➤ Identify some words used to describe spirituality.

a. _____

b. _____

c. _____

d. _____

e. _____

f. _____

g. _____

➤ Individuals' definitions of spirituality are influenced by their own _____, _____, _____, and _____.

➤ Identify the two important characteristics of spirituality.

a. _____

b. _____

➤ Define *religion:* _____

_____

_____

➤ Identify a problem when interchanging the terms *spirituality* and *religion:* _____

_____

_____

The Spiritual Dimension

➤ Briefly explain the spirituality model developed by Farran, et al (1989): _____

_____

_____

_____

➤ When illness, loss, or pain affects a person, energy is depleted, and one's spirit is affected. How this influences a person's motivation to get well, participation in recovery, and ability to change is underestimated.

➤ Briefly explain spiritual development: _____

_____

_____

_____

Critical Thinking and Spirituality

➤ Briefly explain clinical intuition as described by Young (1987): _____

_____

_____

_____

➤ Benner's description of the healing relationship happens when _____, _____, and _____.

➤ Rew (1989) describes a relationship between spirituality and intuition. Briefly explain: _____

_____

_____

Spiritual Health

➤ Define *spiritual health:* _____

_____

_____

➤ Identify how the following age-groups grow spiritually:

Children _____

_____

Adults _____

_____

Older adults _____

_____

Spiritual Problems

➤ Spiritual distress develops as a person seeks to _____

_____

_____.

➤ Briefly explain each of the following causes of spiritual distress:

Acute illness _____

_____

_____

_____

Chronic illness _____

_____

_____

_____

Terminal illness _____

_____

_____

_____

Individuation _____

_____

_____

_____

Near-death experience _____

_____

_____

_____

Religious Problems

➤ Explain how the following can affect the client's sense of well-being:

Change in denominational membership or religious conversion _____

_____

_____

_____

Intensification of adherence to beliefs _____

_____

_____

_____

Loss or questioning of faith _____

_____

_____

_____

▌ NURSING PROCESS AND SPIRITUALITY

➤ An element of quality health care is to exhibit caring for the client so that a relationship of trust forms.

Trust is strengthened when the caregiver _____

_____and _____.

➤ Briefly explain shared community and compassion:

_____

_____

_____

_____

Assessment

➤ List seven questions that may provide information about the client's spiritual health in the following dimensions:

Belief and meaning _____

_____

_____

Authority and guidance _____

_____

_____

_____

Experience and emotion _____
_____
_____
_____

Fellowship and community _____
_____
_____
_____

Ritual and practice _____
_____
_____
_____

Courage and growth _____
_____
_____
_____

Vocation and consequences _____
_____
_____
_____

Nursing Diagnosis

➤ When reviewing a spiritual assessment and integrating the information into an appropriate nursing diagnosis, the nurse should consider the client's current health status from a holistic perspective, with spirituality as the unifying principle.
➤ State the defining characteristics for the nursing diagnosis spiritual well-being: _____
_____
_____
_____
_____
_____

Planning

➤ Identify the three goals for spiritual caregiving.

a. _____
b. _____
c. _____

Implementation

➤ Briefly explain the following interventions and how they are helpful in maintaining or promoting a client's spiritual health:

Establishing presence _____
_____
_____
_____

Supporting a healing relationship _____
_____
_____
_____
_____

Support systems _____
_____
_____
_____

Prayer _____
_____
_____
_____

Diet therapies _____
_____
_____

Supporting rituals _____
_____
_____
_____

Evaluation

➤ Give some examples of evaluative measures used to achieve outcomes in spiritual health: _____

_____

_____

_____

_____

_____

_____

REVIEW QUESTIONS

(The student should select the appropriate answer and cite the rationale for choosing that particular answer.)

1. When planning care to include spiritual needs for a client of the Moslem faith, the religious practices the nurse should understand include all of the following *except:*
   √a. A priest be present to conduct rituals
   b. Strength gained through group prayer
   c. Family members as a source of comfort
   d. Faith healing providing psychological support

Answer (   ) Rationale: _____

_____

_____

2. Mrs. McCarthy, a Roman Catholic, has delivered a premature infant with multiple health problems. The religious practices of this family would include which of the following:
   a. Transplantation of organs is prohibited
   b. A priest must remain with the sick infant
   c. Blood transfusions cannot be given
   √d. Infant baptism is performed when life is endangered

Answer (   ) Rationale: _____

_____

_____

3. When consulting with the dietary department regarding meals for a client of the Hindu religion, which of the following dietary items would *not* be included on the meal trays?
   √a. Meats
   b. Dairy products
   c. Vegetable entrees
   d. Fruits

Answer (   ) Rationale: _____

_____

_____

4. If an Islamic client dies, the nurse should be aware of what religious practice?
   √a. Only relatives and friends may touch the body.
   b. Members of a ritual burial society cleanse the body.
   c. Last rites are mandatory.
   d. The body is always cremated.

Answer (   ) Rationale: _____

_____

_____

5. If a nurse were to use a nursing diagnosis to relate concerns about spiritual health, which of the following would be used?
   √a. Spiritual distress
   b. Inability to adjust
   c. Lack of faith
   d. Religious dilemma

Answer (   ) Rationale: _____

_____

_____

6. Mr. Phillips was recently diagnosed with a malignant tumor. The staff had observed him crying on several occasions, and now he cries as he reads from his Bible. Interventions to help Mr. Phillips cope with his illness would include:
   a. Asking the hospital chaplain to visit him daily
   b. Engaging Mr. Phillips in diversional activities to reduce feelings of hopelessness
   √c. Supporting his use of inner resources by providing time for meditation
   d. Praying with Mr. Phillips as often as possible

Answer (   ) Rationale: _____

_____

_____

Chapter 26

Coping With Loss, Death, and Grieving

The nurse helps clients to understand and accept loss within the context of their culture so that life can continue.

PRELIMINARY READING

Chapter 26, pp. 457-476

COMPREHENSIVE UNDERSTANDING

■ LOSS, DEATH, GRIEF, AND NURSING

➤ While caring for clients and their families, nurses experience personal loss as client-family-nurse relationships end through transfer, discharge, recovery, or death.

➤ Development of a philosophy of life helps nurses function supportively during difficult times.

➤ The nurse utilizes knowledge of the concepts of loss and grief to creatively apply interventions to promote

_____, prevent _____,

and support _____ clients.

Loss

➤ Define *loss:*_____

_____

_____

➤ List and briefly describe the five categories of loss.

a. _____

_____

b. _____

_____

c. _____

_____

d. _____

_____

e. _____

_____

Grief, Mourning, and Bereavement

➤ Define the following:

Grief _____

_____

Mourning _____

_____

Bereavement _____

_____

➤ List four tasks to be accomplished by the grieving person to facilitate healthy adjustment.

a. _____

b. _____

c. _____

d. _____

➤ Define *anticipatory grief:* _____

_____

_____

➤ Define *disenfranchised grief:* _____

_____

_____

Concepts and Theories of the Grieving Process

➤ List the phases of the grieving process proposed by each of the following theorists:

ENGLE

a. _____

b. _____

c. _____

KUBLER-ROSS

a. _____

b. _____

c. _____

d. _____

e. _____

RANDO

a. _____

b. _____

c. _____

NURSING PROCESS AND GRIEF

Assessment

➤ The nurse should avoid assuming that a particular behavior indicates grief and allow persons to share what is happening in their own ways.

➤ Assessment of the client and family begins by exploring

_____

_____.

➤ The nurse assesses how the client _____

reacting rather than how the client _____ reacting.

➤ The following factors influence the way any individual responds to loss. Briefly explain each one:

Personal characteristics _____

_____

_____

_____

_____

Nature of relationships _____

_____

_____

_____

_____

Social support system _____

_____

_____

_____

_____

_____

Nature of the loss _____

_____

_____

_____

_____

_____

Cultural and spiritual beliefs _____

_____

_____

_____

_____

_____

_____

Loss of personal life goals _____

_____

_____

_____

_____

_____

➤ List and briefly define the six dimensions of hope described by Dufault and Martocchio.

a. _____

_____

b. _____

_____

c. _____

_____

d. _____

_____

e. _____

_____

f. _____

_____

➤ List the characteristics of dysfunctional grief for an actual or perceived loss: _____

_____

_____

_____

_____

_____

_____

➤ List the emotions, behaviors, and physical symptoms of a client and family that may indicate grief.

Emotions: _____

_____

_____

_____

Behaviors: _____

_____

_____

_____

Physical symptoms: _____

_____

_____

_____

➤ List five risk factors that increase a person's potential for suffering psychological or physical illness during bereavement.

a. _____

b. _____

c. _____

d. _____

e. _____

➤ Nurses who are not aware of their own grief issues have difficulty relating to clients as unique individuals.

Nursing Diagnosis

➤ Identify the seven behavioral signs of dysfunctional grief.

a. _____

b. _____

c. _____

d. _____

e. _____

f. _____

g. _____

➤ As the clients' conditions worsen, the nurse makes diagnoses relevant to basic needs.

Planning

➤ Grieving has therapeutic value, enabling people to work through their losses, recollect their thoughts and feelings, and resume life with new insights and direction.

➤ List four goals appropriate for a client dealing with loss.

a. _____

b. _____

c. _____

d. _____

➤ List the three most crucial needs of the dying client.

a. _____

b. _____

c. _____

Implementation

➤ Nursing care of the grieving client begins with establishing the significance of the loss.

➤ The nurse observes the response to loss and then attempts to identify the client's strengths in dealing with it.

➤ The nurse must schedule adequate private time with the client and family to promote open communication, accomplishing the following goals:

a. _____

b. _____

c. _____

➤ Communication is blocked by _____,

_____, or _____.

➤ The nurse supports hope by helping the client ____

_____, _____, and _____.

➤ Refusal to die or accept the feeling of helplessness is a motivator.

➤ Identify the early signs of hopelessness and despair:

_____

_____

_____

_____

_____

_____

_____

➤ Nursing interventions focus on promoting a sense of identity, dignity, and self-esteem.

➤ Identify nursing interventions that promote dignity

and self-esteem: _____

_____

_____

_____

_____

_____

_____

_____

➤ As clients and their families begin to confront their losses, it is important for the nurse to encourage a return to their normal life-styles within the limits of the situation.

➤ Briefly summarize the nursing care of dying clients and their families within the following contexts:

Promotion of comfort _____

_____

_____

_____

_____

Maintenance of support _____

_____

_____

_____

_____

Prevention of loneliness and isolation

_____

_____

_____

_____

_____

_____

Promotion of spiritual comfort _____

_____

_____

_____

_____

_____

_____

Support for the grieving family _____

_____

_____

_____

_____

_____

Hospice care _____

_____

_____

_____

_____

_____

_____

➤ Care after death includes caring for the body with dignity and sensitivity. Identify the physiological changes after death and state the nursing interventions to min-

imize: _____

_____

_____

_____

_____

_____

_____

➤ Identify how the nurse experiences bereavement overload and how the nurse may deal with this:

_____

_____

_____

_____

_____

_____

_____

Evaluation

➤ Grieving is an individual process, and resolution of loss does not follow a set schedule.
➤ The care of the dying client requires the nurse to evaluate the client's level of comfort with illness and the client's quality of life.

REVIEW QUESTIONS

(The student should select the appropriate answer and cite the rationale for choosing that particular answer.)

1. Which statement about loss is accurate?
   a. Loss is only experienced when there is an actual absence of something valued.
   b. The more an individual has invested in what is lost, the less the feeling of loss.
   ✓c. Loss may be maturational, situational, or both.
   d. The degree of stress experienced is unrelated to the type of loss.

Answer ( ) Rationale: _____

_____

_____

2. The state of thought, feeling, and activity after a loss is:
   a. Grief
   b. Mourning
   ✓c. Bereavement
   d. Anticipatory grief

Answer ( ) Rationale: _____

_____

_____

3. The developmental stage at which the child is first able to understand logical explanations about death is:
   a. Toddlerhood
   b. Preschool-age
   ✓c. School-age
   d. Adolescence

Answer ( ) Rationale: _____

_____

_____

4. Which statement about bereavement is accurate?
   a. Recovery from grief occurs more rapidly when the death is sudden and unanticipated.
   b. Persons experiencing grief consistently use the support provided by others.
   ✓c. Resolution depends on the meaning of the loss and the situation surrounding the loss.
   d. Persons experiencing less visible or invisible losses tend to receive greater social support.

Answer ( ) Rationale: _____

_____

_____

5. A hospice program emphasizes:
   a. Curative treatment and alleviation of symptoms
   ✓b. Palliative treatment and control of symptoms
   c. Hospital-based care
   d. Prolongation of life

Answer ( ) Rationale: _____

_____

_____

6. Engel's theory of grieving:
   a. Focuses on behavior
   b. Defines loss as death
   ✓c. Includes a bargaining stage
   ✓d. Has a process-oriented framework

Answer ( ) Rationale: _____

_____

_____

7. Trying questionable and experimental forms of therapy is a behavior that is characteristic of which stage of dying?
   a. Anger
   b. Depression
   ✓c. Bargaining
   d. Acceptance

Answer ( ) Rationale: _____

_____

_____

8. Which of the following is an appropriately stated nursing diagnosis for a grieving client?
   a. Grieving related to colon cancer
   b. Dysfunctional grieving related to failure to resolve the grieving process after wife's death 2 months ago
   ✓c. Social isolation related to inability to pursue valued community activities
   ✓d. Spiritual distress related to loss of leg

Answer ( ) Rationale: _____

_____

_____

9. All of the following are crucial needs of the dying client *except:*
   a. Control of pain
   b. Preservation of dignity and self-worth
   c. Love and belonging
   ✗d. Freedom from decision-making

Answer ( ) Rationale: _____

_____

_____

10. Nursing care for the grieving client should begin with:
   ✓a. Establishing the significance of the loss for the client
   b. Clarifying for the client how behaviors reflect feelings
   c. Interpreting the meaning of the client's feelings to him or her
   ✓d. Letting the client know that his or her feelings are understood

Answer ( ) Rationale: _____

_____

_____

11. Which of the following is *not* part of the nurse's role after the death of the client:
   ✓a. Insist that the family view the body to say "good-bye" even if they are reluctant
   b. Place the body in a supine position to make it look as natural and comfortable as possible
   c. Insert the client's dentures to maintain normal facial features
   ✓d. Discuss organ donation with the family if the client is a medically suitable donor

Answer ( ) Rationale: _____

_____

_____

Chapter 27

Basic Human Needs: Individual and Family

The extent to which basic needs are met determines a person's level of health and position on the health-illness continuum.

PRELIMINARY READING

Chapter 27, pp. 477-494

COMPREHENSIVE UNDERSTANDING

■ THE INDIVIDUAL

➤ Define:

Basic human needs _____

_____

_____

_____

Maslow's hierarchy of basic human needs _____

_____

_____

_____

➤ Build the hierarchy of human needs by listing the five levels of basic needs identified by Maslow.

a. _____

b. _____

c. _____

d. _____

e. _____

■ PHYSIOLOGICAL NEEDS

➤ Physiological needs have the highest priority in Maslow's hierarchy.

➤ An individual who has several unmet needs generally seeks to fulfill physiological needs first.

Oxygen

➤ Oxygen is the most essential physiological need.

➤ Define *anaerobic metabolism:* _____

_____

Fluids

➤ The human body requires a balance between intake and output of fluids.

➤ Clients of any age can have unmet fluid needs, but the very young and the very old have the greatest risk.

➤ Briefly explain how the following indicate unmet fluid needs:

Dehydration _____

_____

Edema _____

_____

Nutrition

➤ The human body has an essential need for nutrients, although it can survive without food longer than it can without fluids.

Temperature

➤ The body can function normally within only a narrow temperature range, 37° C (98.6° F) ±1°C. Body temperatures outside this range can result in injuries, permanent effects such as brain damage, or death.

➤ Explain an adaptive response to an increase in temperature: _____

_____

➤ Prolonged exposure to heat increases the body's metabolic activity and increases tissue oxygen demand.

Elimination

➤ The elimination of waste materials is one of the body's metabolic processes.

➤ Waste products are eliminated by the _____,

_____, _____, and _____.

Shelter

➤ Although most people have some kind of shelter, sometimes it is substandard and does not offer full protection.

➤ When assessing whether a client is meeting shelter needs, the nurse identifies the following risks factors:

_____

_____

_____

_____

_____

_____

Rest

➤ The amount of sleep a person gets varies, depending

on _____, _____, _____,

_____, and _____.

Sex

➤ Sex is considered by Maslow to be a basic physiological need that generally takes priority over higher level needs.

➤ Sexual needs and the manner in which they are met

are influence by _____, _____,

_____, _____,

_____ and _____.

■ SAFETY AND SECURITY NEEDS

➤ Safety and security needs are next in priority after the client's physiological needs.

Physical Safety

➤ Maintaining physical safety involves reducing or eliminating threats to body or life.

➤ Meeting physical safety needs sometimes takes precedence over meeting a physiological need.

Psychological Safety

➤ To be safe and secure psychologically, a person must understand what to expect from others, including family members and health care professionals.

■ LOVE AND BELONGING NEEDS

➤ The need for love and belonging arises after _____

_____ and _____

needs are met because _____

_____

_____.

■ ESTEEM AND SELF-ESTEEM NEEDS

➤ The need for self-esteem is linked to the desire for

_____, _____, _____,

_____, _____, and _____.

➤ If clients' self-concepts are changed by illness or injury, nursing care involves improving self-concept and body image.

■ NEED FOR SELF-ACTUALIZATION

➤ When people have met all the lower level needs, it is by self-actualization that they achieve their fullest potential.

➤ Self-actualized people have a mature, multidimensional personality.

➤ Identify six characteristics indicating that an individual has achieved self-actualization.

a. _____

b. _____

c. _____

d. _____

e. _____

f. _____

■ APPLICATION OF BASIC NEEDS THEORY

➤ The nurse needs to apply the basic needs theory in practice, focusing on the needs of the individual rather than on rigid adherence to Maslow's theory.

Relationships Among Needs

➤ In some situations it is unrealistic to expect a client's basic needs to be fulfilled in the fixed hierarchical order. Give two examples.

a. _____

b. _____

Simultaneous Meeting of Needs

➤ After identifying clients' specific needs, the nurse generally has to set priorities to help them meet these needs. Give two examples.

a. _____

b. _____

Factors Influencing Need Priorities

➤ List four factors that influence need priorities.

a. _____

b. _____

c. _____

d. _____

■ THE FAMILY

➤ Identify the three important attributes that characterize contemporary families:

a. _____

b. _____

c. _____

Current Trends

➤ Identify at least four current trends that challenge the

family: _____

_____

_____

_____

_____

_____

➤ Explain the following threats and concerns facing the family:

Changing economic status _____

_____

_____

_____

Homelessness _____

_____

_____

_____

Family violence _____

_____

_____

Human immunodeficiency virus _____

_____

_____

_____

Definition: What Is a "Family"?

➤ The family can be defined as _____,

_____, or as a _____.

➤ To effectively provide care, nurses must understand that individual attitudes about family are deeply ingrained and deserve respect.

➤ To provide individualized care, the nurse understands that families take many forms and have diverse cultural and ethnic orientations.

➤ The nurse must think of the family as a set of _____

_____

or as a network of _____.

Family Forms

➤ Define *family forms*: _____

_____

■ THEORETICAL APPROACHES: AN OVERVIEW

➤ Summarize the following three general perspectives when working with or studying families:

Functional theory, or functionalism _____

_____

_____

_____

_____

_____

Social conflict approach _____

_____

_____

_____

_____

_____

Symbolic interaction _____

_____

_____

_____

_____

■ GENERAL SYSTEMS THEORY
Family as an Open Social System

➤ The family is viewed as an open social system that

exists and interacts with the larger systems (_____

_____) of the community.

➤ The family system consists of interrelated parts (___

_____) that form a variety

of interaction patterns (_____).

Structure

➤ Structure and function are closely related and continually interact with one another.

➤ Structure is based on organization, the _____

_____.

➤ Structure may enhance or detract from the family's ability to respond to stressors. Briefly explain the following:

Rigid structure _____

_____

_____

_____

Open structure _____

_____

_____

_____

Function

➤ Family functioning focuses on the processes used by the family to achieve its goals.

➤ Identify these processes: _____

_____

_____

_____

_____

_____

_____

▌ DEVELOPMENTAL STAGES

➤ Societal changes and an aging population have precipitated changes in the stages and transitions in the family life cycle.

Family and Health

➤ The health of the family is influenced by its relative position in society.

➤ Identify the variables that affect the structure, function,

and health of a family: _____

_____

_____

_____

➤ The family strongly influences the health behaviors of its members. In turn the health status of each individual influences how the family unit functions and its ability to achieve goals.

➤ Family environment is crucial because health behavior reinforced in early life has a strong influence on later health practices.

Attributes of "Healthy" Families

➤ The crisis-proof or effective family is able to integrate the need for stability with the need for growth and change.

➤ Define *family hardiness:* _____

_____

_____

_____

▌ FAMILY NURSING

➤ The goal of family nursing is to _____

_____

_____

_____.

➤ Identify the three levels and focuses proposed for family nursing practice.

a. _____

b. _____

c. _____

Family as Context

➤ The primary focus of the family as context is _____

_____

_____.

Family as Client

➤ The primary focus of the family as client is _____

_____

_____.

▌ NURSING PROCESS FOR THE FAMILY

➤ Three beliefs underlie the family approach to the nursing process. Name them.

a. _____

b. _____

c. _____

Assessment

➤ Areas to include in the family assessment are: ____

_____

_____

_____

_____

_____

_____

Nursing Diagnosis

➤ Nursing diagnoses often focus on the family's ability to cope with its current situation, whether it is an acute illness, an anticipated developmental transition, or negative behaviors that are threatening short-term or long-term health.

Planning

➤ Collaboration with family members is an essential component during the planning stage.
➤ Give two examples of expected outcomes for each of the following:

Family as client _____

_____

_____

Family as context _____

_____

_____

_____

Implementation

➤ Interventions are strategies that help families adjust goals or are the processes by which the family attains them.

➤ Family interventions include nursing actions that

increase _____,

remove _____,

and do _____.

Health Promotion

➤ Define the characteristics of a strong family: ____

_____

_____

_____

_____

➤ Health promotion behaviors that the nurse needs to encourage are often tied to the developmental stage of the family.
➤ Family strengths include _____,

_____, _____,

_____, and _____.

Evaluation

➤ When family as context is the focus, evaluation

emphasizes _____.
➤ When the family receives care as the client, the measure

of family health is _____.
➤ Give at least two examples of the evaluative measures for the following:

Family as client _____

_____

_____

_____

Family as context _____

_____

_____

_____

REVIEW QUESTIONS

(The student should select the appropriate answer and cite the rationale for choosing that particular answer.)

1. Which statement about the hierarchy of basic needs is incorrect?
   a. Priorities assigned to basic human needs are the same for all individuals.
   b. Unmet needs place the individual at risk for illness.
   c. Environmental and social factors may influence the ability to meet needs.
   d. Hospitalized clients have basic needs that are actually or potentially unmet.

Answer ( ) Rationale: _____

_____

_____

2. In developing a care plan, the nurse would first consider the client's need for:
   a. Oxygen
   b. Self-respect
   c. Elimination of wastes
   d. Freedom from harm

Answer ( ) Rationale: _____

_____

_____

3. Mrs. Grant, an active client, is mentally ill. She has been assigned to a student who is learning communication techniques. Mrs. Grant fasted in preparation for just-completed laboratory tests and has had no breakfast. What concept should the student consider at this point?
   a. Active patients need safety measures.
   b. Love and belonging needs rank after physical needs.
   c. Communication is more important than food.
   d. The client's self-esteem will be enhanced by the student-client relationship.

Answer ( ) Rationale: _____

_____

_____

4. Kathy, a 16-year-old adolescent in her second month of pregnancy, is admitted to the hospital for nausea and vomiting. She states that she is having difficulty communicating with her parents and believes no one cares about her. In which category are her needs not being met?
   a. Physiological
   b. Safety and security
   c. Love and belonging
   d. Self-esteem

Answer ( ) Rationale: _____

_____

_____

5. Family functioning can best be described as:
   a. The processes that a family uses to meet its goals
   b. The way family members communicate with each other
   c. Interrelated with family structure
   d. Adaptive behaviors that foster health

Answer ( ) Rationale: _____

_____

_____

6. Family structure can best be described as:
   a. A basic pattern of predictable stages
   b. Flexible patterns that contribute to adequate functioning
   c. The pattern of relationships and ongoing membership
   d. A complex set of relationships

Answer ( ) Rationale: _____

_____

_____

7. The majority of families today:
   a. Consist of a mother, father, and one or more children
   b. Include stepchildren
   c. Include a woman who works outside the home
   d. Are very similar to families of the past

Answer ( ) Rationale: _____

_____

_____

8. Which of the following is *not* true of the crisis-proof, or effective family? The family:
   a. Is able to integrate the need for stability with the need for growth
   b. Has a flexible structure that allows for adaptation of tasks
   c. Has a passive orientation in responding to stressful events
   d. Displays a sense of control over the outcome of life events

Answer ( ) Rationale: _____

_____

_____

9. When planning care for a client and using the concept of family as client, the nurse:
   a. Understands that the client's family will always be a help to the client's health goals.
   b. Considers the developmental stage of the client and not the family
   c. Realizes that cultural background is an important variable when assessing the family
   d. Includes only the client and his or her significant other

Answer ( ) Rationale: _____

_____

_____

10. Interventions used by the nurse when providing care to a rigidly structured family include:
   a. Exploring with them the benefits of moving toward more flexible modes of action
   b. Attempting to change the family structure
   c. Providing solutions for problems as they arise
   d. Administering nursing care in a manner that provides minimal opportunity for change

Answer ( ) Rationale: _____

_____

_____

CLINICAL SITUATIONS

1. Describe how the concept of the family as client differs from the concept of the family as context. In what situations would each be a more appropriate focus?

_____

_____

_____

_____

_____

_____

_____

_____

_____

_____

2. Imagine one of your clients is a young child with a contagious illness. List some of the suggestions you might give the parents to deal with the care of the child and to provide a positive family life for the client's siblings. How would your approach differ if the child were from a single-parent family?

_____

_____

_____

_____

_____

_____

_____

_____

_____

_____

_____

Chapter 28

Conception Through Preschool

The nurse must have a clear understanding of normal or expected growth and behavior in early developmental stages to guide and promote normalcy and to detect and prevent abnormalities.

PRELIMINARY READING

Chapter 28, pp. 496-527

COMPREHENSIVE UNDERSTANDING

▮ GROWTH AND DEVELOPMENT THEORY

➤ Human growth and development are orderly, predictable processes beginning with conception and continuing until death.

➤ All persons progress through definite phases of growth and development, but the pace and behavior of this progression are highly individualized.

➤ The ability to progress through each developmental phase influences the holistic health of the individual.

➤ A developmental perspective helps the nurse understand why commonalities and variations exist and how they influence health.

Definitions

➤ A person experiences quantitative and qualitative changes in growth and development. Summarize the following:

Physical growth _____

_____

_____

Development _____

_____

_____

Maturation _____

_____

_____

_____

Critical periods of development _____

_____

_____

_____

_____

▮ PRINCIPLES OF GROWTH AND DEVELOPMENT

➤ List three commonalities of growth and development applicable to all people.

a. _____

b. _____

c. _____

➤ List the seven basic principles of growth and development.

a. _____

b. _____

c. _____

d. _____

e. _____

f. _____

g. _____

▮ STAGES OF GROWTH AND DEVELOPMENT

➤ Although chronological division is arbitrary, it is based on the timing and sequence of developmental tasks that the individual must accomplish to progress to the next stage.

Major Factors Influencing Growth and Development

➤ The human being is a complex, open system influenced by natural forces from within and from the environment. Give two examples of each.

Forces of nature: _____

_____

_____

External forces: _____

_____

_____

■ THEORIES OF HUMAN DEVELOPMENT

➤ Briefly explain the developmental focus of each of the following theorists:

Freud _____

_____

_____

_____

Erickson _____

_____

_____

_____

Maslow _____

_____

_____

_____

Piaget _____

_____

_____

_____

Kohlberg _____

_____

_____

_____

_____

■ SELECTING A DEVELOPMENTAL FRAMEWORK FOR NURSING

➤ Identify the advantages of using a developmental approach in delivering nursing care: _____

_____

_____

_____

_____

■ CONCEPTION
Intrauterine Life

➤ Summarize the events that occur during intrauterine life in regard to the following:

Fertilization _____

_____

_____

Zygote _____

_____

Blastocyst _____

_____

Implantation _____

_____

_____

Trimesters _____

_____

➤ List the two common causes of intrauterine health problems.

a. _____

_____

b. _____

_____

Physical Development

➤ Explain the developmental process and health concerns for the following trimesters (see table, top of next page):

Trimesters	Developmental Process	Health Concerns
First trimester		
Second trimester		
Third trimester		

Cognitive Development

➤ Identify two prenatal events that are related to cognitive development: _____

_____

_____

Psychosocial Development

➤ The biochemical environment is influenced by the mother. Her emotional and physical states may have significant psychosocial consequences for the unborn child.

▌ TRANSITION FROM INTRAUTERINE TO EXTRAUTERINE LIFE

➤ _____,

_____, and

_____ influence adjustment to the external environment.

Physical Health Concerns

➤ An immediate assessment of the neonate's condition is performed because the first concern is the

_____.

➤ Briefly explain the three priority physical health needs of the neonate.

Airway: _____

_____

_____

_____

Body temperature: _____

_____

_____

Prevention of infection: _____

_____

_____

_____

➤ List the five physiological parameters evaluated through the Apgar assessment.

a. _____

b. _____

c. _____

d. _____

e. _____

Psychosocial Concerns

➤ What two factors are most important in promoting closeness of the parents and the neonate? _____

_____

_____

_____

➤ Define *bonding:* _____

_____

❚ HEALTH PROMOTION FOR THE NEONATE

➤ Summarize the developmental stages of the neonate:

_____

_____

_____

_____

Physical Development

➤ Identify the normal characteristics of the newborn:

Height _____ Weight _____

Head circumference _____

Vital signs _____

Physical characteristics _____

_____

_____

Neurological function _____

_____

Behavioral characteristics _____

_____

➤ Infant behavior is characterized by five distinct states that are highly influenced by environmental stimuli. List them.

a. _____

b. _____

c. _____

d. _____

e. _____

➤ Identify the neonatal testing that is done routinely:

_____

_____

Cognitive Development

➤ Early cognitive development begins with innate behavior, reflexes, and sensory functions.

➤ Identify the sensory functions that contribute to cognitive development in the newborn: _____

_____

_____

Psychosocial Development

➤ Explain the interactions that foster deep attachment between the infant and the parents: _____

_____

_____

❚ HEALTH PROMOTION FOR THE INFANT

➤ Infancy is the period from _____ to _____.

Physical Development

➤ Summarize the normal characteristics of the infant.

Physical growth: _____

_____

_____

_____

Vital signs: _____

_____

_____

_____

Gross motor: _____

_____

_____

_____

Fine motor: _____

_____

_____

Nutrition: _____

_____

_____

_____

Dentition: _____

_____

_____

_____

Immunizations: _____

_____

_____

_____

Cognitive Development

➤ Summarize the cognitive development of an infant:

_____

_____

_____

_____

Psychosocial Development

➤ During the first year, infants begin to differentiate themselves from others as separate beings capable of acting on their own.
➤ Erickson describes the psychosocial developmental

  crisis for the infant as _____ vs. _____.
➤ Identify the experiences that contribute to psychosocial development and that are appropriate at this

  stage: _____

_____

_____

_____

_____

_____

Perception of Health

➤ The foundation for children's perceptions of their health status is laid early in life.
➤ Internal body sensations and experiences with the outside world affect self-perceptions.

▍ HEALTH PROMOTION FOR THE TODDLER

➤ Toddlerhood ranges from _____ to _____.

Physical Development

➤ Summarize the normal characteristics of the toddler.

  Self-care activities: _____

_____

_____

_____

  Motor skills: _____

_____

_____

_____

  Vital sign: _____

_____

  Head circumference: _____

_____

  Weight: _____ Height: _____

Physiological anorexia: _____

Nutrition: _____

_____

_____

_____

Cognitive Development

➤ Summarize preoperational thought stage (Piaget):

_____

_____

_____

_____

_____

➤ Toddlers recognize that they are separate beings from their mothers, but they are unable to assume the view of another.
➤ Describe the moral development: _____

_____

_____

_____

Psychosocial Development

➤ Identify the psychosocial development stage, according to Erickson: _____

_____.

➤ Explain the parental implications for the following developmental states:

  Independence _____

_____

_____

  Social interactions _____

_____

_____

  Play _____

_____

_____

  Safety issues _____

_____

_____

Perception of Health

➤ Children increasingly recognize internal body sensations but have difficulty pinpointing their location.

➤ Children who deviate radically from their usual patterns of eating, sleeping, or playing require assessment to determine if these alterations result from illness.

➤ Children begin to internalize the labels that parents or health care professionals give to the somatic stages.

■ HEALTH PROMOTION FOR THE PRESCHOOLER

➤ The preschool period refers to _____.

Physical Development

➤ Summarize the normal characteristics of the preschooler.

Vital signs: _____

Weight: _____ Height: _____

Nutrition: _____

_____

_____

Coordination: _____

_____

_____

Cognitive Development

➤ Preschoolers continue to master the preoperational stage of cognition.

➤ The first phase of this period, _____ (2 to 4 years), is characterized by _____

_____

_____.

➤ Define *artificialism:* _____

_____

_____

_____

➤ Summarize the intuitive phase (4 years): _____

_____

_____

➤ The greatest fear of this age-group is _____.

➤ Summarize their moral development: _____

_____

_____

Psychosocial Development

➤ The world of preschoolers expands beyond the family into the neighborhood where children meet other children and adults.

➤ Identify some dependent behaviors reverted to during stress or illness: _____

_____

_____

➤ Summarize the pattern of play for the preschooler:

_____

_____

_____

_____

_____

_____

_____

Perception of Health

➤ Parental beliefs about health, children's bodily sensations, and their ability to perform usual daily activities help children develop attitudes about their health.

■ HOSPITALIZATION AND ILLNESS

➤ Hospitalization and illness are stressful experiences, primarily because of _____,

_____, and altered _____.

■ NURSING PROCESS AND THE CHILD

Assessment

➤ Briefly explain the factors that influence a child's reaction to illness and hospitalization.

Development age: _____

_____

_____

_____

_____

_____

Response to hospitalization: _____

_____

_____

_____

_____

_____

History of previous illness, hospitalization, and separation: _____

_____

_____

_____

_____

Medical history: _____

_____

_____

_____

_____

Perception of illness: _____

_____

_____

_____

_____

_____

Support persons: _____

_____

_____

_____

_____

_____

Nursing Diagnosis

➤ Assessment reveals how the child will cope with hospitalization and if this experience will result in other health problems.

Planning

➤ List the six goals to include when planning care for a hospitalized child:

_____

_____

_____

_____

_____

_____

Implementation

➤ List the guidelines that should be followed to minimize a child's separation anxiety:

_____

_____

_____

_____

_____

_____

_____

_____

_____

_____

_____

_____

_____

_____

➤ Identify at least four actions that may facilitate establishing trust with the child and family:

_____

_____

_____

_____

_____

_____

_____

➤ List the common fears among the following age-groups:

Birth to 3 months _____

_____

4 to 12 months _____

_____

1 to 3 years _____

_____

3 to 6 years _____

_____

➤ List four nursing actions to minimize fear in the hospitalized child:

_____

_____

_____

_____

➤ List at least five guidelines to minimize children's physical development associated with hospitalization:

_____

_____

_____

_____

_____

_____

_____

_____

➤ List at least five guidelines to foster normal growth and development in the hospitalized child:

_____

_____

_____

_____

_____

_____

_____

_____

➤ List at least six guidelines when planning play for the hospitalized child:

_____

_____

_____

_____

_____

_____

_____

_____

_____

_____

_____

_____

Evaluation

➤ List three expected outcomes for a child experiencing fear:

_____

_____

_____

_____

_____

REVIEW QUESTIONS

(The student should select the appropriate answer and cite the rationale for choosing that particular answer.)

1. Which statement about human growth and development is accurate?
   a. Growth and development processes are unpredictable.
   b. Growth and development begins with birth and ends after adolescence.
   c. All individuals progress through the same phases of growth and development.
   d. All individuals accomplish developmental tasks at the same pace.

Answer (   ) Rationale: _____

_____

_____

2. A critical period of development is:
   a. Cephalocaudal and proximodistal growth
   b. The 9-month prenatal period of neurological development
   c. The time between conception and medical confirmation of a pregnancy
   d. A specific time during which the environment has its greatest effect on the individual

Answer ( ) Rationale: _____

_____

3. The most common causes of damage to the fetal central nervous system during the third trimester are:
   a. Noxious agents and poor maternal nutrition
   b. Viral infection and maternal stress
   c. Bacterial infection and maternal drug abuse
   d. Maternal tobacco and alcohol abuse

Answer ( ) Rationale: _____

_____

4. Common care of the umbilical cord stump includes all of the following *except:*
   a. Application of antibacterial agent such as triple dye
   b. Application of alcohol with each diaper change
   c. Application of sterile dressing or bandage
   d. Folding the diaper to avoid contact with the stump

Answer ( ) Rationale: _____

_____

5. A neonate receives an Apgar score of 4, 1 minute after birth, and a score of 6, 5 minutes after birth. These Apgar scores indicate that the neonate is:
   a. Adjusting well to extrauterine life
   b. Experiencing little difficulty adjusting to extrauterine life
   c. Experiencing moderate difficulty adjusting to extrauterine life
   d. Experiencing severe distress

Answer ( ) Rationale: _____

_____

6. Which neonatal assessment finding would be considered abnormal?
   a. Cyanosis of the hands and feet during activity
   b. Palpable anterior and posterior fontanels
   c. Soft protuberant abdomen
   d. Sporadic asymmetrical limb movements

Answer ( ) Rationale: _____

_____

7. Infants normally double their birth weight by:
   a. 3 months
   b. 6 months
   c. 9 months
   d. 1 year

Answer ( ) Rationale: _____

_____

8. Which statement about infant cognitive development is accurate?
   a. Sensory stimuli are less important than food for healthy development.
   b. Hospitalized infants require continuous stimuli to enhance cognitive development.
   c. By 12 months, infants are able to comprehend simple commands.
   d. By 12 months, infants continue to have difficulty localizing and discriminating sounds.

Answer ( ) Rationale: _____

_____

9. The mother of a 2-year-old expresses concern that her son's appetite has diminished and that he seems to prefer milk to other solid foods. Which response by the nurse reflects knowledge of principles of communication and nutrition?
   a. "Oh, I wouldn't be too worried; children tend to eat when they're hungry. I just wouldn't give him dessert unless he eats his meal."
   b. "That is not uncommon in toddlers. You might consider increasing his milk to 2 quarts per day to be sure he gets enough nutrients."
   c. "Have you considered feeding him when he doesn't seem interested in feeding himself?"
   d. "A toddler's rate of growth normally slows down. It's common to see a toddler's appetite diminish in response to decreased calorie needs."

Answer ( ) Rationale: _____

_____

10. To stimulate cognitive and psychosocial development of the toddler, it is important for parents to:
    a. Set firm and consistent limits
    b. Foster sharing of toys with playmates and siblings
    c. Provide clarification about what is right and wrong
    d. Limit confusion by restricting exploration of the environment

Answer ( ) Rationale: _____

_____

CLINICAL SITUATIONS

1. Sara is a 1-week-old newborn hospitalized for low birth weight status. What measures can the nurse use to help develop attachment between Sara and her family (mother, father, and 4-year-old brother)?

_____

_____

_____

_____

_____

_____

_____

_____

_____

2. Steven is a 4-year-old boy admitted to the hospital for open heart surgery in 2 days. Describe the approach the nurse should use to prepare him for the procedures and care measures involved with surgery and to help him cope with the required separation from his family and home environment.

_____

_____

_____

_____

_____

_____

_____

_____

_____

Chapter

29 | School Age Through Adolescence

School-age children and adolescents lead demanding, challenging lives. The developmental changes between ages 6 and 18 are diverse and span all areas of growth and development.

PRELIMINARY READING

Chapter 29, pp. 528-548

COMPREHENSIVE UNDERSTANDING

■ SCHOOL-AGE CHILD

➤ The school-age years range from _____ to _____.
➤ The school and home influence growth and development, requiring adjustment by the parents and child.
➤ Parents must learn to allow their child to make decisions, accept responsibility, and learn from life's experiences.
➤ Identify the stressors commonly encountered by

school-age children: _____

_____

_____

_____

_____

_____

_____

_____

_____

_____

Physical Development

➤ Summarize the normal characteristics of the school-age child.

Height and weight: _____

_____

Cardiovascular functioning: _____

_____

_____

_____

Neuromuscular functioning: _____

_____

_____

_____

Nutrition: _____

_____

_____

_____

_____

_____

Skeletal growth: _____

_____

_____

_____

_____

_____

Cognitive Development

➤ Cognitive changes provide the school-age child with the ability to think in a logical manner about the here and now but not about abstraction.
➤ Define the newly developing cognitive skills.

Concrete operations: _____

_____

_____

_____

Decanter: _____

_____

_____

_____

_____

Conservation: _____

_____

_____

Seriation: _____

_____

_____

_____

Classification: _____

_____

_____

_____

➤ Identify techniques that adults can use to help children improve their problem-solving abilities:

_____

_____

_____

_____

_____

➤ Summarize language growth during middle childhood:

_____

_____

_____

_____

Psychosocial Development

➤ The developmental task for school-age children is

_____vs. _____.

➤ Summarize the psychosocial development in relation to the following:

Moral development _____

_____

_____

_____

_____

Peer relationships _____

_____

_____

_____

_____

Sexual identity _____

_____

_____

_____

Self-concept and health _____

_____

_____

_____

_____

Specific Health Concerns of the School-Age Child

➤ _____ and _____ are the leading causes of death or injury.

➤ Infections account for nearly 80% of all childhood illnesses; respiratory infections are the most prevalent.

➤ Identify the specific health concerns of children living

in poverty: _____

_____

_____

_____

_____

_____

_____

_____

➤ Identify at least five health promotion activities appropriate for school-age children.

a. _____

b. _____

c. _____

d. _____

e. _____

■ PREADOLESCENT

➤ Preadolescence refers to _____.

➤ Physically, preadolescence begins _____

_____.

➤ Explain ego ideal: _____

_____

∎ ADOLESCENT

➤ Adolescence is the period of development _____

_____

_____.

➤ Define *puberty,* and explain the changes that occur at

this time: _____

_____

_____

_____.

Physical Changes and Sexual Maturation

➤ List the four major physical changes associated with sexual maturation.

a. _____

_____

b. _____

_____

c. _____

_____

d. _____

➤ Summarize the weight and skeletal changes that occur

at this time: _____

_____

_____

_____

_____

➤ Explain the effects of physical changes on peer inter-

actions: _____

_____

_____

_____

➤ Identify the changes that occur during puberty in relation to the following:

Timing _____

_____

_____

Sequence _____

_____

_____

Hormonal changes _____

_____

_____

Cognitive Development

➤ Changes that occur within the mind and the widen-
ing social environment of the adolescent result in

_____, the highest level of
intellectual development.

➤ During this period of cognitive development, the
adolescent develops the ability to solve problems
through logical operations.

➤ For the first time the young person can move beyond
the physical or concrete properties of a situation and
use reasoning powers to understand the abstract.

➤ Elkind describes two characteristics of cognitive
function. Briefly explain each one.

Imaginary audience: _____

_____

_____

Personal fable: _____

_____

_____

_____

➤ Adolescents have the capability to think as well as
adults but do not have experiences on which to
build.

➤ Summarize the language skills of the adolescent:

_____

_____

_____

_____

Psychosocial Development

➤ The search for _____ is the major
task of adolescent psychosocial development.

➤ Teenagers must establish close peer relationships or
remain socially isolated.

➤ Explain identity vs. role confusion (Erickson): _____

_____

_____

_____

➤ Behaviors indicating negative resolution are _____

_____

_____ .

➤ Explain the following components of total identity:

Sexual identity _____

_____

_____

Group identity _____

_____

_____

Family identity _____

_____

_____

Vocational identity _____

_____

_____

Health identity _____

_____

_____

Moral identity _____

_____

_____

Define Erickson's "psychosocial moratorium":

_____

_____

_____

_____

Specific Health Concerns of the Adolescent Period

➤ Identify the leading cause of death among adolescents

and its sources: _____

_____

➤ During adolescence, substance abuse is a major concern. Adolescents at risk are _____

_____

_____ .

➤ Suicide is the third leading cause of death among adolescents. List the six warning signs of suicide for this group.

a. _____

b. _____

c. _____

d. _____

e. _____

f. _____

➤ In formation of healthy habits of daily living, emphasis is on exercise, sleep, nutrition, and stress-reduction habits.

➤ _____ ,

_____ , and

_____ expectations contribute to early heterosexual and homosexual relations.

➤ Briefly explain the two prominent consequences of adolescent sexual activity.

Sexually transmitted disease (STD): _____

_____

_____

_____

Pregnancy: _____

_____

_____

_____

_____

➤ Identify the health promotion and illness prevention programs for the adolescent.

Accidental deaths: _____

_____

Substance abuse: _____

_____

Sex education: _____

_____

Minority adolescent: _____

_____

_____

_____

∎ NURSING PROCESS

Assessment

➤ List the five areas for nursing assessment of the school-age child and adolescent:

_____

_____

_____

_____

_____

Nursing Diagnosis

➤ List at least five potential diagnoses for the adolescent

client: _____

_____

_____

_____

_____

Planning

➤ The planning phase must directly involve the adolescent and his or her parent in goal-setting.
➤ Planning must also show consideration for social and psychological nursing problems that accompany physical nursing problems.

Implementation

➤ The nurse needs to develop an individual plan for a healthy life-style and follow through with health promotion strategies.

Evaluation

➤ List three expected outcomes for the adolescent with altered health maintenance.

a. _____

b. _____

c. _____

REVIEW QUESTIONS

(The student should select the appropriate answer and cite the rationale for choosing that particular answer.)

1. Which of the following is true of the developmental behaviors of school-age children?
   a. Formal and informal peer group membership is the key in forming self-esteem.
   b. Fears center around the loss of self-control.
   c. Positive feedback from parents and teachers is crucial to development.
   d. A full range of defense mechanisms is used including rationalization and intellectualization.

Answer ( ) Rationale: _____

_____

_____

2. Which statement about physical development in the school-age child is accurate?
   a. The rate of growth during early school years is more rapid than during the preschool period.
   b. Fine motor skills are more refined than gross motor skills.
   c. Girls begin changes associated with puberty as early as age 9.
   d. Regular measurement of height and weight is less important than it is during other developmental stages.

Answer ( ) Rationale: _____

_____

_____

3. The most common nutritional deficiencies during the school-age period include:
   a. Calcium, vitamin C, and B complex vitamins
   b. Iron, calcium, and vitamin A
   c. Iron and vitamin K
   d. Calcium, vitamin D, and vitamin C

Answer ( ) Rationale: _____

_____

_____

4. The leading cause of death in school-age children is:
   a. Accident
   b. Infectious disease
   c. Cancer
   d. Suicide

Answer ( ) Rationale: _____

_____

_____

5. The transition period between childhood and adolescence is:
   a. Pubescence
   b. Late childhood
   c. Transescence
   d. All of the above

Answer (   ) Rationale: _____

_____

_____

6. Which statement about puberty growth changes is correct?
   a. The timing of pubertal growth changes is the same in most females.
   b. The time when sexual changes begin is more significant than their pattern of onset.
   c. The sequence of pubertal growth changes is the same in most individuals.
   d. Growth changes result from pituitary secretion of gonadotropin-releasing hormones.

Answer (   ) Rationale: _____

_____

_____

7. Adolescents have mastered age-appropriate sexuality when they feel comfortable with their sexual:
   a. Behaviors
   b. Choices
   c. Relationships
   d. All of the above

Answer (   ) Rationale: _____

_____

_____

8. The leading cause of death for adolescents is:
   a. Motor vehicle accidents
   b. Drug abuse
   c. Suicide
   d. Infectious disease

Answer (   ) Rationale: _____

_____

_____

9. According to Piaget, the school-age child is in the third stage of cognitive development, which is characterized by:
   a. Conventional thought
   b. Concrete operations
   c. Identity versus role diffusion
   d. Postconventional thought

Answer (   ) Rationale: _____

_____

_____

10. According to Erickson, the developmental task of adolescence is:
    a. Autonomy versus shame and doubt
    b. Self-identity versus role confusion
    c. Industry versus inferiority
    d. Role acceptance versus role confusion

Answer (   ) Rationale: _____

_____

_____

11. All of the following are warning signals that a teenager is considering suicide *except:*
    a. Poor grades in school
    b. Loss of appetite
    c. Increased sleepiness
    d. Verbalization of suicidal thoughts

Answer (   ) Rationale: _____

_____

_____

CLINICAL SITUATIONS

1. Andrew, a 16-year-old, confides to the school nurse, "All my friends are having sex, but I am not sure I am ready, especially since I read about a teenage boy who died from AIDS." How should the nurse counsel him?

_____

_____

_____

_____

_____

_____

_____

_____

2. Chip is a 7-year-old who fractured his right arm while climbing a tree. He lives with his parents and his 4-year-old brother. The pediatric nurse practitioner is responsible for Chip's follow-up care.

a. What physical characteristics should be evaluated (based on Chip's age)?

_____

_____

_____

_____

_____

_____

b. According to Freud, what is Chip's developmental stage, and what developmental skills are affected by his injury?

_____

_____

_____

_____

_____

_____

c. According to Erickson, what conflict is commonly experienced by children Chip's age, and what anticipatory guidance can the nurse offer?

_____

_____

_____

_____

_____

_____

_____

_____

Chapter 30 | Young and Middle Adult

Young and middle adulthood is a period of challenges, rewards, and crises.

PRELIMINARY READING

Chapter 30, pp. 549-567

COMPREHENSIVE UNDERSTANDING

▌MATURITY AND ADULTHOOD
➤ Briefly describe the characteristics of the mature adult:

_____

_____

_____

_____

▌YOUNG ADULT
Theories of Young Adulthood
➤ List and briefly describe the five phases of young and middle adult development described by Levinson.

a. _____

_____

b. _____

_____

c. _____

_____

d. _____

_____

e. _____

_____

➤ Theorists propose that intellectual and moral development differ between men and women.
➤ According to Gilligan, what constitutes women's primary developmental issue? _____

_____

_____

➤ Identify the developmental issues concerning males:

_____

_____

➤ Describe the developmental tasks of the young adult proposed by Diekelmann.

a. _____

b. _____

c. _____

d. _____

e. _____

▌MIDDLE ADULT
➤ In middle adulthood, the individual makes lasting contributions through involvement with others.
➤ High self-esteem, a favorable body image, and a positive attitude toward physiological changes are fostered

when adults engage in _____,

_____, _____, and

_____ practices that promote vigorous, healthy bodies.

Theories of Middle Adulthood
➤ According to Erickson, the primary developmental

task of the middle years is _____.

Briefly explain this stage: _____

_____

_____

_____

➤ Identify Havighurst's proposed seven developmental tasks for the middle adult.

a. _____

b. _____

c. _____

d. _____

e. _____

f. _____

g. _____

■ THE NURSING PROCESS AND YOUNG AND MIDDLE ADULTHOOD

Assessment

Young Adult

➤ Identify the personal life-style assessment of a young adult: _____

_____

_____

_____

_____

_____

_____

➤ Briefly explain the cognitive development in the following areas:

Educational experiences _____

_____

_____

_____

Life experiences _____

_____

_____

_____

Occupational opportunities _____

_____

_____

_____

➤ The emotional health of the young adult is related to the individual's ability to address and resolve personal and social tasks. Explain the patterns of the following age-groups:

23 to 28 _____

_____

29 to 34 _____

_____

35 to 43 _____

_____

➤ The young adult must make decisions concerning career, marriage, and parenthood. Briefly explain the general principles involved.

Career: _____

_____

_____

_____

_____

_____

Sexuality: _____

_____

_____

Four phases of the childbearing cycle

_____

_____

_____

_____

_____

_____

_____

_____

_____

Lactation _____

_____

_____

_____

Types of families:

Singlehood _____

_____

_____

_____

Five tasks to be completed prior to marriage

_____

_____

_____

_____

_____

Six tasks to be accomplished in the establishment of a household

_____

_____

_____

_____

_____

_____

Three developmental stages of a marital relationship

_____

_____

_____

Parenthood _____

_____

_____

_____

_____

HEALTH CONCERNS

➤ Briefly explain the risk factors for young adults.

Violent death: _____

_____

_____

Substance abuse: _____

_____

_____

Pregnancies: _____

_____

_____

STDs: _____

_____

_____

Environmental and occupational risks: _____

_____

_____

_____

➤ Life-style habits such as _____,

_____, _____, and

_____ increase the risk of future illness.

➤ _____ is a man's, woman's, or couple's involuntary inability to conceive.

➤ The psychosocial concerns of the young adult are often related to stress, such as job or family. Briefly explain each one.

Job stress: _____

_____

_____

_____

Family stress: _____

_____

_____

_____

PREGNANT WOMAN AND CHILDBEARING FAMILY

➤ Explain the physiological changes that occur during the following:

Prenatal care _____

_____

_____

_____

_____

_____

First trimester _____

_____

_____

_____

_____

_____

Second trimester _____

_____

_____

_____

_____

Third trimester _____

_____

_____

_____

_____

Puerperium _____

_____

_____

_____

_____

➤ Explain the cognitive changes that occur during pregnancy.

Sensory perception: _____

_____

_____

_____

_____

➤ Explain the psychosocial changes that occur during

pregnancy: _____

_____

_____

_____

_____

Middle Adult

➤ Briefly explain the major physiological changes that occur between 40 and 65 years of age:

_____

_____

_____

_____

_____

_____

_____

_____

_____

_____

_____

_____

_____

➤ Define *menopause:* _____

_____

_____

_____

➤ Define *climacteric:* _____

_____

_____

_____

➤ Changes in the cognitive function are rare except in cases of illness or trauma.
➤ Summarize the psychosocial development of the middle adult in the following areas:

Career transition _____

_____

_____

_____

Sexuality _____

_____

_____

_____

Singlehood _____

_____

_____

Marital changes _____

_____

_____

Family transitions _____

_____

_____

Care of aging parents _____

_____

_____

HEALTH CONCERNS

➤ The following are the physiological concerns for the middle adult. Briefly explain each one:

Stress _____

_____

_____

_____

_____

Chronic illness _____

_____

_____

_____

_____

_____

Levels of wellness _____

_____

_____

Positive health habits _____

_____

_____

_____

_____

➤ Summarize the two psychosocial concerns of the middle adult.

Anxiety: _____

_____

_____

_____

Depression: _____

_____

_____

_____

Nursing Diagnosis

➤ Identify five potential nursing diagnoses for the young or middle adult:

_____

_____

_____

_____

_____

Planning

➤ When providing nursing care for young and middle adults, the nurse must recognize that the needs of clients, families, and communities are interconnected.

➤ State four health maintenance goals for the young and middle adult.

a. _____

b. _____

c. _____

d. _____

Implementation

➤ Identify three interventions for the following:

Changing Health Habits _____

_____

_____

_____

_____

Health Promotion _____

_____

_____

_____

_____

Stress Reduction _____

_____

_____

_____

_____

Evaluation

➤ Each young or middle adult has different health goals.
➤ List two expected outcomes for a young or middle adult with altered health maintenance:

_____

_____

REVIEW QUESTIONS

(The student should select the appropriate answer and cite the rationale for choosing that particular answer.)

1. According to Erickson's developmental theory, the primary developmental task of the middle years is to:
   a. Achieve generativity
   b. Achieve intimacy
   c. Establish a set of personal values
   d. Establish a sense of personal identity

   Answer ( ) Rationale: _____

   _____

   _____

2. The greatest cause of illness and death in the young adult population is:
   a. Sexually transmitted disease
   b. Violence
   c. Cardiovascular disease
   d. Substance abuse

   Answer ( ) Rationale: _____

   _____

   _____

3. Psychosocial changes of pregnancy commonly involve all of the following areas *except:*
   a. Body image
   b. Anxiety and depression
   c. Role changes
   d. Sexuality

   Answer ( ) Rationale: _____

   _____

   _____

4. Which physiological change would be a normal assessment finding in a middle adult?
   a. Increased breast size
   b. Abdominal tenderness and organomegaly
   c. Increased anteroposterior diameter of thorax
   d. Reduced auditory acuity

   Answer ( ) Rationale: _____

   _____

   _____

5. Which statement about behavior and habits is incorrect?
   a. Habits often meet a basic need for the person.
   b. Any change in habits or behavior creates stress.
   c. Habits can be stress-reduction mechanisms.
   d. Nurses are able to change clients' habits.

   Answer ( ) Rationale: _____

   _____

   _____

6. Larry, age 18 years, just graduated from high school. To achieve a "personal identity" according to Levinson's theory on young adulthood he would engage in which of the following behaviors?
   a. Attend a local college and live with his parents
   b. Marry his high-school sweetheart
   c. Follow his parents' advice regarding major decisions
   d. Obtain a job and live away from home

   Answer ( ) Rationale: _____

   _____

   _____

7. Developmental tasks of early adulthood include all of the following *except:*
   a. Establishing an intimate relationship
   b. Developing financial stability
   c. Selecting an occupation
   d. Assuming care of aged parents

   Answer ( ) Rationale: _____

   _____

   _____

8. Which of the following characteristics would the nurse have to consider in planning care for a client in middle adulthood?
   a. Declining sexual interest
   b. Declining motor coordination
   c. Decreasing creativity
   d. Declining thinking ability

   Answer ( ) Rationale: _____

   _____

   _____

9. In planning patient education for Mrs. Smith, a 45-year-old woman who had an ovarian cyst removed, which of the following facts is true about the sexuality of the middle-age adult?
   a. Menstruation ceases after menopause.
   b. Estrogen is produced after menopause.
   c. After reaching climacteric, a male is unable to father a child.
   d. With removal of the ovarian cyst, pregnancy cannot occur.

Answer (   ) Rationale: _____

_____

_____

CLINICAL SITUATIONS

1. During a routine prenatal visit, Suzanne, a 23-year-old primigravida (pregnant for the first time) woman asks the nurse, "Why do I need to come in every month, especially since I feel fine and no one in my family has ever experienced any pregnancy problems? I just cannot find the time, since I have a full-time job and we are in the process of building a new home." Describe how the nurse should respond to her question.

_____

_____

_____

_____

_____

_____

_____

_____

_____

2. Mrs. Charis, 53 years old, is admitted to the hospital for a hysterectomy to treat cervical cancer. She has been married for 30 years and has three children, 17 to 24 years old. She describes her husband as her "best friend" and tells the nurse she is preparing to send her youngest child to college this fall. Mrs. Charis has smoked approximately five cigarettes per day for the past 35 years.
   a. What major task would concern Mrs. Charis as an individual in her middle years? What effect could her current health status have on task achievement?

   _____

   _____

   _____

   _____

   _____

   _____

   _____

   b. What stage of family development are the Charises experiencing? What feelings might parents experience during this stage? What behaviors or activities are characteristic of this stage?

   _____

   _____

   _____

   _____

   _____

   c. Formulate four nursing diagnoses applicable to Mrs. Charis.

   _____

   _____

   _____

   d. State four goals for Mrs. Charis' care during hospitalization.

   _____

   _____

   _____

   _____

31 | Older Adult

Older adulthood traditionally begins after retirement, usually between 65 and 75 years of age.

PRELIMINARY READING

Chapter 31, pp. 568-592

COMPREHENSIVE UNDERSTANDING

➤ Nursing assessment of an older adult (Lueckenotte) takes into account the following points. Briefly explain each one:

The interrelationship between physical and psychosocial aspects of aging _____

_____

_____

_____

_____

_____

_____

The effects of disease and disability on functional status

_____

_____

_____

_____

_____

The decreased efficiency of homeostatic mechanisms

_____

_____

_____

_____

_____

_____

The lack of standards for health and illness norms

_____

_____

_____

_____

_____

_____

▌ TERMINOLOGY
➤ Define:

Geriatrics _____

_____

_____

Gerontology _____

_____

_____

Gerontology nursing _____

_____

_____

▌ MYTHS AND STEREOTYPES
➤ Identify at least five myths and/or stereotypes of the older adult:

_____

_____

_____

_____

_____

➤ Define *ageism:* _____

_____

_____

_____

■ NURSES' ATTITUDES TOWARD OLDER ADULTS

➤ Negative attitudes may result in a reduction in clients' sense of security, adequacy, and well-being.

➤ The nurse must clarify personal attitudes and values about older adults to provide the most effective care.

➤ Nurses who work with older adults must collect complete assessment data, including clients' _____,

_____, and _____.

➤ The nurse's interventions should attempt to incorporate the client's _____ or _____.

■ THEORIES OF AGING

➤ Aging is not a simple progression, so there is no universally accepted theory that can predict and explain the complexities of older adults.

Biological Theories

➤ Give a short description of the following theories:

Free radical theory _____

_____

_____

_____

_____

Cross-link theory _____

_____

_____

_____

_____

Immunological theory _____

_____

_____

_____

_____

Psychosocial Theories

➤ List the four basic concepts of the disengagement theory.

a. _____

b. _____

c. _____

d. _____

➤ Describe the following theories:

Activity theory _____

_____

_____

_____

_____

Continuity theory _____

_____

_____

_____

_____

_____

■ GROWTH AND DEVELOPMENT

➤ List the seven developmental tasks of the older adult.

a. _____

b. _____

c. _____

d. _____

e. _____

f. _____

g. _____

■ COMMUNITY-BASED AND INSTITUTIONAL HEALTH CARE SERVICES

➤ Briefly explain the following health services that are used by the older population:

Home care _____

_____

_____

Day care _____

_____

_____

Respite care _____

_____

_____

Long-term care _____

_____

_____

Hospice care _____

_____

THE NURSING PROCESS AND OLDER ADULTS

 Assessment

PHYSIOLOGICAL CHANGES

➤ Identify the physiological changes that occur in the older adult with regard to the following:

General survey _____

_____

_____

_____

Integumentary system _____

_____

_____

_____

_____

Head and neck _____

_____

_____

_____

_____

Thorax and lungs _____

_____

_____

_____

Heart and vascular system _____

_____

_____

_____

_____

Breasts _____

_____

_____

_____

_____

Gastrointestinal system and abdomen _____

_____

_____

_____

_____

Reproductive system _____

_____

_____

_____

_____

Urinary system _____

_____

_____

_____

_____

Musculoskeletal system _____

_____

_____

_____

_____

Neurological system _____

_____

_____

_____

_____

COGNITIVE CHANGES

➤ The structural and physiological changes occurring in the brain during aging do not necessarily affect the adaptive and functional abilities.

➤ Define *dementia:* _____

_____

➤ Identify the three stages of Alzheimer's disease.

a. _____

b. _____

c. _____

➤ Identify some behavioral responses of a client with Alzheimer's disease: _____

_____

_____

_____

_____

➤ Define *multiinfarct dementia:* _____

_____

➤ Multiinfarct dementia may be related to vascular disorders in the brain. List the conditions from which it results: _____

_____

_____

_____

_____

_____

_____

_____

➤ Define *delirium:* _____

_____

_____

➤ Long-term abuse of alcohol and drugs can affect cognitive functioning. Identify the effects:

_____

_____

_____

_____

_____

➤ Define the following:

Wernicke's syndrome _____

_____

_____

Korsakoff's syndrome _____

_____

_____

Confabulation _____

_____

_____

PSYCHOSOCIAL CHANGES

➤ List at least five areas to be addressed when counseling an older adult about retirement:

_____

_____

_____

_____

_____

➤ Briefly describe the four types of social isolation experienced by older adults.

Attitudinal: _____

_____

_____

Presentational: _____

_____

_____

Behavioral: _____

_____

_____

Geographical: _____

_____

_____

➤ Briefly describe the sexual changes that occur in the older adult: _____

_____

_____

_____

_____

➤ List four factors to assess when assisting older adults with housing needs:

a. _____

b. _____

c. _____

d. _____

- A common misconception is that death of an older adult is a blessing and the culmination of a full life.
- Many dying older adults still have goals, and they are not emotionally prepared to die.

HEALTH MAINTENANCE
- Summarize the physiological health concerns of the following:

Cardiovascular problems _____
_____
_____
_____
_____
_____

Cancer _____
_____
_____
_____
_____
_____

Arthritis _____
_____
_____
_____
_____
_____

Sensory impairments _____
_____
_____
_____
_____
_____

Dental problems _____
_____
_____

- List the four major causes of death in older adults:
  a. _____
  b. _____
  c. _____
  d. _____
- Briefly explain the drug effects commonly seen in adults over 65: _____
_____
_____
_____

- Briefly explain the nutritional needs of the older adult:
_____
_____
_____
_____
_____

- The primary benefits of exercise include maintaining and strengthening functional ability and promoting a sense of enhanced wellness.
- The nurse should plan an exercise program that meets physical needs while allowing for physical impairments.

Nursing Diagnosis

- Data regarding the physiological, cognitive, and psychosocial status of the older adult yield actual or high-risk problems. Identify at least five nursing diagnoses:
_____
_____
_____
_____

- Analysis of data requires consideration of individual strengths and limitations, as well as the older client's perception of health status.

Planning

- A care plan for the older adult focuses on activities to prevent, improve, reduce, or eliminate problems.
- Consideration by the nurse of the experiences of a lifetime, as well as values and sociocultural patterns developed, should serve as the basis for planning individual care.

Implementation

Health Promotion

➤ Increasing scientific evidence suggests that life-style choices influence overall health status and longevity, even when changes are made in late life.

Home Safety

➤ List six environmental factors used to promote a client's safety in the home:

_____

_____

_____

_____

_____

_____

Psychosocial Support

➤ Briefly describe the seven techniques used to maintain the psychosocial health of the older adult.

Therapeutic communication: _____

_____

_____

Touch: _____

_____

_____

Reality orientation: _____

_____

_____

Resocialization: _____

_____

_____

Validation therapy: _____

_____

_____

Reminiscence: _____

_____

_____

Body-image interventions: _____

_____

_____

Medication Use

➤ List the strategies used to reduce an adverse medication reaction in the older adult:

_____

_____

_____

_____

_____

_____

_____

_____

_____

_____

Evaluation

➤ The frequency of evaluation with an older adult is highly individual. Change is often slow and subtle. Thus infrequent or frequent evaluations may be performed.

➤ List four expected outcomes for the older client with impaired physical mobility:

a. _____

b. _____

c. _____

d. _____

REVIEW QUESTIONS

(The student should select the appropriate answer and cite the rationale for choosing that particular answer.)

1. Which statement about older adults is accurate?
   a. Most older adults are institutionalized.
   b. Most older adults live on a fixed income.
   c. Most older adults cannot learn to care for themselves.
   d. Most older adults have no sexual desire.

Answer (   ) Rationale: _____

_____

_____

2. Which statement describing delirium is correct?
   a. Illusions and hallucinations may be experienced by persons with delirium.
   b. The onset of delirium is slow and insidious.
   c. Symptoms of delirium are stable and unchanging.
   d. Symptoms of delirium are irreversible.

Answer (   ) Rationale: _____

_____

_____

3. Mr. Waycome is a 56-year-old business executive showing behavioral changes over the past few years. Mr. Waycome is hesitant in responding to questions posed by his co-workers. He misses regularly scheduled weekly meetings. His secretary must constantly remind him about scheduled appointments and must find his reading glasses, pens, papers, and briefcase. Lately he has come to work without showering, shaving, or changing clothes from the previous day. Mr. Waycome's behaviors are characteristic of which stage of irreversible dementia (Alzheimer's disease)?
   a. Final or terminal
   b. Later
   c. Advanced
   d. Early

Answer (   ) Rationale: _____

_____

_____

4. Multiinfarct dementia is associated primarily with:
   a. Substance abuse
   b. Infectious processes
   c. Cardiac disorder
   d. Vascular disorders

Answer (   ) Rationale: _____

_____

_____

5. Nutritional needs of the older adult:
   a. Are exactly the same as those of young and middle adults
   b. Include increased amounts of vitamin C, vitamin A, and calcium
   c. Include increased kilocalories to support metabolism and activity
   d. Include increased proteins and carbohydrates

Answer (   ) Rationale: _____

_____

_____

6. Recalling the past to assign new meaning to experiences is:
   a. Validation therapy
   b. Reminiscence
   c. Body image therapy
   d. Confabulation

Answer (   ) Rationale: _____

_____

_____

7. Attitudinal isolation occurs when the older adult is rejected from social interactions because of:
   a. Physical appearance
   b. Unacceptable behavior
   c. A bias toward the aged
   d. Physiological impairments

Answer (   ) Rationale: _____

_____

_____

8. The nurse should use which intervention to facilitate reality orientation for the older adult client?
   a. Make decisions for him concerning health practices
   b. Ignore rambling conversation and unrealistic talk
   c. Let him know when he is confused or uses incorrect words
   d. Include information such as time, place, and name in the conversation

Answer (   ) Rationale: _____

_____

_____

9. Ms. Dale states that she does not need the TV turned on because she cannot see very well. Visual changes in older adults include all of the following *except:*
   a. Decreased visual acuity
   b. Decreased accommodation to darkness
   c. Double vision
   d. Sensitivity to glare

Answer (   ) Rationale: _____

_____

_____

10. Mr. DeLone states that he is worried about his parents' plans to retire. All of the following would be appropriate responses regarding retirement of the elderly *except:*
   a. Positive adjustment is often related to how much a person planned for the retirement.
   b. Retirement for most represents a sudden shock that is irreversibly damaging to self-image and self-esteem.
   c. Reactions to retirement are influenced by the importance that has been attached to the work role.
   d. Retirement may affect an individual's physical and psychological functioning.

Answer (   ) Rationale: _____

_____

_____

CLINICAL SITUATIONS

1. You suspect that an older adult client is having difficulty adjusting to his impending retirement. What do you need to know about his developmental task achievement before you develop a nursing care plan aimed at assisting him with this transition?

_____

_____

_____

_____

_____

_____

_____

_____

_____

_____

2. You are conducting a health history on a 77-year-old man who tells you he is having an increasingly difficult time with constipation. What normal, age-related physical changes are likely to be contributing to his constipation?

_____

_____

_____

_____

_____

_____

_____

_____

Chapter

32

Vital Signs

As indicators of health status, vital signs demonstrate the effectiveness of circulation, respiratory rate, and oxygen saturation.

PRELIMINARY READING

Chapter 32, pp. 594-639

COMPREHENSIVE UNDERSTANDING

▮ GUIDELINES FOR TAKING VITAL SIGNS

➤ Identify the guidelines that assist the nurse to incorporate vital sign measurement into practice.

a. _____

b. _____

c. _____

d. _____

e. _____

f. _____

g. _____

h. _____

i. _____

j. _____

k. _____

l. _____

▮ BODY TEMPERATURE

Physiology

➤ The body temperature is the difference between the

_____ and the

amount _____.

➤ Define *core temperature*: _____

_____

➤ Identify the sites of temperature measurement:

_____

_____.

➤ Average, normal temperatures vary depending on the measurement site.

➤ Measurement of the pulmonary artery temperature is the standard against which all other sites are judged for accuracy.

Regulation

➤ The balance of body temperature is precisely regulated by physiological and behavioral mechanisms.

➤ Briefly summarize how neural and vascular mechanisms control body temperature: _____

_____

_____

_____

_____

➤ List four sources, or mechanisms, for heat production.

a. _____

b. _____

c. _____

d. _____

➤ Explain the following mechanisms of body heat loss and give an example of each:

Radiation _____

_____

_____

_____

Conduction _____

_____

_____

_____

Convection _____

_____

_____

_____

Evaporation _____

_____

_____

_____

Diaphoresis _____

_____

_____

_____

➤ Briefly explain the skin's role in temperature regulation.

Insulation of the body: _____

_____

_____

_____

Vasoconstriction: _____

_____

_____

_____

Temperature sensation: _____

_____

_____

_____

➤ Identify four factors that must be present for a person to control body temperature.

a. _____

b. _____

c. _____

d. _____

Factors Affecting Body Temperature

➤ Changes in body temperature within the normal range occur when the relationship between heat production and heat loss is altered by physiological or behavioral variables. Summarize the following variables:

Age _____

_____

_____

_____

Exercise _____

_____

_____

_____

Hormone level _____

_____

_____

_____

Circadian rhythm _____

_____

_____

_____

Stress _____

_____

_____

_____

Environment _____

_____

_____

_____

Temperature Alterations

➤ Changes in body temperature can be related to

_____, _____,

_____, or any combination of these alterations.

➤ Hyperpyrexia, or fever, occurs because _____

_____

_____.

➤ Summarize the alteration in the hypothalamic set point that causes a true fever: _____

_____

_____

_____

_____

➤ Explain how a fever works as an important defense mechanism: _____

_____

_____

➤ Explain how a fever serves a diagnostic purpose:

_____

_____

_____

➤ Explain how a fever affects metabolism: _____

_____

_____

_____

➤ Define and explain the causes of heat exhaustion:

_____

_____

➤ Define and explain the causes of hyperthermia:

_____

_____

➤ Define and explain the causes of heatstroke:

_____

_____

➤ Define and explain the causes of hypothermia:

_____

_____

■ NURSING PROCESS AND THERMOREGULATION

➤ Independent measures can be implemented to increase or minimize heat loss, to promote heat conservation, and to increase comfort.

Assessment

➤ List at least five assessment areas for temperature measurement:

_____

_____

_____

_____

_____

➤ State the formulas for the following conversions:

Fahrenheit to centigrade _____

_____

Centigrade to Fahrenheit _____

_____

➤ Identify the three types of thermometers.

a. _____

b. _____

c. _____

_____

Nursing Diagnosis

➤ Identify three nursing diagnoses related to thermoregulation:

a. _____

b. _____

c. _____

_____

Planning

➤ Clients at high risk for alterations in body temperature require an individualized care plan directed at maintaining normothermia and reducing risk factors.

➤ The care plan for clients with actual temperature alterations focuses on restoring normothermia, minimizing complications, and promoting comfort.

Implementation

Hyperthermia

➤ The procedures used to intervene and treat an elevated temperature depend on the fever's cause; its adverse effects; and its strength, intensity, and duration.

➤ Fever therapy reduces _____,

increases _____, and prevents complications.

➤ Give three examples of each type of therapy.

Pharmacological: _____

_____

_____

Nonpharmacological: _____

_____

_____

➤ Identify an independent and dependent nursing

intervention to control shivering: _____

_____

_____

_____

Heatstroke

➤ The best treatment for heatstroke is prevention. Give five examples of prevention for heatstroke:

_____

_____

_____

_____

_____

➤ What is the first aid and emergency treatment for

heatstroke? _____

_____

_____

_____

Hypothermia

➤ Identify the five preventive measures for hypothermia:

_____

_____

_____

_____

_____

➤ Summarize the treatment for hypothermia:

_____

_____

_____

_____

_____

_____

Evaluation

➤ After any intervention, the nurse measures the client's temperature to evaluate it for any change.

➤ Other evaluative measures are _____

and _____.

■ PULSE

➤ Define *pulse:* _____

_____

Physiology and Regulation

➤ Define:

Stroke volume _____

Cardiac output _____

➤ _____, _____,

and _____ factors regulate the strength of heart contractions and its stroke volume.

Assessment of Pulse

➤ Identify the two most common peripheral pulse sites to assess.

a. _____

b. _____

➤ Identify the five major parts of the stethoscope.

a. _____

b. _____

c. _____

d. _____

e. _____

Character of the Pulse

➤ List four characteristics to identify during peripheral pulse assessment. By using an asterisk, specify the two characteristics when assessing an apical pulse.

a. _____

b. _____

c. _____

d. _____

➤ Define the following:

Tachycardia _____

_____

Bradycardia _____

_____

Dysrhythmia _____

_____

■ NURSING PROCESS AND PULSE DETERMINATION

➤ Pulse assessment determines the general state of cardiovascular health and the response to other system imbalances.

➤ The nurse evaluates client outcomes by assessing the

pulse _____, _____,

_____, and _____

following each intervention.

■ RESPIRATION

➤ Define the following:

Respiration _____

_____

Ventilation _____

_____

Diffusion _____

_____

Hypoxemia _____

_____

Tidal volume _____

_____

Eupnea _____

_____

➤ The most important factor in the control of ventilation

is the level of _____.

➤ Inspiration is a _____ process,

and expiration is a _____ process.

➤ Identify three conditions that may affect ventilatory movements.

a. _____

b. _____

c. _____

Assessment of Respirations

➤ Accurate measurement requires _____

and _____ of the chest wall movement.

➤ List three objective measurements used in respiratory status assessment:

a. _____

b. _____

c. _____

➤ The respiratory processes of diffusion and perfusion can be evaluated by measuring the oxygen saturation of the blood.

➤ The saturation of arterial blood is _____,

and venous blood is _____.

■ NURSING PROCESS AND RESPIRATORY VITAL SIGNS

➤ Vital sign measurement of respiratory rate, pattern, and depth, along with Svo_2, allows the nurse to assess ventilation, diffusion, and perfusion.

➤ The nurse evaluates client outcomes by assessing the

_____, _____, _____,

and _____ following each intervention.

■ BLOOD PRESSURE

➤ Define the following terms:

Blood pressure _____

_____

Systolic _____

_____

Diastolic _____

_____

Physiology of Arterial Blood Pressure

➤ Blood pressure is reflected by the following. Briefly explain each:

Cardiac output _____

_____

_____

Peripheral resistance _____

_____

_____

Blood volume _____

_____

_____

Viscosity _____

_____

_____

Elasticity _____

_____

_____

Factors Influencing Blood Pressure

➤ List six factors that influence blood pressure.

a. _____

b. _____

c. _____

d. _____

e. _____

f. _____

Hypertension

➤ Identify the criteria for the diagnosis of hypertension

in an adult: _____

_____

➤ List five risk factors that are linked to hypertension:

a. _____

b. _____

c. _____

d. _____

e. _____

Hypotension

➤ Identify the criteria for the diagnosis of hypotension

in an adult: _____

_____

_____

_____

Assessment of Blood Pressure

➤ Identify two methods for measuring blood pressure.

a. _____

b. _____

➤ Identify the two types of sphygmomanometers, and list their advantages and disadvantages:

_____

_____

_____

_____

➤ Define the following:

Orthostatic, or postural, hypotension _____

_____

_____

_____

_____

Korotkoff sounds, first _____,

second _____,

third _____,

fourth _____,

and fifth _____

➤ During the initial assessment the nurse should obtain

and record the blood pressure in _____ arms.

➤ The American Heart Association recommends two numbers for a blood pressure measurement. Define each.

Systolic: _____

Diastolic: _____

➤ Identify five common mistakes in measurement:

_____

_____

_____

_____

_____

➤ Explain the rationale for the use of an ultrasonic

stethoscope: _____

_____

➤ List two methods the nurse may use to assess blood pressure when Korotkoff sounds are not audible with

the standard stethoscope: _____

_____

_____

_____

➤ Describe auscultatory gap: _____

_____

_____

_____

➤ Identify the five reasons why the measurement and interpretation of blood pressure in infants and children is difficult:

_____

_____

_____

_____

_____

➤ Identify the advantage and disadvantage of using auto-

matic blood pressure devices: _____

_____

_____

_____

➤ List the benefits of blood pressure self-measurement.

a. _____

b. _____

c. _____

d. _____

NURSING PROCESS AND BLOOD PRESSURE DETERMINATION

➤ The assessment of blood pressure along with pulse assessment is used to evaluate the general state of cardiovascular health and responses to other system imbalances.
➤ The nurse evaluates client outcomes by assessing the blood pressure following each intervention.

RECORDING VITAL SIGNS

➤ In addition to the actual vital sign values, the nurse records in the nurses' notes any accompanying or precipitating symptoms.
➤ The nurse needs to document any intervention initiated as a result of a vital sign measurement.

REVIEW QUESTIONS

(The student should select the appropriate answer and cite the rationale for choosing that particular answer.)
1. The skin plays a role in temperature regulation by:
 a. Insulating the body
 b. Constricting blood vessels
 c. Sensing external temperature variations
 d. All of the above

Answer (   ) Rationale: _____

_____

_____

2. Which of the following sites most accurately reflects the core body temperature?
 a. Oral
 b. Tympanic
 c. Axillary
 d. Skin

Answer (   ) Rationale: _____

_____

_____

3. The nurse bathes the client who has a fever with cool water. The nurse does this to increase heat loss by means of:
 a. Radiation
 b. Convection
 c. Condensation
 d. Conduction

Answer (   ) Rationale: _____

_____

_____

4. The nurse is assessing a client who she suspects has the nursing diagnosis: hyperthermia related to vigorous exercise in hot weather. In reviewing the data the nurse knows that the most important sign of heat stroke is:
 a. Confusion
 b. Hot, dry skin
 c. Excess thirst
 d. Muscle cramps

Answer (   ) Rationale: _____

_____

_____

5. Which of the following statements about pulse regulation is inaccurate?
 a. The medulla regulates heart rate through sympathetic and parasympathetic stimulation.
 b. The heart maintains a relatively constant blood flow despite heart rate variations.
 c. Mechanical, neural, and chemical factors influence heart contractions.
 d. The pulse rate provides a direct measurement of cardiac output.

Answer (   ) Rationale: _____

_____

_____

6. When a client's condition suddenly deteriorates, where is the best pulse assessment site?
 a. Radial
 b. Apical
 c. Carotid
 d. Femoral

Answer (   ) Rationale: _____

_____

_____

7. When the nurse takes the client's radial pulse, he notes a dysrhythmia. His most appropriate action is:
 a. Inform the physician immediately.
 b. Wait 5 minutes and retake the radial pulse.
 c. Take the pulse apically for 1 full minute.
 d. Check the client's record for the presence of a previous dysrhythmia.

Answer (   ) Rationale: _____

_____

_____

8. Mr. Wienski is obese. If the nurse takes his blood pressure using a standardized sized blood pressure cuff, the blood pressure reading will be:
   a. Falsely low
   b. Accurate
   ✓c. Falsely high
   d. Indistinct

Answer ( ) Rationale: _____

_____

_____

9. The most important factor controlling ventilation in the typical adult in the arterial blood is:
   ✓a. Oxygen
   ✓b. Carbon dioxide
   c. pH
   d. Hemoglobin

Answer ( ) Rationale: _____

_____

_____

10. The nurse is auscultating Mrs. McKinnon's blood pressure. The nurse inflates the cuff to 180 mm Hg. At 156 mm Hg, the nurse hears the onset of a tapping sound. At 130 mm Hg the sound changes to a murmur or swishing. At 100 mm Hg the sound momentarily becomes sharper, and at 92 mm Hg it becomes muffled. At 88 mm Hg the sound disappears. Mr. McKinnon's blood pressure is:
    a. 180/92
    b. 180/130
    ✓c. 156/88
    d. 130/88

Answer ( ) Rationale: _____

_____

_____

CLINICAL SITUATIONS

1. A 72-year-old homeless woman has been brought into the emergency department by police who report she was found wandering incoherently in the middle of the street. The temperature outside is –21.0° F, and it has been snowing for 2 hours. In what order should the nurse obtain the vital signs? What method should be used to obtain each vital sign? What factors place this client at risk for impaired temperature regulation?

_____

_____

_____

_____

_____

_____

_____

_____

2. A hospitalized client is admitted for pneumonia, has a tympanic temperature of 100.2° F, a pulse of 84, blood pressure of 130/84, respirations of 22, and an Sao_2 of 98%. Explain the rationale for your anticipated interventions for this client.

_____

_____

_____

_____

_____

_____

_____

_____

_____

_____

Chapter
33

Physical Examination and Health Assessment

The skills of physical assessment and examination provide nurses with powerful tools to detect subtle as well as obvious changes in a client's health.

PRELIMINARY READING

Chapter 33, pp. 640-739

COMPREHENSIVE UNDERSTANDING

■ PURPOSES OF PHYSICAL EXAMINATION

➤ List the five nursing purposes for performing a physical assessment.

a. _____

b. _____

c. _____

d. _____

e. _____

Gathering a Health History

➤ The main objective of interacting with clients is to find out what is central to their concerns and to help them find solutions.

Developing Nursing Diagnoses and a Care Plan

➤ After collecting a history, the nurse conducts a physical

examination to _____, _____,

or _____ the existing database.

➤ A complete assessment is needed to form a definitive diagnosis.
➤ The nurse learns to group significant findings into patterns of data that reveal actual or high-risk nursing diagnoses.
➤ The baseline is _____.

Managing Client Problems

➤ The nurse's success in giving care depends on the ability to recognize change in status and to modify therapies so that the clients gain the most desirable outcome.
➤ Physical assessment skills allow the nurse to

_____ and _____.

Evaluating Nursing Care

➤ Physical assessment skills enhance the evaluation of

nursing measures through monitoring _____

and _____ outcomes of care.

■ CULTURAL SENSITIVITY

➤ How members of different cultures behave influences their willingness to assume responsibility for their health and their tendency to seek professional health care.

■ INTEGRATION OF PHYSICAL ASSESSMENT WITH NURSING CARE

➤ Whether a complete or partial physical assessment is performed, an examination should be integrated into routine care.

■ SKILLS OF PHYSICAL ASSESSMENT
Inspection

➤ Define *inspection*: _____

_____.

➤ List six principles to facilitate accurate inspection of body parts.

a. _____

b. _____

c. _____

d. _____

e. _____

f. _____

Palpation

➤ Define *palpation*: _____

_____.

➤ Identify the parts of the hand used to assess each of the following:

Temperature _____

Pulsations _____

Vibrations _____

Turgor _____

➤ Briefly explain the following:

Light palpation _____

_____

Deep palpation _____

_____

Percussion

➤ Identify the information that is obtained through percussion: _____

_____

➤ Explain the two types of percussion:

Direct _____

_____

Indirect _____

_____

➤ Percussion produces five types of sounds. Identify them.

a. _____

b. _____

c. _____

d. _____

e. _____

Auscultation

➤ Define *auscultation:* _____

_____

➤ Briefly explain the following characteristics of sound:

Frequency _____

Loudness _____

Quality _____

Duration _____

Olfaction

➤ Olfaction helps the nurse detect abnormalities that cannot be recognized by any other means.

I PREPARATION FOR EXAMINATION

➤ List at least three environmental factors that the nurse should attempt to control before performing a physical examination.

a. _____

b. _____

c. _____

Client

➤ Briefly explain the following preparation before an examination:

Physical _____

_____

_____

Psychological _____

_____

_____

_____

Assessment of Age-Groups

➤ List at least six variations in the nurse's individual style that are appropriate when examining children:

_____

_____

_____

_____

_____

_____

_____

_____

_____

➤ List at least five variations in the nurse's individual style that are appropriate when examining older adults:

_____

_____

_____

_____

_____

_____

_____

_____

_____

ORGANIZATION OF THE EXAMINATION

➤ List eight principles to follow for a well-organized examination:

_____

_____

_____

_____

_____

_____

_____

_____

GENERAL SURVEY

➤ List three assessment components of the general survey:

a. _____

b. _____

c. _____

General Appearance and Behavior

➤ Summarize the 14 specific observations of the client's general appearance and behavior:

a. _____

b. _____

c. _____

d. _____

e. _____

f. _____

g. _____

h. _____

i. _____

j. _____

k. _____

l. _____

m. _____

n. _____

Vital Signs

➤ Assessment of vital signs is the first part of the physical assessment.

Height, Weight, and Circumference

➤ A person's general level of health can be reflected in the ratio of height and weight.
➤ List three actions that should be taken to ensure accurate weight measurement of a hospitalized client.

a. _____

b. _____

c. _____

➤ A chest circumference can be compared with the head circumference to rule out problems in head or chest size.

SKIN, HAIR, AND NAILS

➤ The skin provides the body's _____ and _____ and acts as a sensory organ for_____, _____, _____, and _____.

➤ The physical assessment skills of _____, _____, and _____ are used to assess the integument's function and integrity.

Skin

➤ Assessment of the skin can reveal a variety of conditions including changes in _____, _____, _____, _____, and _____.

➤ List at least four risks for skin lesions in the hospitalized client:

_____

_____

_____

_____

➤ For each skin color variation, identify the mechanism producing color change, common causes of the variation, and optimal sites for assessment. (See table, top of next page.)

Skin Color	Mechanisms	Causes	Assessment Sites
Cyanosis			
Pallor			
Jaundice			
Erythema			

➤ Define *hyperpigmentation* and *hypopigmentation*:

_____

_____

_____

_____

➤ Define *moisture:* _____

_____

➤ The temperature of the skin depends on the amount of

_____ circulating through the dermis.

➤ The character of the skin's surface and the feel of

deeper portions are its _____.

➤ Define *skin turgor* and describe normal findings:

_____

_____

➤ Petechiae are _____

_____

_____

_____.

➤ Identify the two causes of edema.

a. _____

b. _____

➤ List at least six criteria for lesion assessment.

a. _____

b. _____

c. _____

d. _____

e. _____

f. _____

➤ Briefly describe the following primary skin lesions:

Macule _____

Papule _____

Nodule _____

Tumor _____

Wheal _____

Vesicle _____

Pustule _____

Ulcer _____

Atrophy _____

Hair and Scalp

➤ Describe the difference between terminal hair and vellus hair:

_____

_____

➤ When inspecting the hair, the nurse notes the

_____, _____, _____,

_____, _____, and _____.

➤ Define *alopecia:* _____

_____

➤ Name the three types of lice.

   a. _____

   b. _____

   c. _____

Nails

➤ When inspecting the nail bed, the nurse notes the

   _____, _____, _____,

   _____, _____, _____,

   and _____.

➤ The nurse palpates the nail base to determine _____

   _____

   _____.

➤ Briefly describe the following abnormalities of the nail bed:

Clubbing _____

_____

Beau's lines _____

_____

Koilonychia _____

_____

Splinter hemorrhages _____

_____

Paronychia _____

_____

▮ HEAD AND NECK
Head

	Inspection	Palpation	Percussion	Auscultation
Head				

Eyes

	Inspection	Palpation	Percussion	Auscultation
Visual Acuity				
Visual Fields				
Extraocular Movements				
Visual Fields				

EXTERNAL EYE STRUCTURES

	Inspection	Palpation	Percussion	Auscultation
Eyebrows				
Eyelids				
Lacrimal Apparatus				
Conjunctivae and Sclerae				
Corneas, Pupils, and Irises				

➤ Define the following eye abnormalities:

Exophthalmos _____

Strabismus _____

Ears

	Inspection	Palpation	Percussion	Auscultation
External Ear				
Middle Ear				
Inner Ear				

➤ Identify the mechanisms for sound transmission.

a. _____

b. _____

c. _____

d. _____

e. _____

➤ The three types of hearing loss are _____,

_____, and _____.

➤ Define *ototoxicity:* _____

_____

Nose and Sinuses

	Inspection	Palpation	Percussion	Auscultation
Nose				
Sinuses				

Mouth and Pharynx

	Inspection	Palpation	Percussion	Auscultation
Lips				
Buccal Mucosa, Gums, and Teeth				
Tongue and Floor of Mouth				
Palate				
Pharynx				

Neck

	Inspection	Palpation	Percussion	Auscultation
Neck Muscles				
Lymph Nodes				
Thyroid Gland				
Carotid Artery and Jugular Vein				
Trachea				

■ THORAX AND LUNGS

➤ Accurate physical assessment of the thorax and lungs requires review of the ventilatory and respiratory functions of the lung.

	Inspection	Palpation	Percussion	Auscultation
Posterior Thorax				
Lateral Thorax				
Anterior Thorax				

➤ Define the following:

Vocal or tactile fremitus _____

_____

_____

_____

➤ Identify the normal breath sounds and where they are

located: _____

_____

_____

_____

➤ Complete the following table of adventitious breath
sounds:

Sound	Auscultation Site	Cause	Character
Crackles			
Rhonchi			
Wheezes			
Pleural Friction Rub			

■ HEART

➤ The assessment of the heart function involves a review of signs and symptoms from the nursing history, pulse assessment, and direct examination of the
heart.

➤ Answer the following questions:

What is the PMI? _____

_____

Where is the PMI normally located in the infant and

young child? _____

_____

_____

Where is the PMI located in the older child and adult?

_____

_____

_____

_____

What techniques may be used to locate the PMI?

_____

_____

➤ Define what occurs during the two phases of the cardiac cycle.

Systole: _____

_____

_____

_____

Diastole: _____

_____

_____

_____

➤ Define the following heart sounds:

S1 _____

S2 _____

S3 _____

S4 _____

	Inspection	Palpation	Percussion	Auscultation
Heart				

➤ Define *dysrhythmia:* _____

_____

➤ Define *murmur:* _____

_____

➤ List the six factors to be assessed when a murmur is detected.

a. _____

b. _____

c. _____

d. _____

e. _____

f. _____

■ VASCULAR SYSTEM

➤ Examination of the vascular system includes measurement of the blood pressure and a thorough assessment of the integrity of the peripheral vascular system.

	Inspection	Palpation	Percussion	Auscultation
Carotid Arteries				
Jugular Veins				
Peripheral Arteries				
Peripheral Veins				
Lymphatic System				

▌ BREASTS

➤ It is important to examine the breasts of female and male clients.

➤ Briefly explain the proper technique for palpating the breast tissue: _____

_____

_____

_____

	Inspection	Palpation	Percussion	Auscultation
Breasts				

➤ List seven characteristics that should be included when describing an abnormal breast mass:

_____

_____

_____

_____

_____

_____

_____

▌ ABDOMEN

➤ The abdominal examination includes an assessment of the lower GI tract in addition to the liver, stomach, uterus, ovaries, kidneys, and bladder.

	Inspection	Auscultation	Percussion	Palpation
Abdomen				
Liver				

➤ Describe four techniques used to help the client relax during abdominal assessment.

a. _____

b. _____

c. _____

d. _____

➤ Define the following:

Hernias _____

_____

Distention _____

_____

Peristalsis _____

_____

Paralytic ileus _____

_____

Borborygmi _____

_____

Rebound tenderness _____

_____

Aneurysm _____

_____

■ FEMALE GENITALIA AND REPRODUCTIVE TRACT

➤ Briefly explain the preparation of a client for a complete examination of the genitalia and reproductive

tract: _____

_____

_____

_____

_____

	Inspection	Palpation	Percussion	Auscultation
External Genitalia				
Cervix				
Vagina				

▌MALE GENITALIA

➤ An examination of the male genitalia includes assessment of the external genitalia and the inguinal ring and canal.

	Inspection	Palpation	Percussion	Auscultation
Penis				
Scrotum				
Inguinal Ring and Canal				

▌RECTUM AND ANUS

	Inspection	Palpation	Percussion	Auscultation
Rectum and Anus				

▌MUSCULOSKELETAL SYSTEM

➤ The assessment of musculoskeletal function focuses on determining range of joint motion, muscle strength and tone, and joint and muscle condition.

	Inspection	Palpation	Percussion	Auscultation
Joint Motion				

➤ Define *hypertonicity* and *hypotonicity:* _____

_____

_____

▌NEUROLOGICAL SYSTEM

➤ The neurological system is responsible for many functions including _____

_____.

Mental and Emotional Status

➤ There are five areas that Folstein's mini-mental state tool assesses. Name them.

_____

_____

_____

_____

_____

➤ An alteration in mental or emotional status may reflect a disturbance in cerebral functioning.
➤ List three factors that may change cerebral function.

a. _____

b. _____

c. _____

➤ Define *delirium* and list the clinical criteria for it:

_____

_____

_____

_____

_____

➤ The level of consciousness exists along a continuum, from full awakening, alertness, and cooperation to unresponsiveness to any form of external stimuli.
➤ Identify the tool and the three factors to assess consciousness:

_____

_____

_____

_____

_____

➤ Behavior, moods, hygiene, grooming, and choice of dress reveal pertinent information about mental status.
➤ Explain the function of the cerebral cortex in language:

_____

_____

_____

_____

➤ There are two types of aphasia. Describe each one.

Receptive: _____

_____

_____

Expressive: _____

_____

_____

_____

Intellectual Function

➤ Intellectual function includes the following. Briefly explain how each is assessed.

Memory: _____

_____

Knowledge: _____

_____

Abstract thinking: _____

_____

Association: _____

_____

Judgment: _____

Cranial Nerve Function

➤ Identify the 12 cranial nerves:

_____   _____

_____   _____

_____   _____

_____   _____

_____   _____

_____   _____

Sensory Function

➤ The sensory pathways of the central nervous system conduct sensations of _____,

_____, _____,

_____, and _____.

➤ Summarize how a nurse would assess the client's sensory function: _____

_____

_____

_____

Motor Function

➤ Identify the functions of the cerebellum:

_____

_____

_____

➤ Describe the maneuvers used to assess balance and gross motor function

a. _____

b. _____

c. _____

Reflexes

➤ Eliciting reflex reactions allows the nurse to assess the integrity of sensory and motor pathways of the reflex arc and specific spinal cord segments.

➤ Briefly explain the two categories of normal reflexes:

_____

_____

_____

_____

REVIEW QUESTIONS

(The student should select the appropriate answer and cite the rationale for choosing that particular answer.)

1. The component that should receive the highest priority before a physical examination is:
   a. Preparation of the environment
   b. Preparation of the equipment
   c. Physical preparation of the client
   d. Psychological preparation of the client

Answer ( ) Rationale: _____

_____

2. To promote psychological comfort of the female client during the physical examination, the female nurse would:
   a. Ask the client to use the bathroom
   b. Assemble the necessary equipment
   c. Ask a third person to be present
   d. Explain each step of the examination

Answer ( ) Rationale: _____

_____

3. The nurse assesses the skin turgor of the client by:
   a. Grasping a fold of skin on the back of the hand and releasing
   b. Palpating the skin with the dorsum of the hand
   c. Pressing the skin for 5 seconds, releasing, and noting each centimeter of depth
   d. Inspecting the buccal mucosa with a penlight

Answer ( ) Rationale: _____

_____

4. All of the following are part of the assessment of appearance and behavior *except:*
   a. Signs of distress
   b. Height and weight
   c. Hygiene and grooming
   d. Mood and affect

Answer ( ) Rationale: _____

_____

5. While examining Mr. Parker, the nurse notes a circumscribed elevation of skin filled with serous fluid on his upper lip. The lesion is 0.4 cm in diameter. This type of lesion is called a:
   a. Macule
   b. Nodule
   c. Vesicle
   d. Pustule

Answer ( ) Rationale: _____

_____

6. The notes indicate that PERRLA has been recorded on the assessment sheet for Mrs. Stone. PERRLA refers to:
   a. The condition of larcimal apparatus
   b. The condition of conjunctiva and sclera
   c. The pupillary reflexes to light and accommodation
   d. The visualization of the internal eye structures

Answer ( ) Rationale: _____

_____

7. The nurse inspects the client's buccal mucosa for:
   a. Pallor
   b. Striae
   c. Epistaxis
   d. Hemoptysis

Answer ( ) Rationale: _____

_____

8. When assessing the client's thorax, the nurse should:
   a. Complete the left side and then the right side
   b. Change position of the stethoscope between inspiration and expiration
   c. Compare symmetrical areas from side to side
   d. Begin with the posterior lobes on the right side

Answer ( ) Rationale: _____

_____

9. In a client with pneumonia, the nurse hears low-pitched, continuous musical sounds over the bronchi on expiration. These sounds are called:
   a. Crackles
   b. Rhonchi
   c. Wheezes
   d. Friction rubs

Answer ( ) Rationale: _____
_____
_____

10. To locate the PMI (point of maximal impulse), the nurse would place the stethoscope at the:
    a. Fourth to fifth intercostal space at the left midclavicular line
    b. Third to fourth intercostal space, left of the right midclavicular line
    c. Second intercostal space on the right side
    d. Second intercostal space on the left side

Answer ( ) Rationale: _____
_____
_____

11. The second heart (S2) sound occurs when:
    a. The mitral and tricuspid valves close
    b. There is rapid ventricular filling
    c. Systole begins
    d. The aortic and pulmonic valves close

Answer ( ) Rationale: _____
_____
_____

12. Mr. Smith is an 85-year-old man with a history of cerebrovascular disease. Which of the following will the nurse perform when examining Mr. Smith's carotid arteries?
    a. Vigorous palpation of the arteries
    b. Simultaneous assessment of both arteries
    c. Auscultation of left and right carotid pulses
    d. Measurement of carotid arterial pressures

Answer ( ) Rationale: _____
_____
_____

13. While examining Mrs. Boyd's breasts, the nurse explains the techniques of breast self-examination. Palpation of breast tissue is best performed while one is:
    a. Standing with the arm raised
    b. Lying prone
    c. Sitting with shoulders back
    d. Standing and bending at the waist

Answer ( ) Rationale: _____
_____
_____

14. What is the correct order of the physical examination of the abdomen?
    a. Inspection, palpation, percussion, auscultation
    b. Inspection, auscultation, palpation, percussion
    c. Palpation, percussion, inspection, auscultation
    d. Inspection, palpation, auscultation, percussion

Answer ( ) Rationale: _____
_____
_____

15. A client who understands written and verbal speech but who cannot write or speak appropriately has:
    a. Sensory aphasia
    b. Receptive aphasia
    c. Motor aphasia
    d. Mental retardation

Answer ( ) Rationale: _____
_____
_____

CLINICAL SITUATIONS

1. Mr. Leonard enters the clinic with a history of weight loss and general fatigue. Describe three body systems that may be involved. What questions might you ask the client to discover the primary system involved?

_____

_____

_____

_____

_____

_____

_____

_____

2. What physical examination measures might you use to evaluate abdominal pain, oral hygiene, and application of a cast to the arm?

_____

_____

_____

_____

_____

_____

_____

_____

_____

_____

Chapter 34 | Infection Control

In all settings, clients and their families must be able to recognize sources of infections and to institute protective measures.

PRELIMINARY READING

Chapter 34, pp. 741-788

COMPREHENSIVE UNDERSTANDING

■ NATURE OF INFECTION

➤ An infection is an _____

_____ .

➤ Define *asymptomatic:* _____

_____

Chain of Infection

➤ List the six elements (in the chain) required to produce an infection:

a. _____

b. _____

c. _____

d. _____

e. _____

f. _____

➤ Microorganisms include _____,

_____, _____, and _____.

➤ Define:

Resident organisms _____

_____

Transient microorganisms _____

_____

➤ The potential for microorganisms or parasites to cause disease depends on four factors. Name them.

a. _____

b. _____

c. _____

d. _____

➤ Define *reservoir:* _____

_____

➤ Define *carriers:* _____

_____

➤ To thrive, organisms require the following. Briefly explain each one.

Food: _____

Oxygen: _____

Water: _____

Temperature: _____

pH: _____

Light: _____

➤ Microorganisms can exit through a variety of sites. Briefly explain each one.

Skin and mucous membranes: _____

_____

_____

_____

Respiratory tract: _____

_____

_____

_____

Urinary tract: _____

_____

_____

_____

Gastrointestinal tract: _____

_____

_____

_____

Reproductive tract: _____

_____

_____

_____

Blood: _____

_____

_____

_____

➤ List the four major routes through which microorganisms are transmitted from the reservoir to the host.

a. _____

b. _____

c. _____

d. _____

➤ The most common mode of transmission is _____

_____.

➤ Organisms can enter the body through _____

_____.

➤ Define *susceptibility:* _____

_____

_____

➤ Define *virulent:* _____

_____

▌ THE INFECTIOUS PROCESS

➤ The severity of the client's illness depends on the

_____, the

_____, and _____.

➤ Describe the two types of infections.

Localized: _____

_____

Systemic: _____

_____

Defenses against Infection

➤ Explain the normal body defenses against infection.

Normal flora: _____

_____

_____

_____

_____

Body system defenses: _____

_____

_____

_____

_____

Inflammation: _____

_____

_____

_____

_____

➤ For each body system or organ, identify at least one defense mechanism and the primary action to prevent infection.

System/Organ	Defense Mechanism	Action
Skin		
Mouth		
Respiratory Tract		
Urinary Tract		
Gastrointestinal Tract		

➤ Define *inflammation:* _____

_____

➤ The inflammatory response includes the following. Briefly explain:

Vascular and cellular responses _____

_____

_____

_____

Inflammatory exudate _____

_____

_____

_____

_____

Tissue repair _____

_____

_____

_____

_____

➤ Define *immune response:* _____

_____

_____

➤ After an antigen enters the body, it travels in the blood or lymph and initiates the following responses. Briefly explain:

Cell-mediated immunity _____

_____

_____

_____

_____

Humoral immunity _____

_____

_____

_____

_____

➤ Define *complement:* _____

_____

➤ Define *interferon:* _____

_____

Nosocomial Infections

➤ Define *nosocomial infections:* _____

_____

➤ Define the following types of nosocomial infections:

Iatrogenic _____

_____

Exogenous _____

_____

Endogenous _____

_____

➤ Identify at least three factors increasing a hospitalized client's risk of acquiring a nosocomial infection.

a. _____

b. _____

c. _____

■ CONCEPT OF ASEPSIS

➤ Asepsis is _____

_____.

➤ Describe the two types of aseptic techniques.

Medical: _____

_____

Surgical: _____

_____

➤ Identify when each type of technique is considered contaminated.

Medical: _____

_____

Surgical: _____

_____

■ THE NURSING PROCESS IN INFECTION CONTROL

Assessment

➤ The nurse assesses the client's _____,

_____, and _____.

➤ Knowing the factors that increase susceptibility or risk for infection, the nurse is better able to plan preventive therapy that includes aseptic technique.

Status of Defense Mechanisms

➤ Identify at least four risk factors of each.

Inadequate primary defenses: _____

_____

_____

_____

Inadequate secondary sources: _____

_____

_____

_____

➤ The following factors influence client susceptibility. Explain each one.

Age: _____

_____

_____

_____

Nutritional status: _____

_____

_____

_____

Heredity: _____

_____

_____

Disease process: _____

_____

_____

Medical therapy: _____

_____

_____

_____

Clinical Appearance

➤ Describe the clinical appearance of each type of infection.

Local: _____

_____

_____

_____

_____

Systemic: _____

_____

_____

_____

_____

➤ Describe how an infection is manifested in an older

adult: _____

_____

_____

_____

Laboratory Data

➤ List at least five laboratory values that may indicate infection:

_____

_____

_____

_____

_____

Clients with Infection

➤ The ways that infection affects the client's and family's

needs may be _____,

_____, _____,

_____, or _____.

Nursing Diagnosis

➤ The nurse may diagnose a risk for infection or make diagnoses that result from the effects of infection on health status.

Planning

➤ List four common goals for the client with an actual or potential risk for infection.

a. _____

b. _____

c. _____

d. _____

Implementation

➤ List the two major nursing responsibilities for controlling infection.

a. _____

_____

b. _____

_____

➤ List five ways a nurse may prevent an infection from developing or spreading.

a. _____

b. _____

c. _____

d. _____

e. _____

Medical Asepsis

➤ The nurse follows certain principles and procedures to prevent infection and to control its spread. Briefly explain each one.

Control or elimination of infectious agents: _____

_____

_____

_____

_____

_____

_____

Control or elimination of reservoirs: _____

_____

_____

_____

_____

_____

Control of portals of exit: _____

_____

_____

_____

_____

_____

Control of transmission (handwashing): _____

_____

_____

_____

_____

_____

_____

Control of portals of entry: _____

_____

_____

_____

_____

_____

Protection of the susceptible host (isolation practices):

_____

_____

_____

_____

_____

_____

Protection for personnel (barrier projections):

Gowns _____

_____

_____

_____

Masks _____

_____

_____

_____

Gloves _____

_____

_____

_____

Protective eyewear _____

_____

_____

_____

Specimen collection _____

_____

_____

_____

Bagging articles or linen _____

_____

_____

_____

Transporting clients _____

_____

_____

➤ Place an X under the barriers required to maintain protective asepsis for each category-specific isolation technique in the following:

Type of Isolation	Room	Gown	Gloves	Mask
Strict				
Content				
Respiratory				
Enteric Precautions				
Tuberculosis Isolation				
Drainage and Secretion Precautions				
Universal Blood and Body Fluid Precautions				
Care of the Severely Compromised Client				

Role of the Infection Control Professional

➤ List eight responsibilities of the infection control professional.

a. _____

b. _____

c. _____

d. _____

e. _____

f. _____

g. _____

h. _____

Infection Prevention and Control for Hospital Personnel

➤ List the OSHA guidelines that were established to protect employees.

a. _____

b. _____

c. _____

d. _____

e. _____

Client Education

➤ List the topics the nurse needs to discuss with the client in relation to infection-control practices.

a. _____

b. _____

c. _____

d. _____

e. _____

f. _____

Surgical Asepsis

➤ Surgical asepsis requires the _____
_____
_____
_____.

➤ List three teaching points to reduce the risk of client-associated contamination during sterile procedures or treatments.

a. _____
_____

b. _____
_____

c. _____
_____

➤ List the seven principles of surgical asepsis.

a. _____

b. _____

c. _____

d. _____

e. _____

f. _____

g. _____

➤ List and briefly explain the nine steps of the nurse performing a sterile procedure.

a. _____

_____

_____

b. _____

_____

_____

c. _____

_____

_____

d. _____

_____

_____

e. _____

_____

_____

f. _____

_____

_____

g. _____

_____

_____

h. _____

_____

_____

i. _____

_____

_____

Evaluation

➤ The nurse documents the client's responses to therapies for infection control.
➤ A clear description of any signs and symptoms of systemic or local infection is necessary to give all nurses a baseline for comparative evaluation.
➤ List three expected outcomes for clients with a risk for infection:

a. _____

b. _____

c. _____

REVIEW QUESTIONS

(The student should select the appropriate answer and cite the rationale for choosing that particular answer.)

1. Of the following, which is not an element in the development or chain of infection?
   a. Infectious agent or pathogen
   b. Reservoir for pathogen growth
   c. Means of transmission
   d. Formation of immunoglobulin

Answer ( ) Rationale: _____

_____

_____

2. Pathogenic organisms include all of the following *except:*
   a. Bacteria
   b. Leukocytes
   c. Viruses
   d. Fungi

Answer ( ) Rationale: _____

_____

_____

3. The best definition of the action of normal flora is:
   a. Participates in maintaining a person's health by inhibiting multiplication of disease-causing microorganisms
   b. Affects the methods of transmission of disease
   c. Assists with the formation of antibodies
   d. Assists with the digestion and absorption of nutrients

Answer ( ) Rationale: _____

_____

_____

4. The severity of a client's illness will depend on all of the following *except:*
   a. Extent of infection
   b. Pathogenicity of the microorganism
   c. Susceptibility of the host
   d. Incubation period

Answer ( ) Rationale: _____

_____

_____

5. Which of the following clients would be at risk for infection related to inadequate primary defenses?
   a. Chronic smoker
   b. Client with anemia
   c. Client with leukopenia
   d. Client taking steroids

Answer ( ) Rationale: _____

_____

_____

6. Which of the following best describes an iatrogenic infection?
   a. Results from a diagnostic or therapeutic procedure
   b. Occurs when clients are infected with their own organisms as a result of immunodeficiency
   c. Involves an incubation period of 3 to 4 weeks before being detected
   d. Results from an extended infection of the urinary tract

Answer (   ) Rationale: _____

_____

_____

7. All of the following are part of the nurse's role in infection control *except:*
   a. Recognizing the signs and symptoms of infection
   b. Collecting specimens of drainage from infected wound sites
   c. Deciding on the appropriate antibiotic to be administered to the client
   d. Supporting the client's body defense mechanisms

Answer (   ) Rationale: _____

_____

_____

8. Which of the following is *not* part of the role of the infection control department?
   a. Reviewing infection control policies and procedures
   b. Performing venipunctures on clients to obtain blood cultures
   c. Investigating outbreaks of infection
   d. Providing input regarding the selection of client care products

Answer (   ) Rationale: _____

_____

_____

9. The nurse sets up a nonbarrier sterile field on the client's overbed table. In which instance is the field contaminated?
   a. The nurse keeps the top of the table above his or her waist.
   b. Sterile saline solution is spilled on the field.
   c. Sterile objects are kept within a 1-inch border of the field.
   d. The nurse, who has a cold, wears a double mask.

Answer (   ) Rationale: _____

_____

_____

10. What should the nurse do when opening a sterile package wrapped in linen or paper on a flat surface?
    a. Check the package to be sure it is no more than 1 week past the expiration date.
    b. Open the outer flap toward the body.
    c. Reach across the sterile field to stabilize the first side flap.
    d. Allow the last flap to fall flat on the surface.

Answer (   ) Rationale: _____

_____

_____

11. The primary reason for gowning during protective asepsis is to:
    a. Keep warm because the isolation room is usually cool.
    b. Ensure that the client is not exposed to the organisms on the nurse's uniform.
    c. Maintain a sterile environment when providing client care.
    d. Prevent soiling of clothing during contact with the client.

Answer (   ) Rationale: _____

_____

_____

12. When a client on respiratory isolation must be transported to another part of the hospital, the nurse:
    a. Places a mask on the client before leaving the room.
    b. Obtains a physician's order to prohibit the client from being transported.
    c. Advises other health team members to wear masks and gowns when coming in contact with the client.
    d. Instructs the client to cover the mouth and nose with a tissue when coughing or sneezing.

Answer (   ) Rationale: _____

_____

_____

CLINICAL SITUATIONS

1. Explain the elements of the CDC recommendations for a two-tier approach to isolation. How do these tiers differ? Which diseases require increased protective measures?

_____

_____

_____

_____

_____

_____

_____

_____

_____

_____

_____

2. Mr. Jones is an 86-year-old client whose diagnosis includes vomiting and diarrhea, presumed secondary to *Staphylococcus aureus*. Develop a discharge teaching plan.

_____

_____

_____

_____

_____

_____

_____

_____

_____

_____

_____

_____

Chapter 35 | Administration of Medications

The nurse is responsible for understanding a drug's action and its side effects, administering it correctly, monitoring the client's response, and helping the client self-administer drugs correctly and knowledgeably.

PRELIMINARY READING

Chapter 35, pp. 789-867

COMPREHENSIVE UNDERSTANDING

■ DRUG NOMENCLATURE AND FORMS

➤ A drug, or medication, is a substance used in the

_____, _____, _____,

_____ or _____ .

Names

➤ A single medication may have four different names. Define each one.

Chemical name _____

Generic name _____

Official name _____

Trade name _____

Classification

➤ A drug classification indicates _____

_____

_____ .

Drug Forms

➤ The form of the drug determines its _____

_____ .

■ DRUG LEGISLATION AND STANDARDS

Drug Standards

➤ Identify and briefly explain the five accepted drug standards that must be met.

a. _____

_____

b. _____

_____

c. _____

_____

d. _____

_____

e. _____

_____

Legislation and Control

➤ Explain the Pure Food and Drug Act of 1906:

_____

_____

_____

➤ Federal, state, and local legislation governs nursing practice, including the administration of medications.

➤ _____ define and set limits on the scope of a nurse's professional functions and responsibilities.

➤ Before assuming the responsibility of administering IV medications, the nurse should be aware of the

_____ .

➤ Identify the role of the nurse when administering controlled substances: _____

_____

Nontherapeutic Drug Use

➤ Identify the ethical and legal obligations of the nurse when caring for clients with drug abuse or

drug dependency: _____

_____

_____

_____

➤ Identify at least five factors that lead to nontherapeutic drug use:

_____

_____

_____

_____

_____

_____

▮ NATURE OF DRUG ACTIONS

➤ A drug does not create a function in a tissue or organ but rather alters physiological functions.

Mechanism of Action

➤ Define *mechanism of actions:* _____

_____

_____

➤ The most common mechanism of drug action is

_____.

Pharmacokinetics

➤ Define *pharmacokinetics:* _____

_____

_____

_____

Absorption

➤ Define *absorption:* _____

_____

_____

➤ Briefly explain the following factors influencing drug absorption:

Route of administration _____

_____

_____

_____

Ability of a drug to dissolve _____

_____

_____

_____

Conditions of site _____

_____

_____

_____

_____

Distribution

➤ The rate and extent of distribution depend on the physical and chemical properties of the drug and the physiological makeup of the person taking the drug.

▮ BODY WEIGHT AND COMPOSITION

➤ A direct relationship exists between the amount of drug administered and the amount of body tissue in which it is distributed. Give two examples:

_____

_____

_____

_____

_____

▮ CIRCULATORY DYNAMICS

➤ Drugs pass more easily from interstitial to intravascular spaces than they do between body compartments.
➤ The concentration of a drug at a specific site depends on:

_____

_____

_____

_____

➤ Identify two biological barriers to the passage of drugs:

a. _____

_____

b. _____

_____

I PROTEIN BINDING
➤ The degree to which drugs bind to serum protein, such as albumin, affects drug distribution.

Metabolism
➤ Define *biotransformation*, and identify where it occurs:

_____

_____

_____

_____

Excretion
➤ After drugs are metabolized, they exit the body

through the _____,

_____, _____,

_____, and _____.

➤ Identify the main organ for drug excretion, and explain what happens if this organ function declines:

_____

_____

_____

➤ Define the following predicted or unintended effects of drugs:

Therapeutic effects _____

_____

_____

Side effects _____

_____

_____

Toxic effects _____

_____

_____

Idiosyncratic reactions _____

_____

_____

Allergic reactions _____

_____

_____

Drug tolerance _____

_____

_____

Drug interactions _____

_____

_____

Drug Dose Responses
➤ When a medication is prescribed, the goal is to achieve a constant blood level within a safe therapeutic range.
➤ Repeated doses are required to achieve a constant therapeutic concentration of a medication because a portion of a drug is always being excreted.
➤ Define:

Serum concentration _____

_____

Serum half-life _____

_____

➤ Explain the following time intervals of drug actions:

Onset of drug action _____

_____

Peak action _____

_____

Duration of action _____

_____

Plateau _____

_____

➤ Identify the route that is the ideal way to achieve a constant therapeutic drug level:

_____

I FACTORS INFLUENCING DRUG ACTIONS
➤ Explain the following factors that affect drug actions:

Genetic differences _____

_____

_____

_____

Physiological variables _____

_____

_____

_____

Environmental conditions _____

_____

_____

_____

Psychological factors _____

_____

_____

_____

Diet _____

_____

_____

_____

ROUTES OF ADMINISTRATION
➤ The route chosen for administering a drug depends on its properties and desired effect as well as the client's physical and mental condition.

Oral Routes
➤ The oral route is the easiest and the most commonly used route.
➤ List the three types of oral routes; explain how the oral routes are used; and identify the effects of using these routes:

_____

_____

_____

_____

_____

_____

Parenteral Routes
➤ The parenteral route involves giving a drug through injection into body tissues.
➤ List the four major types of parenteral injections.

a. _____

b. _____

c. _____

d. _____

➤ Define the advanced techniques of medication administration.

Epidural: _____

_____

_____

Intrathecal: _____

_____

_____

Intraosseous: _____

_____

_____

Intraperitoneal: _____

_____

_____

Intrapleural: _____

_____

_____

Intraarterial: _____

_____

_____

Intracardiac: _____

_____

_____

Intraarticular: _____

_____

_____

Topical Administration
➤ Drugs applied to the skin and mucous membranes principally have local effects.
➤ Identify the five methods for applying medications to mucous membranes.

a. _____

b. _____

c. _____

d. _____

e. _____

Inhalation

➤ Explain the following types of inhalations:

Nasal _____

_____

Oral _____

_____

Endotracheal, or tracheal _____

_____

Intraocular

➤ Intraocular administration involves inserting a medication disk, similar to contact lens, into the client's eye.

■ SYSTEMS OF DRUG MEASUREMENT

➤ The following are measurements used in drug therapy. Briefly explain their basic units:

Metric system _____

_____

_____

Apothecary system _____

_____

_____

Household measurements _____

_____

_____

Solutions

➤ Define:

A solution _____

Concentration _____

■ CONVERTING MEASUREMENT UNITS

Conversions within One System

➤ Indicate which direction the decimal point is moved for the following mathematical calculations in the metric system:

Division _____

Multiplication _____

Conversion between Systems

➤ To make actual drug calculations, it is necessary to work with units in the same measurement system.
➤ Before making a conversion, the nurse compares the measurement system available with that ordered.
➤ Complete the following measurement equivalents:

Metric	Apothecary	Household
1 ml	_____ minims	_____ drops
_____ ml	_____ fluid drams	1 tablespoon
30 ml	_____ fluid ounce(s)	_____ tablespoon
_____ ml	_____ fluid ounce(s)	1 cup
_____ ml	1 pint	_____ pint
_____ ml	_____ quart	1 quart

➤ Complete the following conversions:

100 mg = _____ g

2.5 L = _____ ml

500 ml = _____ L

15 mg = _____ gr

30 gtt = _____ ml

gr ⅙ = _____ mg

Dosage Calculations

➤ Write out the formula applied to determine the correct dose when preparing solid or liquid forms of medications: _____

_____

➤ Define the following:

Dose ordered _____

_____

Dose on hand _____

_____

Amount on hand _____

_____

Pediatric Dosages

➤ Write out the formula applied to accurately calculate pediatric dosages:

_____

_____

ADMINISTERING MEDICATIONS

➤ The nurse giving the medications bears responsibility and accountability for the accuracy of the five rights.

Physician's Role

➤ Identify the primary responsibilities of the physician in giving medications to clients:

_____

_____

_____

_____

Types of Orders

➤ Briefly explain the four common types of medication orders.

Standing: _____

_____

PRN: _____

_____

Single (one-time): _____

_____

Stat: _____

_____

Prescriptions

➤ List the five parts of a prescription.

a. _____

b. _____

c. _____

d. _____

e. _____

Pharmacist's Role

➤ Identify the primary responsibility of the pharmacist in the administration of medications:

_____

_____

_____

Distribution Systems

➤ List the three medication distribution systems and their pros and cons:

_____

_____

_____

_____

Nurse's Role

➤ Summarize the nurse's primary responsibilities when administering medications:

_____

_____

_____

_____

_____

NURSING PROCESS AND MEDICATIONS

Assessment

➤ List the nine areas for nursing assessment and the rationale for obtaining this information before medication administration.

a. _____

_____

b. _____

_____

c. _____

_____

d. _____

_____

e. _____

_____

f. _____

_____

g. _____

_____

h. _____

_____

i. _____

_____

Nursing Diagnosis

➤ Assessment provides data on the client's condition, ability to self-administer drugs, and drug use patterns, which can be used to determine actual or potential problems with drug therapy.

Planning

➤ The nurse organizes care activities to ensure that safe administrative techniques are used.
➤ Identify the four goals that the nurse or client needs to meet before administration of medications:

a. _____

_____

b. _____

_____

c. _____

_____

d. _____

_____

Implementation

➤ The transcribed order includes the _____.
➤ The nurse who administers the wrong medication or an incorrect dosage is legally responsible for the error.

➤ Briefly explain the following:

Accurate dosage calculation and measurement

_____

_____

Correct administration _____

_____

Recording drug administration _____

_____

HEALTH PROMOTION THROUGH CLIENT TEACHING

➤ List six guidelines to ensure proper use and storage of drugs in the home.

a. _____

_____

b. _____

_____

c. _____

_____

d. _____

_____

e. _____

_____

f. _____

_____

MAINTAINING CLIENTS' RIGHTS

➤ Briefly summarize the Patient's Bill of Rights related to drug administration:

_____

_____

_____

_____

_____

_____

Evaluation

➤ The nurse monitors a client's response to medications by knowing the therapeutic action and common side effects of each medication.

➤ Identify five evaluative measures to identify actual outcomes related to the following:

Route of administration _____

_____

_____

Therapeutic effect _____

_____

_____

Safety and comfort _____

_____

_____

Client teaching _____

_____

_____

Self-administration _____

_____

_____

▮ MEDICATION DELIVERY

➤ List the "five rights" of medication delivery.

a. _____

b. _____

c. _____

d. _____

e. _____

▮ MEDICATION ERRORS

➤ Define *medication error,* and explain how it can occur:

_____

_____

_____

_____

▮ SPECIAL CONSIDERATIONS FOR ADMINISTERING MEDICATIONS TO SPECIFIC AGE-GROUPS

Infants and Children

➤ Identify the appropriate nursing action used in administering medications to an infant or child:

_____

_____

_____

_____

Older Adults

➤ List the five patterns of drug use by the elderly client, and briefly explain each one.

a. _____

_____

b. _____

_____

c. _____

_____

d. _____

_____

e. _____

_____

▮ ORAL DRUG ADMINISTRATION

➤ Unless the client has impaired gastrointestinal functioning or is unable to swallow, an oral medication is the safest and easiest to give.

➤ To protect the client against possible aspiration, the

nurse does _____

_____

_____

_____ .

▮ ADMINISTRATION OF INJECTIONS

➤ Each type of injection requires certain skills to ensure that the drug reaches the proper location.

Syringes

➤ Identify the three major types of syringes.

a. _____

b. _____

c. _____

Needles

➤ Name the three factors that must be considered in selecting a needle for an injection:

a. _____

_____

b. _____

_____

c. _____

_____

Disposable Injection Units

➤ Identify the advantages of using the Tubex or Carpuject injection systems:

_____

_____

Preparing an Injection from an Ampule

➤ An ampule is _____.
➤ The procedure for withdrawal of medications from ampules is outlined in Procedure 35-2.

Preparing an Injection from a Vial

➤ A vial is a _____.
➤ The vial is a closed system, and air must be injected into it to permit easy withdrawal of the solution.
➤ The procedure for withdrawal of medications from vials is outlined in Procedure 35-2.

Mixing Medications

➤ If two drugs are compatible, it is possible to mix them together into one injection if the total dosage is within the accepted limits.

Mixing Medications from Two Vials

➤ List the three principles to follow when mixing medications from two vials:

a. _____

_____

b. _____

_____

c. _____

_____

Mixing Medications from One Vial and One Ampule

➤ When mixing medications from an ampule and a vial, which medication should be prepared first?

_____

_____

Preparing Insulin

➤ Insulin is classified by its rate of action as _____

_____, _____,

and _____.

➤ List the simple guidelines for mixing two kinds of insulin in the same syringe.

a. _____

b. _____

➤ List the steps the nurse or client follows to prepare insulin from two vials.

a. _____

b. _____

c. _____

d. _____

e. _____

f. _____

Administering Injections

➤ List eight techniques used to minimize client discomfort associated with injections.

a. _____

_____

b. _____

_____

c. _____

_____

d. _____

_____

e. _____

_____

f. _____

_____

g. _____

_____

h. _____

_____

Subcutaneous Injections

➤ The best sites for SQ injections include _____

_____, _____,

and _____.

➤ The site most frequently recommended for heparin injection is _____.

➤ Define:

Hypertrophy _____

_____

Lipodystrophy _____

_____

➤ Identify the maximum amount of water-soluble medication that is given by the SQ route: _____.

➤ State the rule that may be followed to determine if a SQ injection should be given at a 90- or 45-degree angle:

_____

_____

Intramuscular Injections

➤ Identify the major risk of using the IM route:

_____

_____

➤ The angle of insertion for an IM injection is _____ degrees.

➤ Indicate the maximum volume of medication for IM injection in each of the following groups:

Well-developed adult _____

Older children, older adults, or thin adults _____

Older infants and small children _____

▌ SITES

➤ List the assessment criteria for selecting an IM site.

a. _____

b. _____

c. _____

d. _____

➤ Describe the method used for accurately locating the following injection sites:

Vastus lateralis muscle _____

_____

_____

_____

Ventrogluteal muscle _____

_____

_____

_____

Dorsogluteal muscle _____

_____

_____

_____

_____

Deltoid muscle _____

_____

_____

_____

_____

▌ Z-TRACK METHOD

➤ Explain the rationale for using the Z-track method of injection: _____

_____

➤ Describe the procedure for administering an intramuscular injection using the Z-track technique:

_____

_____

▌ AIR-LOCK TECHNIQUE

➤ Describe the procedure for administering an intramuscular injection using the air-lock technique:

_____

_____

_____

Intradermal Injections

➤ Describe the procedure for administering an intradermal injection for skin testing: _____

_____

_____

_____

▌ SAFETY IN ADMINISTERING MEDICATIONS BY INJECTION

➤ List six ways in which a nurse is likely to receive a needlestick injury.

a. _____

b. _____

c. _____

d. _____

e. _____

f. _____

▌ PROTECTING YOURSELF FROM NEEDLESTICK INJURIES

➤ Identify some precautions the nurse should take when administering medications:

Giving medications with safety syringe _____

_____

_____

IV administration _____

_____

_____

_____

_____

LARGE-VOLUME INFUSIONS
➤ Identify the advantage and disadvantage of the large-

volume infusion method: _____

_____

_____

INTRAVENOUS BOLUS
➤ Explain the advantage and disadvantage of the IV

bolus route of administration: _____

_____

_____

VOLUME-CONTROLLED INFUSIONS
➤ List the four advantages of using volume-controlled
infusions.

a. _____

b. _____

c. _____

d. _____

PIGGYBACK IV ADMINISTRATION

➤ Piggyback sets are _____.

INTERMITTENT VENOUS ACCESS
➤ List the three advantages of using intermittent venous access devices.

a. _____

b. _____

c. _____

TOPICAL DRUG APPLICATIONS
Skin Applications
➤ Explain the procedure for administering the following skin applications:

Ointment _____

_____

Lotion _____

_____

Powder _____

_____

Patches _____

_____

Eye Applications
➤ List the four principles for administering eye medications.

a. _____

b. _____

c. _____

d. _____

Ear Instillations
➤ Explain the procedure for administering ear instillations in the following:

Adults _____

_____

Children _____

_____

Nasal Instillations
➤ Explain the procedure for administering nasal instilla-

tions: _____

_____

_____

_____

Vaginal Instillations
➤ Explain the procedure for administering vaginal instil-

lations: _____

_____

_____

_____

Rectal Instillations
➤ Explain the procedure for administering rectal instilla-

tions: _____

_____

_____

_____

_____

ADMINISTERING DRUGS BY INHALATION
➤ To maximize the effect of metered dose inhaler medi-

cations, the nurse advises the client to _____

_____.

Irrigations

➤ List the three principles the nurse follows when performing irrigations.

a. _____

b. _____

c. _____

■ RESTORATIVE CARE: TEACHING CLIENTS TO ADMINISTER INTRAVENOUS THERAPY AT HOME

➤ When receiving home intravenous therapy, client

education should include _____

_____

_____

_____ .

REVIEW QUESTIONS

(The student should select the appropriate answer and cite the rationale for choosing that particular answer.)

1. The study of how drugs enter the body, reach their site of action, are metabolized, and exit from the body is called:
   a. Pharmacology
   b. Pharmacokinetics
   c. Pharmacopeia
   d. Biopharmaceutica

Answer ( ) Rationale: _____

_____

_____

2. Which statement correctly characterizes drug absorption?
   a. Most drugs must enter systemic circulation to have a therapeutic effect.
   b. Mucous membranes are relatively impermeable to chemicals, making absorption slow.
   c. Oral medications are absorbed more quickly when administered with meals.
   d. Drugs administered subcutaneously are absorbed more quickly than those injected intramuscularly.

Answer ( ) Rationale: _____

_____

_____

3. Most drug biotransformation occurs in the:
   a. Kidneys
   b. Blood
   c. Intestines
   d. Liver

Answer ( ) Rationale: _____

_____

_____

4. Which client is at risk for an increase in drug activity or toxicity?
   a. Client W, who has an albumin level within normal limits
   b. Client X, who weighs 20% more than his ideal body weight
   c. Client Y, who has increased glomerular filtration
   d. Client Z, who has liver disease

Answer ( ) Rationale: _____

_____

_____

5. All of the following are examples of mild allergy symptoms that may occur in response to antibiotic therapy *except:*
   a. Urticaria
   b. Rash
   c. Wheezing
   d. Pruritus

Answer ( ) Rationale: _____

_____

_____

6. Onset of drug action would be considered the time it takes for a drug to:
   a. Produce a response
   b. Accelerate the cellular process
   c. Reach its highest effective concentration
   d. Produce blood serum concentration and maintenance

Answer ( ) Rationale: _____

_____

_____

7. Which of the following is not a parenteral route of administration?
   a. Buccal
   b. Subcutaneous
   c. Intramuscular
   d. Intradermal

Answer ( ) Rationale: _____

_____

_____

8. According to the apothecary system, 1 ml is equal to:
   a. 15 minims
   b. 1 teaspoon
   c. 15 drops
   d. 1 tablespoon

Answer ( ) Rationale: _____

_____

_____

9. Dr. Green has ordered Garamycin 25 mg IM. Garamycin is available 40 mg per 1 ml. How many milliliters should the client receive?
   a. 0.5 ml
   b. 6 ml
   c. 0.63 ml
   d. 2 ml

Answer ( ) Rationale: _____

_____

_____

10. A child weighs 12 kg (Body surface area 0.54 m²). Using the body surface area formula, what dose of drug X should the child receive if the normal adult dose of drug X is 300 mg?
    a. 50 mg
    b. 90 mg
    c. 100 mg
    d. 200 mg

Answer ( ) Rationale: _____

_____

_____

11. If a client refuses a medication or is undergoing tests or procedures that result in a missed dose, the nurse will circle the prescribed administration time on the drug record, in addition to:
    a. Discontinuing the order
    b. Charting in the nurses' notes why the medication was not given
    c. Changing the dose times for the client's convenience
    d. Leaving the medication at the bedside for the client to take later

Answer ( ) Rationale: _____

_____

_____

12. The nurse is mixing two medications in one syringe. All of the following apply except:
    a. Do not contaminate one medication bottle with the other medication.
    b. Use a 20-ml syringe to facilitate drawing up and mixing the medication.
    c. Ensure that the final dosage is accurate.
    d. Maintain aseptic technique.

Answer ( ) Rationale: _____

_____

_____

13. The nurse is preparing an insulin injection in which both regular and modified insulin will be mixed. Into which vial should the nurse inject air first?
    a. The vial of modified insulin
    b. The vial of regular insulin
    c. Either vial, as long as modified insulin is drawn up first
    d. Neither vial; it is not necessary to put air into vials before withdrawing medication

Answer ( ) Rationale: _____

_____

_____

14. Which of the following is not an advantage of volume-controlled IV infusions?
    a. Reduces risk of rapid-dose infusion
    b. Allows for administration of drugs that are stable for a limited time in solution
    c. Allows for control of IV intake
    d. Eliminates need for regulation of flow rate

Answer ( ) Rationale: _____

_____

_____

15. Tony Brown, who is 6 years old, has ear drops ordered for pain. To straighten the ear canal before instillation of the drops, the nurse would:
    a. Pull the pinna upward and backward
    b. Pull the pinna downward and backward
    c. Pull the pinna upward and outward
    d. Pull the pinna downward and outward

Answer ( ) Rationale: _____

_____

_____

CLINICAL SITUATIONS

1. Your 73-year-old client is having visual difficulties. What specific interventions should you use to promote compliance and safety in administering medications?

_____

_____

_____

_____

_____

_____

_____

_____

_____

2. How is your nursing approach modified when administering medications to infants and children?

_____

_____

_____

_____

_____

_____

_____

_____

_____

_____

Chapter

36 | Safety

Safety, often defined as freedom from psychological and physical injury, is a basic human need that must be met.

PRELIMINARY READING

Chapter 36, pp. 870-892

COMPREHENSIVE UNDERSTANDING

▮ ENVIRONMENTAL SAFETY

➤ A client's environment includes _____

_____.

➤ List the five characteristics of a safe environment.

a. _____

b. _____

c. _____

d. _____

e. _____

Basic Needs

➤ Identify the four physiological needs that influence a person's safety.

a. _____

b. _____

c. _____

d. _____

▮ OXYGEN

➤ A common environmental hazard in the home is

_____.

➤ Define *carbon monoxide:* _____

_____

Humidity

➤ Define *relative humidity:* _____

_____

➤ Explain what happens to a client when the relative humidity is:

High _____

_____

Low _____

_____

Nutrition

➤ Define *food poisoning:* _____

➤ Identify the assessment criteria for a client with suspected food poisoning: _____

_____

_____

_____

➤ Define *hypothermia:* _____

_____

➤ Identify the clients at high risk for hypothermia:

_____

_____

_____

_____

_____

_____

_____

_____

_____

Reduction of Physical Hazards

➤ List the four physical hazards that contribute to falls:

a. _____

_____

b. _____

_____

c. _____

_____

d. _____

_____

Reduction of Transmission of Pathogens

➤ Define *pathogen:* _____

_____

➤ Identify the most effective method for limiting the

transmission of pathogens: _____

_____

➤ Define *immunization:* _____

_____

➤ Describe the two types of immunity:

Active _____

_____

Passive _____

_____

➤ Describe how the human immunodeficiency virus (HIV) is transmitted and who is at risk:

_____

_____

_____

_____

Pollution Control

➤ A pollutant is _____

_____.

➤ Define the following types of pollution:

Air _____

_____

Land _____

_____

Water _____

_____

Noise _____

_____

➤ Define *sensory overload:* _____

_____

▌ NURSING PROCESS AND SAFETY

Assessment

➤ List five factors that influence a client's safety in the community.

a. _____

b. _____

c. _____

d. _____

e. _____

➤ Identify at least three threats to safety in the following developmental stages:

Infant, toddler, preschooler _____

_____

_____

_____

_____

School-age _____

_____

_____

_____

➤ Describe five measures to reduce the risk of accidents in adolescents.

a. _____

b. _____

c. _____

d. _____

e. _____

➤ Threats to an adult's safety are frequently related to

_____

_____.

➤ The major cause of accidental death in the adult 75

years or older is _____.

➤ Identify the physiological changes that increase the client's risk for injury:

_____

_____

_____

_____

_____

_____

_____

_____

HEALTH CARE AGENCY

➤ List the four major risks to client safety in the health care environment.

a. _____

b. _____

c. _____

d. _____

Nursing Diagnosis

➤ Identify four actual or potential nursing diagnoses for safety risks:

a. _____

b. _____

c. _____

d. _____

Planning

➤ Identify six potential expected outcomes focusing on a client's need for safety.

a. _____

b. _____

c. _____

d. _____

e. _____

f. _____

Implementation

➤ Identify at least four interventions for each of the following developmental age-groups:

Infant, toddler, preschooler _____

_____

_____

_____

_____

School-age _____

_____

_____

_____

_____

Adolescents _____

_____

_____

_____

_____

Adult _____

_____

_____

_____

_____

Older adult _____

_____

_____

_____

ENVIRONMENTAL CONSIDERATIONS

➤ Define *medical asepsis:* _____

_____

➤ Define *surgical asepsis:* _____

_____

➤ Specific safety concerns in the environment consist of

_____, _____, _____,

_____, and _____.

➤ List eight measures to prevent falls in the health care setting:

a. _____

b. _____

c. _____

d. _____

e. _____

f. _____

g. _____

h. _____

➤ A physical restraint is _____

_____ .

➤ List the four purposes for restraints.

a. _____

b. _____

c. _____

d. _____

➤ List eight alternatives to the use of restraints.

a. _____

b. _____

c. _____

d. _____

e. _____

f. _____

g. _____

h. _____

➤ Describe six fire containment guidelines.

a. _____

b. _____

c. _____

d. _____

e. _____

f. _____

➤ A poison is _____

_____ .

➤ List five teaching strategies for prevention of electrical hazards.

a. _____

b. _____

c. _____

d. _____

e. _____

➤ List the measures with which the nurse must be familiar to reduce exposure to radiation:

_____

_____

_____

_____

_____

_____

Evaluation

➤ The nurse continually assesses the client's and family's need for additional support services such as

_____ , _____ ,

_____ , and _____ .

The expected outcomes include a _____ ,

_____ , and _____ .

REVIEW QUESTIONS

(The student should select the appropriate answer and cite the rationale for choosing that particular answer.)

1. Which of the following would most threaten an individual's safety?
   a. 70% humidity
   b. Carbon dioxide
   c. Unrefrigerated fresh vegetables
   d. Lack of water supply

Answer ( ) Rationale: _____

_____

_____

2. The developmental stage which carries the highest risk of injury from fall is:
   a. Preschool
   b. School-age
   c. Adulthood
   d. Older adulthood

Answer ( ) Rationale: _____

_____

_____

3. Mr. Krantz, an 82-year-old client, has just been admitted to your unit. To increase the safety of his environment, all of the following would be appropriate *except:*
   a. Help Mr. Krantz put on rubber-soled shoes for walking.
   b. Remove excess furniture from the room.
   c. Apply a vest restraint at night.
   d. Keep Mr. Krantz's call light within his reach.

Answer (   ) Rationale: _____

_____

_____

4. Mrs. Field falls asleep while smoking in bed and drops the burning cigarette on her blanket. When she awakens, her bed is on fire, and she quickly calls the nurse. On observing the fire, the nurse should immediately:
   a. Report the fire.
   b. Attempt to extinguish the fire.
   c. Assist Mrs. Fields to a safe place.
   d. Close all windows and doors to contain the fire.

Answer (   ) Rationale: _____

_____

_____

5. A mother calls the poison control center and reports that her 2-year-old daughter drank some gasoline, which she found in the garage. What response by the nurse is appropriate?
   a. "Give her a large glass of water to drink."
   b. "Bring her to the emergency room immediately."
   c. "How could you let her get hold of gasoline?"
   d. "Give her 1 tablespoon of ipecac to induce vomiting."

Answer (   ) Rationale: _____

_____

_____

6. Sixteen-year-old Jimmy is admitted to an adolescent unit with a diagnosis of substance abuse. The nurse examines Jimmy and finds that he has bloodshot eyes, slurred speech, and an unstable gait. He smells of alcohol and is unable to answer questions appropriately. The appropriate nursing diagnosis would be:
   a. Self-care deficit related to alcohol abuse
   b. Altered thought processes related to sensory overload
   c. Knowledge deficit related to alcohol abuse
   d. High risk for injury related to impaired sensory perception

Answer (   ) Rationale: _____

_____

_____

7. Mr. Kawakami has become very confused during his hospitalization and has pulled his IV line out twice. The best intervention to provide for Mr. Kawakami's safety would be:
   a. Elbow restraints
   b. A vest restraint
   c. One wrist restraint on the arm with the IV
   d. Bilateral wrist restraints

Answer (   ) Rationale: _____

_____

_____

8. Restraints should be completely removed every:
   a. 8 hours
   b. 4 hours
   c. 2 hours
   d. 30 minutes

Answer (   ) Rationale: _____

_____

_____

9. The majority of childhood fatalities are associated with:
   a. Accidental poisoning
   b. Accidents
   c. Congenital diseases
   d. Infectious diseases

Answer (   ) Rationale: _____

_____

_____

10. If a client receives an electric shock, the nurse's first action should be to:
    a. Assess the client's pulse
    b. Assess the client for thermal injury
    c. Notify the physician
    d. Notify the maintenance department

Answer (   ) Rationale: _____

_____

_____

CLINICAL SITUATIONS

1. Mr. Jones is a disoriented older adult who likes to wander the halls in the long-term care facility where you are assigned. Restraining him adds to his disorientation and causes him to become agitated. Describe alternative nursing measures that could be used to ensure his safety.

_____
_____
_____
_____
_____
_____
_____
_____
_____

2. You are assigned to a pediatric clinic and notice that when Mrs. Lopez arrives she and her three children are all sitting in the front seat and none are using seatbelts. Her 3-month-old infant is being held by her 5-year-old, and her 2-year-old is sitting in the middle. How would you approach her about the hazards of this practice? What interventions are appropriate?

_____
_____
_____
_____
_____
_____
_____
_____
_____

Mobility and Immobility

To maintain optimal physical mobility, the nervous, muscular, and skeletal systems of the body must be intact and functioning.

PRELIMINARY READING

Chapter 37 pp. 893-947

COMPREHENSIVE UNDERSTANDING

■ OVERVIEW OF BODY MECHANICS

➤ Define *body mechanics*: _____

_____

Body Alignment

➤ Define *body alignment*: _____

_____

➤ Correct body alignment reduces _____

_____, maintains,

_____ and contributes _____.

Body Balance

➤ Body balance is achieved when a _____

_____, _____,

and _____.

➤ Balance is required for _____,

_____, _____,

and _____.

➤ The ability to balance can be compromised by

_____, _____,

_____, _____,

and _____.

Coordinated Body Movement

➤ Define *center of gravity*: _____

_____

➤ Define *friction*: _____

_____

➤ List two techniques that minimize friction.

a. _____

b. _____

■ REGULATION OF MOVEMENT

➤ List three systems responsible for coordinating body movements.

a. _____

b. _____

c. _____

Skeletal System

➤ List four functions of the skeletal system.

a. _____

b. _____

c. _____

d. _____

➤ Describe the following:

Long bones _____

_____

Short bones _____

_____

Pathological fractures _____

_____

Joints _____

_____

Synostotic joint _____

_____

Cartilaginous joint _____

_____

Fibrous joint _____

_____

Synovial joint _____

_____

Ligaments _____

Cartilage _____

Skeletal Muscle

➤ Briefly describe how skeletal muscles affect movement: _____

➤ Briefly describe the two types of muscle contractions:
Isotonic _____

Isometric _____

➤ Explain leverage: _____

➤ Define *posture*, and name the associated muscles: _____

➤ Coordination and regulation of different muscle groups depend on the following. Briefly explain each:
Muscle tone _____

Antagonistic muscles _____

Synergistic muscles _____

Antigravity muscles _____

Damage to the central nervous system _____

_____

_____

_____

_____

_____

_____

Direct trauma to the musculoskeletal system _____

_____

_____

_____

_____

_____

■ IMPAIRED MOBILITY

➤ Mobility refers to _____

_____.

Bed Rest

➤ Define *bed rest:* _____

_____

➤ Impaired physical mobility is defined as _____

_____

_____

_____.

Immobility

➤ List four conditions that may result in immobility.

a. _____

b. _____

c. _____

d. _____

➤ List at least two hazards of immobility for each area.

Metabolic: _____

_____

_____

_____

Respiratory: _____

_____

_____

Cardiovascular: _____

_____

_____

Musculoskeletal: _____

_____

_____

_____

Integumentary: _____

_____

_____

_____

Elimination: _____

_____

_____

➤ Identify the most common psychological changes that occur with immobility: _____

_____

_____

_____

■ DEVELOPMENTAL CHANGES

➤ Identify the descriptive characteristics of body alignment and mobility related to the following developmental stages:

Infants _____

_____

_____

_____

Toddlers _____

_____

_____

_____

Preschool and school-age children _____

_____

_____

_____

Adolescents _____

_____

_____

_____

Adults _____

_____

_____

_____

Older adults _____

_____

_____

_____

■ NURSING PROCESS FOR IMPAIRED BODY ALIGNMENT AND MOBILITY

Assessment

➤ Briefly describe the four major areas for assessment of client mobility.

Range of motion: _____

_____

_____

_____

Gait: _____

_____

_____

_____

Exercise and activity tolerance: _____

_____

_____

_____

_____

Body alignment: _____

_____

_____

_____

_____

➤ Describe the six objectives to be achieved during assessment of body alignment.

a. _____

_____

b. _____

_____

c. _____

_____

d. _____

_____

e. _____

_____

f. _____

_____

➤ Briefly describe the physiological hazards of immobility in relation to the following systems:

Metabolic _____

_____

_____

_____

Respiratory _____

_____

_____

_____

_____

Cardiovascular _____

_____

_____

_____

Musculoskeletal _____

_____

_____

_____

_____

Integumentary _____

_____

_____

_____

Elimination _____

_____

_____

_____

➤ List four areas of assessment for the older adult.

a. _____

b. _____

c. _____

d. _____

Nursing Diagnosis

➤ List six actual or potential nursing diagnoses related to body alignment and immobility.

a. _____

b. _____

c. _____

d. _____

e. _____

f. _____

Planning

➤ List 10 goals appropriate for clients with actual or potential positioning and mobility needs.

a. _____

b. _____

c. _____

d. _____

e. _____

f. _____

g. _____

h. _____

i. _____

j. _____

Implementation

➤ List four criteria to be assessed before lifting a client or object.

a. _____

b. _____

c. _____

d. _____

➤ Indicate the correct use for each positioning device listed.

Device	Uses
Pillow	
Footboard	
Trochanter roll	
Sandbag	
Hand-wrist splints	
Trapeze bar	
Restraints	
Side rails	
Bed board	

➤ List the common trouble areas for the clients in the following positions:

Positions *Give a brief description of the position.*	Trouble Areas
Fowler's	a.
	b.
	c.
	d.
	e.
	f.
	g.
Supine	a.
	b.
	c.
	d.
	e.
	f.
	g.
	h.
Prone	a.
	b.
	c.
	d.
Side-lying	a.
	b.
	c.
	d.
	e.
Sims'	a.
	b.
	c.
	d.

➤ List the six general guidelines to apply in any transfer procedure.

a. _____

b. _____

c. _____

d. _____

e. _____

f. _____

➤ List four areas for the nurse to consider to determine if assistance is required when moving a client in bed.

a. _____

b. _____

c. _____

d. _____

➤ Indicate the type of joint and range of motion exercises for the body parts listed in the table below.

➤ List the five steps to be taken by the nurse in preparing to assist the client to walk.

a. _____

b. _____

c. _____

d. _____

e. _____

➤ Describe how a nurse would assist a client with hemiplegia or hemiparesis: _____

_____

_____

➤ Explain the guidelines that would be taught to a client using a single straight-legged cane: _____

_____

_____

_____

➤ Describe the appropriate measurements for axillary crutches: _____

_____

➤ List four crutch safety guidelines to be taught to clients before they are allowed to walk independently.

a. _____

_____

b. _____

_____

c. _____

_____

d. _____

_____

➤ Explain the following crutch gaits:

Tripod position _____

_____

_____

Four-point _____

_____

_____

Body Part	Type of Joint	Type of Movement
Neck		
Shoulder		
Elbow		
Forearm		
Wrist		
Fingers and thumb		
Hip		
Knee		
Ankle and foot		
Toes		

Three-point _____

_____

_____

Two-point _____

_____

_____

Swing-through _____

_____

_____

➤ List the sequence of movement for crutch walking on stairs.

Ascending stairs: _____

_____

_____

_____

Descending stairs: _____

_____

_____

➤ Identify two nursing interventions to meet each of the following goals for the immobilized client:

Maintain optimal nutritional (metabolic) state ____

_____

_____

_____

Promote lung expansion _____

_____

_____

_____

Prevent stasis of pulmonary secretions _____

_____

_____

_____

Maintain patent airway _____

_____

_____

_____

Minimize orthostatic hypotension _____

_____

_____

_____

_____

Decrease cardiac workload _____

_____

_____

_____

Prevent thrombus formation _____

_____

_____

_____

Maintain muscle strength and joint mobility _____

_____

_____

_____

Maintain normal elimination patterns _____

_____

_____

_____

Maintain usual psychosocial state _____

_____

_____

_____

➤ Identify two nursing interventions for the following immobilized clients:

Young child _____

_____

_____

Older adult _____

_____

_____

_____

Evaluation

➤ The optimal outcomes are the client's ability to maintain or improve body alignment and joint mobility.

➤ The nurse evaluates specific interventions designed to

promote _____, improve

_____, and protect _____.

REVIEW QUESTIONS

(The student should select the appropriate answer and cite the rationale for choosing that particular answer.)

1. Which of the following is true of body mechanics?
   a. The narrower the base of support, the greater the stability of the nurse.
   b. The higher the center of gravity, the greater the stability of the nurse.
   c. When friction is reduced between the object to be moved and the surface on which it is moved, less force is required to move it.
   d. Rolling, turning, or pivoting requires more work than lifting.

Answer ( ) Rationale: _____

_____

_____

2. White, shiny, flexible bands of fibrous tissue binding joints together and connecting various bones and cartilage types are known as:
   a. Muscles
   b. Ligaments
   c. Joints
   d. Tendons

Answer ( ) Rationale: _____

_____

_____

3. Mrs. Harper has an increased convexity in the curvature of the thoracic spine. This is known as:
   a. Kyphosis
   b. Torticollis
   c. Lordosis
   d. Scoliosis

Answer ( ) Rationale: _____

_____

_____

4. The nurse would expect all of the following physiological effects of exercise on the body systems *except:*
   a. Decreased cardiac output
   b. Increased respiratory rate and depth
   c. Increased muscle tone, size, and strength
   d. Change in metabolic rate

Answer ( ) Rationale: _____

_____

_____

5. Which of the following is a correctly stated nursing diagnosis for the client who has difficulty with movement?
   a. Needs help to walk related to inflammation of the right knee
   b. Impaired physical mobility related to muscular dystrophy
   c. Activity intolerance related to dislike of exercise
   d. High risk for injury related to lack of knowledge of safe transfer techniques

Answer ( ) Rationale: _____

_____

_____

6. Which of the following is a potential hazard that the nurse should assess for when the client is in the prone position?
   a. Unprotected pressure points at the sacrum and heels
   b. Internal rotation of the shoulder
   c. Increased cervical flexion
   d. Plantar flexion

Answer ( ) Rationale: _____

_____

_____

7. Which of the following is *not* appropriate in performing a three-person carry to transfer a client from bed to a stretcher?
   a. Use three nurses of a similar height.
   b. Place the stretcher parallel to the bed.
   c. Nurses roll client to their chests.
   d. One nurse assumes the leadership role and directs the other two.

Answer ( ) Rationale: _____

_____

_____

8. Movements of the hip include all of the following *except:*
   a. Flexion
   b. Hyperextension
   c. Circumduction
   d. Opposition

Answer (   ) Rationale: _____

_____

_____

9. Which of the following is a physiological effect of prolonged bed rest?
   a. Decrease in urinary excretion of nitrogen
   b. Increase in cardiac output
   c. Decrease in lean body mass
   d. Decrease in lung expansion

Answer (   ) Rationale: _____

_____

_____

10. All of the following measures are used to assess for deep vein thrombosis *except:*
    a. Measure the circumference of each leg daily, placing the tape measure at the midpoint of the knee.
    b. Observe the dorsal aspect of lower extremities for redness, warmth, and tenderness.
    c. Ask the client about the presence of calf pain.
    d. Check for a positive Homans' sign.

Answer (   ) Rationale: _____

_____

_____

11. Which of the following is an appropriate intervention to maintain the respiratory system of the immobilized client?
    a. Turn the client every 4 hours.
    b. Maintain maximum fluid intake of 1500 ml per day.
    c. Apply an abdominal binder continuously while in bed.
    d. Encourage use of an incentive spirometer.

Answer (   ) Rationale: _____

_____

_____

CLINICAL SITUATIONS

1. Mr. Kauffman, who is 69 years of age, is being released from the hospital today. He is going home with his daughter, who will be caring for him. He will be confined to bed. List and discuss the guidelines you will give to Mr. Kauffman's daughter concerning body mechanics.

_____

_____

_____

_____

_____

_____

_____

_____

_____

_____

2. You are caring for an 80-year-old female client with a fractured hip who has been healthy and independent until this hospitalization. What are your priorities for reducing the risk of complications from immobility?

_____

_____

_____

_____

_____

_____

_____

_____

_____

Chapter 38 | Skin Integrity

Impaired skin integrity occurs from prolonged pressure, irritation of the skin, or immobility, leading to the development of pressure ulcers.

PRELIMINARY READING

Chapter 38, pp. 948-992

COMPREHENSIVE UNDERSTANDING

■ ECONOMIC CONSEQUENCES OF PRESSURE ULCERS

➤ Define *pressure ulcer:* _____

_____

_____

➤ Identify the prevalence of pressure ulcers in the following settings:

Acute care setting _____

_____

Restorative care _____

_____

Home care _____

Prediction and Prevention of Pressure Ulcers

➤ List five risk factors for pressure ulcer development.

a. _____

b. _____

c. _____

d. _____

e. _____

■ PRESSURE ULCERS

➤ Define the following terms:

Tissue ischemia _____

_____

_____

_____

Blanching _____

_____

_____

_____

Darkly pigmented skin _____

_____

_____

_____

Capillary closing pressure _____

_____

_____

_____

Normal reactive hyperemia _____

_____

_____

_____

Abnormal reactive hyperemia _____

_____

_____

_____

Risk Factors for Pressure Ulcer Development

➤ Briefly explain the following factors that contribute to increased risk for a pressure ulcer:

Impaired sensory input _____

_____

_____

_____

_____

_____

_____

Impaired motor function _____

_____

_____

_____

_____

_____

Alterations in level of consciousness _____

_____

_____

_____

_____

Casts and traction orthotic devices _____

_____

_____

_____

_____

Contributing Factors to Pressure Ulcer Formation

➤ Describe why each of the following mechanisms contributes to pressure ulcer formation in the "at-risk" client:

Shearing force _____

_____

_____

Moisture _____

_____

_____

_____

Poor nutrition _____

_____

_____

_____

Anemia _____

_____

_____

Fever _____

_____

_____

Infection _____

_____

_____

Impaired circulation _____

_____

_____

_____

Obesity _____

_____

_____

_____

Cachexia _____

_____

_____

_____

Age _____

_____

_____

_____

Pathogenesis of Pressure Ulcers

➤ Identify the three elements for pressure ulcer development.

a. _____

b. _____

c. _____

➤ List the most common sites in which pressure ulcers

develop: _____

_____

_____

_____

➤ Staging systems for pressure ulcers are based on the depth of tissue destroyed. Briefly describe each stage.

I: _____

II: _____

_____

III: _____

_____

IV: _____

_____

➤ Describe the following wound classifications:

Black wounds _____

_____

Yellow wounds _____

_____

Red wounds _____

_____

■ NURSING PROCESS AND PRESSURE ULCERS

Assessment

➤ Identify nursing assessment data for the following dimensions:

Skin _____

_____

_____

_____

_____

_____

Mobility _____

_____

_____

_____

_____

Nutritional status _____

_____

_____

_____

_____

Pain _____

_____

_____

_____

_____

Nursing Diagnosis

➤ List three nursing diagnoses related to impaired skin integrity.

a. _____

b. _____

c. _____

Planning

➤ List six possible goals for the client at risk for pressure ulcers.

a. _____

b. _____

c. _____

d. _____

e. _____

f. _____

Implementation

➤ Nursing interventions focus on _____

_____ or _____

of pressure ulcers.

➤ Briefly explain the three major areas of nursing interventions for the prevention of pressure ulcers.

Hygiene and skin care: _____

_____

_____

_____

_____

_____

Positioning: _____

_____

_____

_____

_____

Support surfaces: _____

_____

_____

_____

_____

➤ Aspects of pressure ulcer treatment include local care of the wound and supportive measures. Briefly explain the following:

Debridement _____

_____

_____

_____

_____

Cleansing _____

_____

_____

_____

_____

_____

Dressing application _____

_____

_____

_____

_____

_____

➤ Define *moist wound-healing,* and list the appropriate steps to take to accomplish it:

_____

_____

_____

_____

_____

_____

_____

_____

_____

➤ Describe two nursing interventions in relation to nutritional status in the treatment of pressure ulcers.

a. _____

b. _____

Evaluation

➤ List three possible outcomes of care for clients with impaired skin integrity:

a. _____

b. _____

c. _____

REVIEW QUESTIONS

(The student should select the appropriate answer and cite the rationale for choosing that particular answer.)

1. Ischemia is defined as:
   a. Increased tissue buildup during the healing process
   b. Deficiency of blood supply to a part
   c. Decreased fluid to the tissues
   d. Increased irritability of nerves

Answer (   ) Rationale: _____

_____

_____

2. Mr. Post is in a Fowler's position to improve his oxygenation status. The nurse notes that he frequently slides down in the bed and needs to be repositioned. Mr. Post is at risk for developing a pressure ulcer on his coccyx because of:
   a. Friction
   b. Shearing force
   c. Maceration
   d. Impaired peripheral circulation

Answer (   ) Rationale: _____

_____

_____

3. Which of the following is not a subscale on the Braden scale for predicting pressure ulcer risk?
   a. Age
   b. Sensory perception
   c. Moisture
   d. Activity

Answer (   ) Rationale: _____

_____

_____

4. Which of the these clients has a nutritional risk for pressure ulcer development?
   a. Client A has an albumin level of 3.5.
   b. Client B has a hemoglobin level within normal limits.
   c. Client C has a protein intake of 0.5 gm per kilogram per day.
   d. Client D has a body weight that is 5% greater than his ideal weight.

Answer (   ) Rationale: _____

_____

_____

5. Mrs. Greer is an immobilized client. Which of the following is not a factor that will increase her risk of pressure development?
   a. Has unrelieved pressure to her hip of greater than 32 mm Hg
   b. Displays reactive hyperemia on her coccyx that lasts for 30 minutes after being turned to her side
   c. Has low intensity pressure over a long period to her heels as a result of elastic stockings
   d. Is positioned so that she has an unequal distribution of body weight

Answer (   ) Rationale: _____

_____

_____

6. Mr. Nguyen has a pressure ulcer on his sacral area. The area is open, and the nurse can see the subcutaneous tissue. What stage is this ulcer?
   a. Stage I
   b. Stage II
   c. Stage III
   d. Stage IV

Answer (   ) Rationale: _____

_____

_____

7. Which of the following is a correctly stated nursing diagnosis for a client with actual or potential skin integrity?
   a. High risk for impaired skin integrity related to possible abdominal surgery in the AM
   b. Impaired skin integrity related to urinary incontinence
   c. Impaired skin integrity related to cerebrovascular accident
   d. High risk for impaired skin integrity related to nurses not adhering to posted turning schedule

Answer (   ) Rationale: _____

_____

_____

8. Which measure should *not* be part of the nursing plan for a client at risk for impaired skin integrity?
   a. Clean skin daily with soap.
   b. Apply zinc oxide to anal area after each episode of fecal incontinence.
   c. Apply polymer filling incontinence briefs as long as client is incontinent of urine.
   d. Keep head of client's bed at no more than a 25-degree angle.

Answer (   ) Rationale: _____

_____

_____

9. Mr. Perkins has a stage II ulcer of his right heel. What would be the most appropriate treatment for this ulcer?
   a. Apply a thick layer of enzymatic ointment to the ulcer and the surrounding skin.
   b. Apply a calcium alginate dressing and change when strike through is noted.
   c. Apply a heat lamp to the area for 20 minutes twice daily.
   d. Apply a hydrocolloid dressing, and change as necessary.

Answer (   ) Rationale: _____

_____

_____

10. The removal of necrotic tissue to allow healthy tissue to regenerate is:
   a. Escharotomy
   b. Sloughing
   c. Debridement
   d. Undermining

Answer (   ) Rationale: _____

_____

_____

CLINICAL SITUATIONS

1. Your client's mobility is severely restricted, and he is receiving a medication that causes peripheral vaso-constriction. What interventions are essential in reducing pressure ulcer formation?

_____

_____

_____

_____

_____

_____

_____

_____

2. You have just admitted a client from a nursing home to your division. On initial assessment, you find a stage II pressure ulcer. How do you determine the type of care and dressing to use with this particular pressure ulcer?

_____

_____

_____

_____

_____

_____

_____

_____

Sensory Alterations

Stimulation comes from many sources inside
and outside the body, particularly through the
senses of sight (visual), hearing (auditory), touch
(tactile), smell (olfactory), and taste (gustatory).

PRELIMINARY READING

Chapter 39, pp. 993-1014

COMPREHENSIVE UNDERSTANDING

■ NORMAL SENSATION

➤ List and briefly explain the 3 functional components
necessary for any sensory experience.

a. _____

_____

_____

b. _____

_____

_____

c. _____

_____

_____

■ SENSORY ALTERATIONS

➤ The types of sensory alterations commonly seen by

the nurse are _____,

_____, and _____.

➤ When a client suffers from more than one sensory
alteration, the ability to function and relate effectively within the environment is seriously impaired.

➤ List eight factors that may influence sensory function.

a. _____

b. _____

c. _____

d. _____

e. _____

f. _____

g. _____

h. _____

Sensory Deficits

➤ Define *sensory deficit:* _____

_____

_____

➤ Clients with sensory deficits may change behavior in
the following ways. Give an example of each:

Adaptive _____

_____

_____

Maladaptive _____

_____

_____

Sensory Deprivation

➤ List the three major types of sensory deprivation,
and give an example of each.

a. _____

_____

_____

b. _____

_____

_____

c. _____

_____

_____

Sensory Overload

➤ Define *sensory overload:* _____

_____

_____

_____

➤ Identify the behavioral changes that are associated with sensory overload:

_____

_____

_____

_____

_____

▌ NURSING PROCESS AND SENSORY ALTERATIONS

) Assessment

➤ Complete the grid by describing at least one assessment technique for the identified sensory function and the behaviors for an adult and child that would indicate a sensory deficit.

Sense	Assessment Technique	Child Behavior	Adult Behavior
Vision			
Hearing			
Touch			
Smell			
Taste			
Position sense			

Health Promotion Habits

➤ The nurse needs to assess the daily routines that clients follow to maintain sensory function. List four questions related to this.

a. _____

_____

_____

b. _____

_____

_____

c. _____

_____

_____

d. _____

_____

_____

➤ The nurse also assesses a client's compliance with routine health screening. List three questions related to this.

a. _____

_____

_____

b. _____

_____

_____

c. _____

_____

_____

Persons at Risk

➤ List three groups that are at high risk for sensory alterations during hospitalization.

a. _____

b. _____

c. _____

Nursing History

➤ List three questions that the nurse may ask the client to get him or her to describe a sensory deficit.

a. _____

_____

_____

b. _____

_____

_____

c. _____

_____

_____

➤ List three questions the nurse may ask the client to elicit knowledge about the onset and duration of the sensory alteration.

a. _____

_____

_____

b. _____

_____

_____

c. _____

_____

➤ Give an example of how a nurse may assess the client's self-rating of a sensory deficit:

_____

_____

_____

_____

Ability to Perform Self-Care

➤ List the client's functional abilities that the nurse may assess:

_____

_____

_____

_____

_____

Environment

➤ The following factors may minimize or heighten sensory alterations. Explain each one:

Hazards _____

_____

_____

_____

_____

Meaningful stimuli _____

_____

_____

_____

Amount of stimuli _____

_____

_____

_____

_____

Socialization

➤ It is important for the nurse to know the client's social skills and level of satisfaction with the support given by family and friends. Identify four questions that would be appropriate in determining these factors.

a. _____

_____

_____

b. _____

_____

_____

c. _____

_____

_____

d. _____

_____

_____

Communication Methods

➤ Clients with existing sensory deficits often develop alternative ways of communicating. Give two examples:

a. _____

_____

b. _____

_____

➤ Define the following types of aphasia:

Expressive _____

_____

_____

Receptive _____

_____

_____

Global _____

_____

_____

➤ To understand the nature of a communication problem, the nurse must know if a client has trouble

_____, _____,

_____, _____,

or _____.

Mental Status

➤ Identify the three dimensions to evaluate when assessing mental status, and give an example of each.

a. _____

_____

_____

b. _____

_____

_____

c. _____

_____

_____

Physical Assessment

➤ To identify sensory deficits, the nurse assesses

_____, _____,

_____, and _____, as well

as the ability to discriminate _____.

Nursing Diagnosis

➤ List 12 actual or potential nursing diagnoses for a client with sensory alterations.

a. _____

b. _____

c. _____

d. _____

e. _____

f. _____

g. _____

h. _____

i. _____

j. _____

k. _____

l. _____

b. _____

c. _____
_____

d. _____
_____

◖ Planning

➤ List eight goals appropriate for clients with sensory alterations.

a. _____

b. _____

c. _____

d. _____

e. _____

f. _____

g. _____

h. _____

◖ Implementation

➤ Nursing interventions are chosen based on the nursing diagnosis and the related factors contributing to the client's problem.

Health Promotion

➤ List four general measures to promote visual function.

a. _____
_____

➤ Identify the common trauma injuries that result in hearing or vision loss in both adults and children.

Adults: _____
_____
_____

Children: _____
_____
_____

➤ Explain the measures to take to maintain sensory function at the highest level with the use of assistive devices.

_____
_____
_____
_____
_____
_____

➤ Complete the grid by filling in the normal physiological changes that occur and citing how the nurse can maximize the loss.

Senses	Physiological Change	Interventions
Vision		
Hearing		
Taste and smell		
Touch		

➤ List three methods to establish a safe environment with regard to the following adaptations:
Visual loss

a. _____

_____

b. _____

_____

c. _____

_____

Reduced hearing

a. _____

_____

b. _____

_____

c. _____

_____

Reduced olfaction

a. _____

_____

b. _____

_____

c. _____

_____

Reduced tactile sensation

a. _____

_____

b. _____

_____

c. _____

_____

➤ Describe six communication methods appropriate for clients with a hearing impairment.

a. _____

b. _____

c. _____

d. _____

e. _____

f. _____

Managing Acute Sensory Deficits

➤ When clients enter acute care settings for therapeutic management of sensory deficits or as a result of traumatic injury, the following approaches are used to maximize sensory function. Briefly explain each:

Orientation to the environment _____

_____

_____

_____

_____

_____

Safety measures _____

_____

_____

_____

_____

_____

Controlling sensory stimuli _____

_____

_____

_____

_____

_____

Maintaining Healthy Lifestyles

➤ After a client has experienced a sensory loss, it becomes important to understand the following. Briefly explain each:

Understanding sensory loss _____

_____

_____

_____

_____

_____

Socialization _____

_____

_____

_____

_____

Promoting self-care _____

_____

_____

_____

_____

_____

Evaluation

➤ List three outcomes of care for clients with a sensory alteration.

a. _____

b. _____

c. _____

REVIEW QUESTIONS

(The student should select the appropriate answer and cite the rationale for choosing that particular answer.)

1. All of the following are true of age-related factors that influence sensory function *except:*
   a. Refractive errors are the most common types of visual disorders in children.
   b. Visual changes in adulthood include presbyopia.
   c. Older adults hear high-pitched sounds the best.
   d. Neonates are unable to discriminate sensory stimuli.

Answer ( ) Rationale: _____

_____

_____

2. Mr. Green, a 62-year-old farmer, has been hospitalized for two weeks for thrombophlebitis. He has no visitors, and the nurse notices that he appears bored, restless, and anxious. The type of alteration occurring because of sensory deprivation is:
   a. Affective
   b. Cognitive
   c. Perceptual
   d. Receptual

Answer ( ) Rationale: _____

_____

_____

3. The nurse assesses a newly admitted client who has a visual deficit. All of the following comments would be appropriate *except:*
   a. "Wearing glasses isn't bad. Lots of people have to do that."
   b. "Rate your eyesight as excellent, good, fair, poor, or bad."
   c. "What problems are you experiencing as a result of your vision loss?"
   d. "How long have you been having problems with your eyesight?"

Answer ( ) Rationale: _____

_____

_____

4. Which of the following would *not* provide meaningful stimuli for a client?
   a. A clock or calendar with large numbers
   b. A television that is kept on all day at a low volume
   c. Family pictures and personal possessions
   d. Interesting magazines and books

Answer ( ) Rationale: _____

_____

_____

5. Clients with existing sensory loss must be protected from injury. What determines the safety precautions taken?
   a. The existing dangers in the environment
   b. The financial availability to make needed safety changes
   c. The nature of the client's actual or potential sensory loss
   d. The availability of a support system to enable the client to exist in his or her present environment

Answer ( ) Rationale: _____

_____

_____

6. Goals for nursing care of clients with actual or potential sensory alterations include all of the following *except:*
   a. Promoting optimal function of existing senses
   b. Preventing additional sensory loss
   c. Promoting the client's acceptance of dependency
   d. Controlling the environment to create meaningful sensory stimuli

Answer ( ) Rationale: _____

_____

_____

7. An appropriate nursing intervention to help a client who has a recent visual impairment is:
   a. Stand on the client's dominant side, approximately one step behind him to assist with walking.
   b. Keep bedside rails up at night.
   c. Provide a night-light with a blue bulb.
   d. Keep necessary objects on the client's bedside table.

Answer ( ) Rationale: _____

_____

_____

8. In communicating with a client who has a hearing impairment, the nurse should:
   a. Be sure the client has glasses on if she or he wears them.
   b. Exaggerate lip movements to facilitate lipreading.
   c. Repeat the conversation if it is not understood at first.
   d. Rely on the client's family to speak for him or her.

Answer ( ) Rationale: _____

_____

_____

9. A client who is unable to name common objects or express simple ideas in words or writing suffers from:
   a. Expressive aphasia
   b. Receptive aphasia
   c. Global aphasia
   d. Mental retardation

Answer ( ) Rationale: _____

_____

_____

10. When ambulating a client with visual impairment, the nurse should:
    a. Stand on the client's dominant side, and grasp the client's arm.
    b. Stand on the client's nondominant side, approximately one step behind the client, grasping the client's arm.
    c. Stand slightly in front of the client, on the client's nondominant side, allowing the client to grasp the nurse's arm.
    d. Stand on the client's dominant side, slightly in front of the client, allowing the client to grasp the nurse's arm.

Answer ( ) Rationale: _____

_____

_____

CLINICAL SITUATIONS

1. Mrs. Wilson enters the community clinic to have her 4-year-old child's hearing tested. As the nurse, you learn that Mrs. Wilson has a 6-year-old and that both children are very active. Approximately 6 months ago the 4-year-old entered the clinic with a ruptured eardrum following a fireworks incident. Describe nursing interventions designed to prevent additional sensory loss for the 4-year-old and the 6-year-old.

_____

_____

_____

_____

_____

_____

_____

_____

_____

2. Mrs. Tillis lives in a two-room apartment on the second floor. During a home visit, you notice there is a single light over the stairwell. The client's apartment is painted in a dull gray, with throw rugs throughout. Mrs. Tillis is 80 years old and lives alone. What recommendations might you make to improve the safety of Mrs. Tillis' environment?

_____

_____

_____

_____

_____

_____

_____

_____

Chapter 40 | Hygiene

Maintenance of personal hygiene is necessary for an individual's comfort, safety, and well-being.

PRELIMINARY READING

Chapter 40, pp. 1016-1087

COMPREHENSIVE UNDERSTANDING

▮ FACTORS INFLUENCING HYGIENIC PRACTICE

➤ The manner in which a person performs personal hygiene can be influenced by the following factors. Briefly explain each:

Body Image _____

_____

_____

_____

Social Practices _____

_____

_____

_____

Socioeconomic Status _____

_____

_____

_____

Knowledge _____

_____

_____

_____

Cultural Variables _____

_____

_____

_____

Personal Preferences _____

_____

_____

_____

Physical Condition _____

_____

_____

_____

_____

▮ TYPES OF HYGIENIC CARE

➤ Identify the types of hygienic care commonly performed.

a. _____

b. _____

c. _____

d. _____

e. _____

▮ CARE OF THE SKIN

➤ Define the following terms related to the skin:

Epidermis _____

_____

Stratum corneum _____

_____

Melanocytes _____

_____

Dermis _____

_____

Sebum _____

_____

Eccrine glands _____

_____

Apocrine glands _____

_____

Cerumen _____

_____

➤ List the functions of the skin:

_____

_____

_____

_____

_____

_____

❚ THE NURSING PROCESS AND SKIN CARE

◗ Assessment

➤ To determine the condition of the skin, the nurse observes the _____,

_____, _____,

_____, _____,

and _____.

➤ List the skin problems influenced by hygienic measures: _____

_____

➤ For each developmental stage, briefly describe normal conditions creating high risk for impaired skin integrity:

Neonate _____

_____

_____

Toddler _____

_____

_____

Adolescent _____

_____

_____

Older adult _____

_____

➤ List six factors to assess to determine a client's ability to perform personal skin care.

a. _____

b. _____

c. _____

d. _____

e. _____

f. _____

➤ Briefly explain the six conditions that place clients at risk for impaired skin integrity.

Immobilization: _____

_____

_____

Reduced sensation: _____

_____

_____

Nutrition and hydration: _____

_____

_____

Secretions and excretions: _____

_____

_____

Vascular insufficiency: _____

_____

_____

External devices: _____

_____

_____

◗ Nursing Diagnosis

➤ List five actual or potential nursing diagnoses for impaired skin integrity.

a. _____

b. _____

c. _____

d. _____

e. _____

Planning

➤ List four goals for clients receiving skin care.

a. _____

b. _____

c. _____

d. _____

Implementation

➤ Describe each therapeutic bath by completing the table below.

➤ List four guidelines the nurse should follow when assisting or providing a client with any type of bath.

a. _____

b. _____

c. _____

d. _____

➤ Define *perineal care,* and name the types of clients who

need it most: _____

_____

_____

➤ A back rub promotes _____,

_____, _____,

and _____.

➤ Provide the rationale for each action included in bathing an infant:

Keeping the infant covered as much as possible:

_____

_____

_____

Using plain water (no soaps) for bathing:

_____

_____

_____

Avoiding use of lotions and oils:

_____

_____

_____

Eliminating use of cotton-tipped swabs for cleansing ears or nares:

_____

_____

_____

Applying alcohol or triple dye to the umbilical cord:

_____

_____

_____

Therapeutic Bath	Purpose	Safety Factors
Sitz Bath		
Hot water tub bath		
Warm water tub bath		
Cool water bath		
Soak		

Drying gently but thoroughly:

_____

_____

_____

➤ List the steps for a sponge bath for newborn infants:

_____

_____

_____

_____

_____

➤ List the steps for a tub bath for infants:

_____

_____

_____

_____

_____

Evaluation

➤ List four outcomes for the client with impaired skin integrity:

a. _____

b. _____

c. _____

d. _____

CARE OF FEET AND NAILS

➤ The feet and nails often require special attention to

prevent _____, _____,

and _____ to tissues.

➤ Name the factors from which problems result:

_____

_____

_____

_____

_____

NURSING PROCESS AND FOOT CARE

Assessment

➤ Assessment of the feet involves a thorough examination

of _____, _____,

_____, and _____.

➤ Identify the characteristics of the following foot and nail problems:

Callus _____

_____

Corns _____

_____

Plantar warts _____

_____

Tinea Pedis _____

_____

Ingrown nails _____

_____

Ram's horn nails _____

_____

Paronychia _____

_____

Foot odors _____

_____

➤ Identify the common foot problems of the older adult:

_____

_____

_____

_____

_____

➤ Briefly explain how footwear may predispose a client

to foot and nail problems: _____

_____

_____

_____

_____

Nursing Diagnosis

➤ List seven actual or potential nursing diagnoses for a client with foot or nail problems.

a. _____

b. _____

c. _____

d. _____

e. _____

f. _____

g. _____

Planning

➤ List four goals for a client receiving nail and foot care.

a. _____

b. _____

c. _____

d. _____

Implementation

➤ List 16 guidelines to include when advising clients with diabetes or peripheral vascular disease about foot care.

a. _____

b. _____

c. _____

d. _____

e. _____

f. _____

g. _____

h. _____

i. _____

j. _____

k. _____

l. _____

m. _____

n. _____

o. _____

p. _____

∎ HEALTH PROMOTION

➤ Many complications can be avoided if clients are motivated to carry out proper foot and nail care as part of their daily hygiene.

Evaluation

➤ List two possible outcomes for a client with alterations in the foot or nails.

a. _____

b. _____

∎ ORAL HYGIENE

➤ Oral hygiene helps maintain _____
_____.

➤ Education about common gum and tooth disorders and methods of prevention can motivate clients to follow good oral hygiene practices.

Health Promotion for Teeth

➤ List the goals of Healthy People 2000.

a. _____

b. _____

c. _____

d. _____

∎ NURSING PROCESS AND ORAL HYGIENE

➤ Clients who do not follow regular oral hygiene practices may have _____
_____
_____
_____.

➤ Complete the grid (top of next page) in relation to the physiological development of the oral cavity.

➤ Explain the rationale for assessing the client's eating patterns:

_____
_____
_____
_____

Developmental Level	Changes
Infant	
18 months to 6 years	
6 to 12 years	
12 to 18 years	
18 to 40 years	
Pregnancy	
40 to 65 years	
65 years and over	

➤ List six questions to ask a client to help assess his or her oral hygiene practices.

a. _____
b. _____
c. _____
d. _____
e. _____
f. _____

➤ Identify five risk factors that predispose a client to oral problems.

a. _____
b. _____
c. _____
d. _____
e. _____

➤ Define the following common oral problems:

Dental caries _____

_____

Plaque _____

_____

Pyorrhea _____

_____

Periodontal disease _____

_____

Halitosis _____

_____

Cheilosis _____

_____

Stomatitis _____

_____

Glossitis _____

_____

Gingivitis _____

_____

Nursing Diagnosis

➤ Identify six actual or potential nursing diagnoses for oral hygiene problems.

a. _____

b. _____

c. _____

d. _____

e. _____

f. _____

Planning

➤ List the goals for clients in need of oral hygiene.

a. _____

b. _____

c. _____

d. _____

Implementation

➤ Briefly explain the following interventions in relation to oral hygiene:

Diet _____

_____

_____

Brushing _____

_____

_____

Fluoride use _____

_____

_____

Flossing _____

_____

_____

_____

Denture care _____

_____

_____

➤ The following clients require special oral hygiene methods because of their level of dependence on the nurse or the presence of oral mucosa problems. Explain why:

Unconscious clients _____

_____

_____

_____

Clients at risk for stomatitis _____

_____

_____

_____

Clients with diabetes _____

_____

_____

_____

Clients with oral infections _____

_____

_____

_____

Evaluation

➤ LIst three outcomes for a client with oral hygiene problems.

a. _____

b. _____

c. _____

HAIR CARE

➤ List five factors that can change the characteristics of the hair.

a. _____

b. _____

c. _____

d. _____

e. _____

NURSING PROCESS AND HAIR CARE

Assessment

➤ Define the following hair and scalp conditions:

Dandruff _____

Ticks _____

Pediculosis _____

Pediculosis capitis _____

Pediculosis corporis _____

Pediculosis pubis _____

Alopecia _____

➤ Describe the changes that occur with hair growth through the following developmental stages:

Infancy _____

Childhood _____

Middle childhood _____

Adolescence _____

Adulthood _____

➤ Identify four physical conditions that would affect self-care ability:

a. _____

b. _____

c. _____

d. _____

Nursing Diagnosis

➤ List five nursing diagnoses related to hair and scalp care.

a. _____

b. _____

c. _____

d. _____

e. _____

Planning

➤ List three goals for a client in need of hair and scalp care.

a. _____

b. _____

c. _____

Implementation

➤ Briefly describe the rationale for the following interventions:

Brushing and combing _____

Shampooing _____

Shaving _____
_____
_____
_____
_____

Mustache and beard care _____
_____
_____
_____
_____
_____

☾ Evaluation

➤ List three outcomes for a client with hair and scalp problems.

a. _____

b. _____

c. _____

■ CARE OF THE EYES, EARS, AND NOSE

➤ Nursing care centers on preventing infection and maintaining the client's normal organ function.

Eyes

➤ Describe hygienic care for the following organs:

Eyes _____
_____
_____

Ears _____
_____
_____

Nose _____
_____
_____

■ NURSING PROCESS AND EYES, EARS, AND NOSE CARE

☾ Assessment

➤ List the assessment criteria for the following:

Eyes _____
_____
_____
_____
_____

Ears _____
_____
_____
_____
_____

Nose _____
_____
_____
_____
_____

➤ List at least two factors to assess about a client's knowledge and use of each sensory aid.

Eyeglasses _____
_____
_____

Contact lenses _____
_____
_____
_____

Artificial eye _____
_____
_____

Hearing aid _____
_____
_____
_____

Nursing Diagnosis

➤ List five potential or actual nursing diagnoses related to an alteration of the sensory organs.

a. _____

b. _____

c. _____

d. _____

e. _____

Planning

➤ List three goals for a client requiring special hygienic care related to the eyes, ears, or nose.

a. _____

b. _____

c. _____

Implementation

➤ Describe the basic eye care for the unconscious client:

_____

_____

_____

_____

➤ Describe the correct procedure for cleaning glasses:

_____

_____

_____

➤ List the four advantages of contact lenses over glasses.

a. _____

b. _____

c. _____

d. _____

➤ List the five common problems for contact lens wearers and the cause of each.

a. _____

b. _____

c. _____

d. _____

e. _____

➤ Identify three conditions in which the client's contact lenses should be removed immediately.

a. _____

b. _____

c. _____

➤ Describe each of the following techniques necessary in caring for an artificial eye:

Removal _____

_____

_____

Cleansing _____

_____

_____

Reinsertion _____

_____

_____

Storage _____

_____

_____

➤ Identify guidelines that should be taught to improve visual health.

a. _____

b. _____

c. _____

d. _____

e. _____

➤ Describe the procedure for removing cerumen from the ear: _____

_____

_____

_____

➤ Describe the following types of hearing aids:

In-the-canal (ITC) _____

_____

_____

_____

In-the-ear (ITE) _____

_____

_____

_____

Behind-the-ear (BTE) _____

_____

_____

_____

➤ Describe three interventions used to remove secretions from the nose.

a. _____

b. _____

c. _____

☾ Evaluation

➤ Identify three outcomes for a client with eyes, ears, or nose problems.

a. _____

b. _____

c. _____

■ CLIENT'S ROOM ENVIRONMENT

Maintaining Comfort

➤ Identify four factors the nurse can control to create a more comfortable environment.

a. _____

b. _____

c. _____

d. _____

Room Equipment

➤ Describe the basic room equipment and the proper use of each:

Overbed table _____

_____

_____

Bedside table _____

_____

_____

Chairs _____

_____

_____

Lights _____

_____

_____

➤ Draw a simple stick figure to illustrate each of the following positions:

Fowler's

Semi-Fowler's

Trendelenburg

Reverse Trendelenburg

➤ Identify the points the nurse should remember when making a client's bed: _____

_____

_____

_____

REVIEW QUESTIONS

(The student should select the appropriate answer and cite the rationale for choosing that particular answer.)

1. Sweat glands, sebaceous glands, and hair follicles are found in which layer of skin?
   a. Epidermis
   b. Dermis
   c. Subcutaneous
   d. Fat

Answer (   ) Rationale: _____

_____

2. Mr. Gray is a 19-year-old client in the rehabilitation unit. He is completely paralyzed below the neck. The most appropriate bath for Mr. Gray is a:
   a. Partial bed bath
   b. Complete bed bath
   c. Sitz bath
   d. Tepid bath

Answer (   ) Rationale: _____

_____

3. All of the following will help maintain skin integrity in the older adult except:
   a. Environmental air that is cold and dry
   b. Use of warm water and mild cleansing agents for bathing
   c. Bathing every other day
   d. Drinking 8-10 glasses of water a day

Answer (   ) Rationale: _____

_____

_____

4. When preparing to give complete AM care to a client, what would the nurse do first?
   a. Gather necessary equipment and supplies
   b. Remove client's gown or pajamas, while maintaining privacy
   c. Assess client's preferences for bathing practices
   d. Lower side rail and assist client in assuming a comfortable position

Answer (   ) Rationale: _____

_____

_____

5. A fungating lesion that appears on the sole of the foot and is caused by papillomavirus is know as:
   a. A callus
   b. A plantar's wart
   c. Athlete's foot
   d. Paronychia

Answer (   ) Rationale: _____

_____

_____

6. Mrs. Veech is a diabetic. Which intervention should be included in her teaching plan regarding foot care?
   a. Use a pumice stone to smooth corns and calluses
   b. File toenails straight across and square
   c. Apply powder to dry areas along the feet and between the toes
   d. Wear elastic stockings to improve circulation

Answer (   ) Rationale: _____

_____

_____

7. Permanent teeth begin to replace deciduous teeth at approximately:
   a. 4 years of age
   b. 5 years of age
   c. 6 years of age
   d. 7 years of age

Answer (   ) Rationale: _____

_____

_____

8. The nurse is performing mouth care for an unconscious client. What should the nurse do first?
   a. Assess for a gag reflex.
   b. Retract upper and lower teeth with a padded tongue blade.
   c. Put client in the Sims' position.
   d. Obtain a portable suction machine.

Answer (   ) Rationale: _____

_____

_____

9. A hair and scalp assessment reveals that John has head lice. An appropriate intervention would be:
   a. Shave hair off affected area.
   b. Place oil on the hair and scalp until all lice are dead.
   c. Shampoo with Kwell and repeat 12 to 24 hours later.
   d. Shampoo with regular shampoo and dry with hairdryer set at the hottest setting.

Answer (   ) Rationale: _____

_____

_____

10. Which of the following is not appropriate for the nurse assisting a client with soft contact lenses?
   a. Add a few drops of sterile saline to the eye before removing the lens.
   b. After sliding the lens off the cornea, pull the upper eyelid down gently to compress the lens.
   c. Rinse lenses with appropriate solution before reinserting.
   d. Position lenses for insertion so that they resemble a bowl that has a lip.

Answer (   ) Rationale: _____

_____

_____

11. After making the bed, the nurse should:
   a. Lower the bed as close to the floor as possible
   b. Secure the call light within the client's reach
   c. Assist the client to a comfortable position
   d. All of the above

Answer (   ) Rationale: _____

_____

_____

CLINICAL SITUATIONS

1. Mrs. Jones, a 70-year-old widow who lives alone, has been admitted to your unit. She is frail and unkempt. Her skin is extremely dry and cracked, with some reddened areas on the sacrum. Describe appropriate nursing interventions you would take in this situation. What other assessments are required?

_____

_____

_____

_____

_____

_____

_____

_____

_____

2. Mrs. Lee, a 50-year-old newly diagnosed diabetic, has long toenails and asks you to cut them. Describe the sequence of actions you would take, and give a rationale for each.

_____

_____

_____

_____

_____

_____

_____

_____

_____

Nutrition

Standards for the Joint Commission on Accreditation of Health Care Organizations require that health care practitioners collaborate with the client and each other to develop, implement, and evaluate a nutritional plan of care.

PRELIMINARY READING

Chapter 41, pp. 1089-1127

COMPREHENSIVE UNDERSTANDING

▮ PRINCIPLES OF NUTRITION

➤ List three requirements of the body for fuel.

a. _____

_____

b. _____

_____

c. _____

_____

➤ Define the following:

Metabolism _____

_____

_____

Anabolism _____

_____

_____

Catabolism _____

_____

_____

Basal metabolic rate (BMR) _____

_____

_____

_____

Nutrients _____

_____

_____

_____

Nutrient density _____

_____

_____

_____

➤ List the six categories of nutrients. Using an asterisk, identify the one that is most important.

a. _____

b. _____

c. _____

d. _____

e. _____

f. _____

Carbohydrates

➤ Each gram of carbohydrate produces _____ kilocalories (kcal).

➤ Identify the three classifications of carbohydrates.

a. _____

b. _____

c. _____

➤ Plants store carbohydrates as _____.

➤ Explain how carbohydrates are stored: _____

_____

_____

_____

➤ Carbohydrate metabolism consists of three main processes. List them.

a. _____

b. _____

c. _____

➤ The recommended range for carbohydrate intake in the diet is _____.

➤ Carbohydrate is the main source of fuel for the

_____, _____,

_____ and _____,

as well as the _____.

Proteins

➤ Proteins provide a source of energy _____ kcal/g and are essential for_____.

➤ The simplest form of protein is _____. Identify two forms of _____

_____.

➤ A complex protein is_____

_____.

➤ Explain the difference between complete and incomplete proteins: _____

_____

_____

_____

➤ Complete the grid below by listing three food sources for each protein classification:

➤ Briefly describe what is meant by each of the following:

Nitrogen balance _____

_____

_____

_____

Negative nitrogen balance _____

_____

_____

_____

Positive nitrogen balance _____

_____

_____

_____

➤ The required daily allowance of protein for an adult is _____.

Lipids

➤ Lipids (fats) are the most calorically dense nutrient, and they provide _____ kcal per gram.

➤ Lipids include fats that are _____ and oils that are _____.

➤ Identify the two basic types of lipids.

a. _____

b. _____

➤ Lipogenesis is _____.

Complete Proteins	Incomplete Proteins

➤ Define the following types of fats and give an example of each:

Saturated _____

_____

_____

Unsaturated _____

_____

_____

Polyunsaturated _____

_____

_____

➤ The body stores energy as _____.

➤ Nutritional guidelines recommend the adult dietary

lipid intake of no more than _____.

Water

➤ Water composes _____
of total body weight.

➤ _____ have the
greatest percentage of total body weight as water, and

_____ people have the least.

➤ Fluid needs are met by _____

and by water produced during _____.

Vitamins

➤ List the water-soluble vitamins: _____

_____.

➤ List the fat-soluble vitamins: _____

_____.

➤ Complete the grid on p. 270 by describing the function of the vitamin, three major food sources, and common manifestations of deficiency.

Minerals

➤ Complete the grid on p. 271 by describing the function of the mineral, three major food sources, and common manifestations of deficiency.

▌ DIGESTION

➤ Digestion of food consists of mechanical breakdown and chemical reactions by which food is reduced to its simplest form.

➤ Enzymes are _____.

➤ The following activities of digestion are interdependent. Explain each one:

Mechanical _____

_____

Chemical _____

_____

Hormonal _____

_____

➤ Match the food substance with the enzyme that aids its digestion.

Substance

a. Protein

b. Carbohydrate

c. Fat

Enzyme

a. Ptyalin _____

b. Pepsin _____

c Lipase _____

d. Polypeptidase _____

e. Amylase _____

f. Sucrase _____

g. Maltase _____

h. Lactase _____

i. Trypsin _____

➤ The major portion of digestion occurs in the

_____.

▌ ABSORPTION

➤ The primary source of absorption is the _____

_____.

➤ Absorption of water is the main function of the ____

_____.

➤ Describe a condition in which intestinal motility is

increased and absorption is decreased _____

_____

_____.

Nutrient	Function	Sources	Effects of Deficiency
B₁			
B₂			
Niacin			
B₆			
Folacin, folic acid, folate			
B₁₂			
Pantothenic acid			
Biotin			
C			
A			
D			
E			
K			

Nutrient	Function	Sources	Effects of Deficiency
Calcium			
Magnesium			
Phosphorus			
Copper			
Fluoride			
Iodine			
Iron			
Zinc			

Metabolism

➤ Explain the two types of metabolism:

Anabolism: _____

_____

_____

Catabolism: _____

_____

_____

_____

Storage

➤ The body's major form of stored energy is _____

_____, which is stored as

_____.

➤ Glycogen is _____

_____.

▮ ELIMINATION

➤ Feces contain _____

_____

_____

_____.

■ NUTRITION AND HEALTH PROMOTION

➤ Current dietary guidelines are based upon valuable scientific evidence, meal planning to provide a nutritionally adequate diet, and levels of intake of specific nutrients to maintain health.

Food Guide Pyramid

➤ Using the space at the bottom of the page, diagram and label the food guide pyramid developed by the U.S. Department of Agriculture (USDA).

Recommended Daily Allowances

➤ Define RDAs: _____

_____

_____

➤ Explain the significance of the National Labeling and

Education Act (NLEA) of 1990: _____

_____

_____

_____

Other Dietary Guidelines

➤ List the seven dietary guidelines for Americans issued by the USDA and the Department of Health and Human Services.

a. _____

_____

b. _____

_____

c. _____

_____

d. _____

_____

e. _____

_____

f. _____

_____

g. _____

_____

Alternative Food Patterns

➤ Define the following vegetarian diets:

Lactovegetarian _____

_____

Ovolactovegetarian _____

_____

Vegans _____

_____

Fruitarian _____

_____

DEVELOPMENTAL VARIABLES IN PROMOTING AND MAINTAINING HEALTHY NUTRITION

Infants

➤ An energy intake of approximately _____ kcal/kg is needed in the first half of infancy and

_____ kcal/kg in the second half.

➤ A full-term newborn is able to digest and absorb

_____

_____.

➤ Amylase is not present until _____ months of age.

➤ Infants need _____ ml/kg/day of fluid.

➤ List four nutrients that must be supplemented in the breast-fed infant.

a. _____

_____

b. _____

_____

c. _____

_____

d. _____

_____

➤ Explain why the following should not be used in infant formula:

Cow's milk _____

_____

Honey and corn syrup _____

_____

➤ List four indications of infant readiness to begin solid foods:

a. _____

b. _____

c. _____

d. _____

Toddlers and Preschoolers

➤ The toddler needs _____ calories but an increased amount of _____ in relation to body weight.

➤ Complete the grid below by indicating the minimum requirements for the toddler and preschooler.

Food Groups	Toddler	Preschool
Milk		
Fruit and vegetable		
Bread and cereal		
Meat		

School-age Children and Adolescents

➤ Complete the grid below by indicating the minimum requirements for school-age children and adolescents.

➤ Identify the common deficiencies in adolescents:

Girls _____

_____

Boys _____

_____

Fast-food eating _____

_____

Intense exercise _____

_____

Pregnancy _____

_____

Young and Middle Adults

➤ Obesity becomes a problem because of _____

_____

_____.

➤ Adult women who use oral contraceptives need extra

_____

_____.

➤ The energy requirements of pregnancy are related to

_____

_____.

➤ Explain the increased amounts of the following items that are required for pregnancy and lactation:

Pregnancy

Calories _____

_____

Calcium _____

_____

Iron _____

_____

Vitamins _____

_____

Fluids _____

_____

Lactation

Calories _____

_____

Protein _____

_____

Calcium _____

_____

Vitamins _____

_____

Fluids _____

_____

Older Adults

➤ List four factors influencing nutritional status of the older adult. Using an asterisk, identify one factor considered to be the most important.

a. _____

_____

_____

b. _____

_____

_____

Food Groups	School-Age Children	Adolescents
Milk		
Fruit and vegetable		
Bread and cereal		
Meat		

c. _____

_____

_____

d. _____

_____

_____

■ NUTRITION AND THE NURSING PROCESS

➤ Close daily contact with clients and their families enables nurses to make observations about their physical status, food intake, weight gain or loss, and responses to therapy.

Assessment

➤ List the four components of a nutritional assessment.

a. _____

b. _____

c. _____

d. _____

➤ Define *anthropometry:* _____

_____

_____

➤ Explain how to measure the following:

Wrist circumference _____

_____

_____

Mid-upper arm circumference _____

_____

_____

Triceps skinfold _____

_____

_____

Mid-upper arm muscle circumference _____

_____

_____

➤ Identify the common laboratory tests used to study

the nutritional status of a client: _____

_____

_____

_____

➤ List the five factors on which dietary history focuses.

a. _____

b. _____

c. _____

d. _____

e. _____

➤ List seven factors influencing dietary patterns.

a. _____

b. _____

c. _____

d. _____

e. _____

f. _____

g. _____

➤ Describe three ways that excessive alcohol ingestion may contribute to nutritional deficiencies.

a. _____

b. _____

c. _____

➤ For each assessment area, list at least two signs of poor nutrition.

General appearance

a. _____

b. _____

General vitality

a. _____

b. _____

Weight

a. _____

b. _____

Hair

a. _____

b. _____

Skin

a. _____

b. _____

Mouth

a. _____

b. _____

Eyes

a. _____

b. _____

Gastrointestinal function

a. _____

b. _____

Cardiovascular function

a. _____

b. _____

Neurological function

a. _____

b. _____

Musculoskeletal function

a. _____

b. _____

➤ List five conditions that predispose a client at risk to nutritional problems.

a. _____

b. _____

c. _____

d. _____

e. _____

➤ Explain why the following postoperative clients are at risk for nutritional problems:

Oral and throat surgery _____

_____

_____

_____

Stomach surgery _____

_____

_____

_____

Intestinal surgery _____

_____

_____

➤ Briefly explain why immobilized clients are at risk for

nutritional problems: _____

_____

_____

_____

Nursing Diagnosis

➤ List three potential or actual nursing diagnoses for altered nutritional status.

a. _____

b. _____

c. _____

Planning

➤ List four goals for a client with nutritional problems.

a. _____

b. _____

c. _____

d. _____

➤ List the five nutrients provided through parenteral nutrition (PN).

a. _____

b. _____

c. _____

d. _____

e. _____

➤ List three goals for a client receiving parenteral nutrition (PN).

a. _____

b. _____

c. _____

Implementation

➤ List three situations that occur in the hospital setting that influence nutritional intake.

a. _____

_____

b. _____

_____

c. _____

_____

➤ List five ways that a nurse can stimulate the client's appetite.

a. _____

_____

b. _____
_____

c. _____
_____

d. _____
_____

e. _____
_____

➤ List three nursing measures to foster an environment conducive to eating.

a. _____

b. _____

c. _____

➤ Identify the diet modifications necessary for the following diseases:

Gastrointestinal _____
_____
_____
_____

Cardiovascular _____
_____
_____
_____

Diabetes _____
_____
_____
_____

Renal _____
_____
_____
_____

Cancer _____
_____
_____
_____

HIV _____
_____
_____
_____

➤ Identify the psychosocial effects of special diets:
_____
_____
_____
_____

➤ Identify three nursing measures for a disabled client.

a. _____

b. _____

c. _____

➤ Identify the dietary counseling a nurse would give to a client being discharged with a diet prescription:
_____
_____
_____
_____

ENTERAL NUTRITION AND TUBE FEEDING

➤ Define *enteral nutrition:* _____
_____

➤ Explain the beneficial effect of enteral feedings as compared with parenteral nutrition:
_____
_____
_____
_____
_____
_____
_____

➤ Identify the clients suitable for the following types of formulas:

Protein _____
_____

Elemental, or peptide based _____
_____

Disease specific _____
_____

➤ Explain the following types of feeding tubes:

Nasogastric _____
_____

Gastrostomy _____

_____

Peg _____

➤ Identify the tube type preferred for enteral tube feedings: _____

➤ The most reliable method to test placement of a small bore feeding tube is _____.

➤ Explain a method that the nurse may use to test placement of a small-bore feeding tube: _____

_____

_____.

➤ List the four major complications of enteral feedings.

a. _____

b. _____

c. _____

d. _____

➤ List the three factors on which safe administration of parenteral nutrition depends:

a. _____

b. _____

c. _____

➤ Define *refeeding syndrome:* _____

_____

_____

_____

➤ Lipid emulsions are _____.

➤ The adverse reactions to lipid emulsion include ___

_____

_____.

➤ Briefly describe the rationale for each action associated with initiation and maintenance of total parenteral nutrition.

Trendelenburg position: _____

_____

_____

_____

Valsalva maneuver: _____

_____

_____

_____

Chest x-ray examination: _____

_____

_____

_____

Sterile technique and dressings: _____

_____

_____

_____

Infusion flow rate: _____

_____

_____

_____

Monitoring blood glucose every four hours: _____

_____

_____

_____

➤ List six potential complications of parenteral nutrition and the symptoms of each.

a. _____

b. _____

c. _____

d. _____

e. _____

f. _____

REVIEW QUESTIONS

(The student should select the appropriate answer and cite the rationale for choosing that particular answer.)

1. Which nutrient is the body's most preferred energy source?
   a. Protein
   b. Fat
   c. Carbohydrate
   d. Vitamin

Answer ( ) Rationale: _____

_____

_____

2. Positive nitrogen balance would occur in which condition?
   a. Infection
   b. Starvation
   c. Burn injury
   d. Pregnancy

Answer ( ) Rationale: _____
_____
_____

3. The major portion of absorption of nutrients occurs in the:
   a. Mouth
   b. Large intestine
   c. Small intestine
   d. Stomach

Answer ( ) Rationale: _____
_____
_____

4. Mrs. Nelson is talking with the nurse about the dietary needs of her 23-month-old daughter, Laura. Which of the following responses by the nurse would be appropriate:
   a. "Use skim milk to cut down on the fat in Laura's diet."
   b. "Laura should be drinking at least 1 quart of milk per day."
   c. "Laura needs fewer calories in relation to her body weight now than she did as an infant."
   d. "Laura needs less protein in her diet now because she isn't growing as fast."

Answer ( ) Rationale: _____
_____
_____

5. During which developmental period are snacks a necessity to compensate for increased growth and caloric needs?
   a. Preschool
   b. School-age
   c. Adolescence
   d. Young adulthood

Answer ( ) Rationale: _____
_____
_____

6. The nurse is evaluating lab results on a newly admitted client. Which of the following would be indicative of a protein deficit?
   a. Elevated hemoglobin level
   b. Decreased hematocrit level
   c. Elevated transferrin level
   d. Decreased albumin level

Answer ( ) Rationale: _____
_____
_____

7. All of the following clients are at risk for alteration in nutrition *except:*
   a. Client J, who is 86 years old, lives alone, and has poorly fitting dentures
   b. Client K, who has been NPO for 7 days following bowel surgery and is receiving 3000 ml, 10% dextrose per day
   c. Client L, whose weight is 10% above his ideal body weight
   d. Client M, who is a 17-year-old woman, weighs 90 lb, and frequently complains about her baby fat

Answer ( ) Rationale: _____
_____
_____

8. Mr. Phillips has just returned to the unit after undergoing eye surgery and has bandages on both eyes. When his lunch tray is delivered, the best intervention for the nurse would be to:
   a. Open all containers and leave, letting him be as independent as possible.
   b. Feed him, allowing sufficient time for tasting, chewing, and swallowing.
   c. Tell him the position of food according to the hours of a clock.
   d. Keep him on a liquid diet until the bandages are removed.

Answer ( ) Rationale: _____
_____
_____

9. Which of the following is the most accurate method of bedside confirmation of placement of a small-bore nasogastric tube?
   a. Auscultate epigastrium for gurgling or bubbling.
   b. Test Ph of withdrawn gastric contents.
   c. Assess client's ability to speak.
   d. Assess the length of the tube that is outside the client's nose.

Answer ( ) Rationale: _____
_____
_____

10. Caring for the client receiving total parenteral nutrition would include all of the following *except:*
    a. Changing infusion tubing every 24 hours
    b. Checking vital signs every four hours
    c. Performing blood glucose monitoring every 6 hours
    d. Changing venipuncture dressing every 24 hours

Answer (   ) Rationale: _____

_____

_____

11. A client who has been hospitalized after experiencing a heart attack will most likely receive a diet consisting of:
    a. Low fat, low sodium, and high carbohydrates
    b. Low fat, high protein, and high carbohydrates
    c. Low fat, low sodium, and low carbohydrates
    d. Liquids for several days, progressing to a soft and then a regular diet

Answer (   ) Rationale: _____

_____

_____

CLINICAL SITUATIONS

1. You are assigned to work in a well-baby clinic. You are doing an assessment on 8-month-old John. His weight is 12 lb. His mother states that he "mostly drinks milk." What additional assessment data do you need to determine the presence of a nutritional deficit.

_____

_____

_____

_____

_____

_____

_____

_____

_____

2. You are receiving a morning report on Mr. Karl. Nasogastric tube feedings have been ordered. The night nurse stated that his abdomen was distended, and she withheld the 0500 feeding. What assessments do you need to make about Mr. Karl's tolerance to the tube feeding, the placement of the tube, and the resumption of tube feedings?

_____

_____

_____

_____

_____

_____

_____

_____

Sleep

Achieving the best possible sleep quality is important for the promotion of good health as well as the recovery of ill individuals.

PRELIMINARY READING

Chapter 42, pp. 1128-1152

COMPREHENSIVE UNDERSTANDING

▮ SLEEP AND REST

➤ Define *rest:* _____

_____

_____

➤ Define *sleep:* _____

_____

_____

_____

Promoting Rest

➤ List three basic conditions required for proper rest.

a. _____

b. _____

c. _____

▮ PHYSIOLOGY OF SLEEP

➤ Sleep is a cyclical, physiological process that alternates with longer periods of wakefulness.

Circadian Rhythms

➤ Define the following cyclical rhythms:

Circadian _____

_____

Infradian _____

_____

Ultradian _____

_____

➤ The fluctuation and predictability of body temperature, heart rate, blood pressure, hormone secretion, sensory acuity, and mood depend on the maintenance of the 24-hour circadian cycle.

➤ List the common symptoms of a disturbance in the

sleep cycle: _____

_____

_____

Sleep Regulation

➤ Sleep involves a sequence of physiological states maintained by highly integrated central nervous system activity that is associated with changes in the

_____, _____,

_____, _____,

_____, and _____ systems.

➤ Complete the grid on the next page comparing the cerebral mechanisms responsible for sleep regulation.

➤ Explain the two phases of sleep:

NREM _____

_____

REM _____

_____

➤ Describe the characteristics of the following stages of sleep:

Stage 1 _____

_____

_____

_____

Stage 2 _____

_____

_____

_____

	Sleep Mechanisms	Arousal Mechanisms
Name		
Anatomical location		
Neurotransmitter		

Stage 3 _____

_____

_____

_____

Stage 4 _____

_____

_____

_____

REM _____

_____

_____

➤ Describe the normal adult sleep pattern: _____

_____

_____

_____

_____

■ FUNCTIONS OF SLEEP

➤ Sleep contributes to physiological and psychological restoration. Explain the following:

Cardiac function _____

_____

_____

_____

Hormones _____

_____

_____

_____

Conservation of energy _____

_____

_____

_____

Cognition _____

_____

_____

_____

Dreams

➤ Explain the functions of dreams: _____

_____

_____

_____

_____

Normal Sleep Requirements and Patterns

➤ Complete the grid listing the normal sleep patterns and rituals for the following developmental stages:

Developmental Stage	Sleep Patterns	Usual Rituals
Neonates		
Infants		
Toddlers		
Preschoolers		
School-age children		
Adolescents		
Young adults		
Middle adults		
Older adults		

∎ FACTORS AFFECTING SLEEP

➤ Physiological, psychological, and environmental factors can alter the quality and quantity of sleep.

Physical Illness

➤ Explain how the following conditions affect sleep:

Discomfort _____

_____

_____

Respiratory disease _____

_____

_____

_____

_____

Coronary artery disease _____

_____

_____

_____

Hypertension _____

_____

_____

Hypothyroidism _____

_____

_____

Hyperthyroidism _____

_____

_____

Nocturia _____

_____

_____

Restless legs syndrome _____

_____

_____

_____

Peptic ulcer disease _____

_____

_____

_____

Drugs and Substances

➤ Sleepiness and sleep deprivation are common side effects of medications. Describe how the following affect sleep:

Hypnotics _____

_____

_____

_____

Diuretics _____

_____

_____

_____

Antidepressants _____

_____

_____

_____

Alcohol _____

_____

_____

_____

Caffeine _____

_____

_____

_____

Beta-blockers _____

_____

_____

_____

Benzodiazepines _____

_____

_____

_____

Narcotics _____

_____

_____

_____

Lifestyle

➤ List four alterations in routine that can disrupt sleep patterns:

a. _____

b. _____

c. _____

d. _____

Usual Sleep Patterns and Excessive Daytime Sleepiness (EDS)

➤ EDS often results in _____,

_____, _____,

and _____.

Emotional Stress

➤ Explain how stress affects sleep: _____

_____

_____

_____

_____

Environment

➤ List and briefly describe three environmental factors that affect sleep.

a. _____

_____

_____

b. _____

_____

_____

c. _____

_____

_____

Exercise and Fatigue

➤ Explain how exercise promotes sleep: _____

_____

_____

_____

Food and Caloric Intake

➤ List and briefly describe five foods that affect sleep.

a. _____

_____

b. _____

_____

c. _____

_____

d. _____

_____

e. _____

_____

❙ SLEEP DISORDERS

➤ List and briefly describe the four major categories of sleep disorders.

a. _____

_____

b. _____

_____

c. _____

_____

d. _____

_____

Insomnia

➤ Define *insomnia:* _____

_____

_____

➤ List two situations that are associated with insomnia.

a. _____

_____

b. _____

_____

Sleep Apnea

➤ Define *sleep apnea:* _____

_____

_____

_____

➤ Define *obstructive sleep apnea:* _____

_____

_____

_____

➤ Define *central sleep apnea:* _____

_____

_____

_____

➤ Identify four treatment modalities for a client with sleep apnea.

a. _____

b. _____

c. _____

d. _____

Narcolepsy

➤ Define *narcolepsy:* _____
_____
_____
_____

➤ Define the following terms related to narcolepsy:

Cataplexy _____
_____
_____
_____

Hypnogic hallucinations _____
_____
_____
_____

➤ Identify the developmental stage in which narcolepsy symptoms first develop: _____
_____

➤ Identify three treatment modalities for the client with narcolepsy.

a. _____

b. _____

c. _____

Sleep Deprivation

➤ List four physiological and four psychological manifestations of sleep deprivation in the grid below.

Parasomnias

➤ Define *parasomnias:* _____
_____

➤ Describe the appropriate position for an infant to promote safe, restful sleep: _____
_____
_____
_____

➤ Define the following parasomnias:

Somnambulism _____
_____

Nocturnal enuresis _____
_____

Bruxism _____
_____

■ NURSING PROCESS AND SLEEP

Assessment

➤ Sleep is a subjective experience.
➤ Assessment is aimed at understanding the characteristics of any sleep problem and the client's usual sleep habits so that ways for promoting sleep can be incorporated into nursing care.

Physiological Symptoms	Psychological Symptoms

➤ List four areas to be assessed when obtaining a sleep history.

a. _____

b. _____

c. _____

d. _____

➤ List and briefly describe the six areas to be assessed with a client who has a sleeping problem.

a. _____

b. _____

c. _____

d. _____

e. _____

f. _____

➤ Give an example of three questions to ask clients with the following sleep disorders:

Insomnia _____

_____

_____

_____

_____

Sleep apnea _____

_____

_____

_____

_____

Narcolepsy _____

_____

_____

_____

_____

➤ List five physiological factors that might interfere with sleep.

a. _____

b. _____

c. _____

d. _____

e. _____

➤ List four life events that might interfere with sleep.

a. _____

b. _____

c. _____

d. _____

➤ List two emotional factors that might interfere with sleep.

a. _____

b. _____

➤ List four bedtime rituals that might interfere with sleep.

a. _____

b. _____

c. _____

d. _____

➤ List three environmental factors that might interfere with sleep.

a. _____

b. _____

c. _____

➤ List four behaviors a client may manifest with sleep deprivation.

a. _____

b. _____

c. _____

d. _____

Nursing Diagnosis

➤ List eight potential or actual nursing diagnoses for a client with a sleep disturbance.

a. _____

b. _____

c. _____

d. _____

e. _____

f. _____

g. _____

h. _____

Planning

➤ List four goals appropriate for a client needing rest or sleep.

a. _____

b. _____

c. _____

d. _____

Implementation

➤ Nursing interventions designed to improve the quality of a person's sleep are largely focused on health promotion.

➤ Clients require a sleeping environment with the following. Give two examples of each:

Room temperature and ventilation

a. _____

b. _____

Control of noise

a. _____

b. _____

Comfortable bed

a. _____

b. _____

Proper lighting

a. _____

b. _____

➤ List three bedtime rituals appropriate for the following:

Infants _____

_____

Toddlers and preschoolers _____

_____

Adults _____

_____

➤ List six comfort measures the nurse may initiate to promote a client's sleep.

a. _____

b. _____

c. _____

d. _____

e. _____

f. _____

➤ The nurse becomes a gatekeeper by postponing or rescheduling visits by family, asking consultants to reschedule visits, or questioning the frequency of certain procedures.

➤ For each of the following situations, give two examples of nursing measures that will promote sleep:

Physiological disturbances

a. _____

_____

b. _____

_____

Stress reduction

a. _____

_____

b. _____

_____

Use of bedtime snacks

a. _____

_____

b. _____

_____

➤ Briefly describe the effect of benzodiazepines in promoting sleep. _____

_____

➤ Identify three types of clients that should not use benzodiazepines, and explain why.

a. _____

b. _____

c. _____

➤ The regular use of sleeping medication can lead to

_____

_____.

➤ Identify eight teaching strategies that the client can use to follow proper sleep hygiene habits at home.

a. _____

_____

b. _____

_____

c. _____

_____

d. _____

_____

e. _____

_____

f. _____

_____

g. _____

_____

h. _____

_____

Evaluation

➤ List three outcomes for a client with a sleep disturbance.

a. _____

b. _____

c. _____

REVIEW QUESTIONS

(The student should select the appropriate answer and cite the rationale for choosing that particular answer.)

1. The 24-hour day-night cycle is known as:
   a. Circadian rhythm
   b. Infradium rhythm
   c. Ultradian rhythm
   d. NonREM rhythm

Answer ( ) Rationale: _____

_____

_____

2. If sleep loss has occurred, in which stage will the sleeper spend most of the night?
   a. Stage 1
   b. Stage 3
   c. Stage 4
   d. REM

Answer ( ) Rationale: _____

_____

_____

3. Mrs. Miller tells the nurse that her 75-year-old mother is experiencing sleep difficulties. Which of the following would be an inappropriate nursing response?
   a. "The total sleep time for the older adult averages 6 to 7 hours distributed throughout the day."
   b. "With increasing age, sleep quality deteriorates."
   c. "The older adult requires more time to fall asleep."
   d. "Generally, the elderly are more difficult to arouse."

Answer ( ) Rationale: _____

_____

_____

4. Which of the following is true of the sleep requirements of infants?
   a. Infants develop a nighttime pattern of sleep by 3 to 4 weeks of age.
   b. Bottle-fed babies usually sleep less than breast-fed babies.
   c. A 6-month-old infant averages 18 hours of sleep per day.
   d. Active infants sleep less than quiet infants.

Answer ( ) Rationale: _____

_____

_____

5. Which of the following substances will promote normal sleep patterns?
   a. L-tryptophan
   b. Beta-blockers
   c. Alcohol
   d. Narcotics

Answer ( ) Rationale: _____

_____

_____

6. All of the following are symptoms of sleep deprivation *except:*
   a. Hyperactivity
   b. Irritability
   c. Rise in body temperature
   d. Decreased motivation

Answer ( ) Rationale: _____

_____

_____

7. Mrs. Peterson complains of difficulty falling asleep, awakening earlier than desired, and not feeling rested. She attributes these problems to leg pain that is secondary to her arthritis. What would be the appropriate nursing diagnosis for her?
   a. Sleep pattern disturbances related to arthritis
   b. Fatigue related to leg pain
   c. Knowledge deficit regarding sleep hygiene measures
   d. Sleep pattern disturbances related to chronic leg pain

Answer (　) Rationale: _____

_____

_____

8. The nurse is planning care for the client with sleep pattern disturbance related to environmental disturbances and sleep habit interruption. Which intervention would be appropriate?
   a. Turn off all lights in the client's room.
   b. Synchronize schedules for medications and treatments to minimize interruptions.
   c. Encourage exercise immediately before bedtime.
   d. Discuss with client the advantages of long-term benzodiazepine use.

Answer (　) Rationale: _____

_____

_____

9. Mr. Jackson expresses concern that his newborn son is sleeping too much. The nurse's initial response should be:
   a. "Don't worry, most newborns sleep a lot."
   b. "You sound concerned; let's examine how many hours he's actually sleeping."
   c. "You need to discuss this with his pediatrician."
   d. "Please have your wife call me to discuss this."

Answer (　) Rationale: _____

_____

_____

10. A nursing care plan for a client with sleep problems has been implemented. All of the following would be expected outcomes *except:*
   a. Client reports no episodes of awakening during the night.
   b. Client falls asleep within 1 hour of going to bed.
   c. Client reports satisfaction with amount of sleep.
   d. Client rates sleep as an 8 or above on the visual analog scale.

Answer (　) Rationale: _____

_____

_____

CLINICAL SITUATIONS

1. You are the nurse working in the outpatient medical clinic for a small community hospital. A patient who has recently been diagnosed with cancer is in for testing and is accompanied by his wife. The patient has had a great deal of pain lately. The wife's appearance is listless. She has difficulty following the conversation with her husband. What areas of assessment would you include for this family? What is the potential sleep problem they may be experiencing?

_____

_____

_____

_____

_____

_____

_____

_____

2. Ms. Sims is a 32-year-old account executive with a major corporation. She has been moving up the corporate ladder for a number of years. She travels frequently, sometimes to Europe. She freely admits that her sleep schedule is erratic because of frequent, late evening meetings. She has trouble falling asleep at night because she is so "wound up." She knows that she needs to be getting more sleep. "I just don't feel that well in the morning. It takes me awhile to get energized." Ms. Sims drinks at least 10 cups of coffee daily. What factors in Ms. Sim's history suggest a sleep disturbance problem may exist? What additional factors would you like to assess about her? Develop a plan of care based on your findings.

_____

_____

_____

_____

_____

_____

_____

_____

_____

Chapter 43 | Comfort

Pain is subjective. No two persons experience pain in the same way, and no two painful events create identical responses or feelings.

PRELIMINARY READING

Chapter 43, pp. 1153-1190

COMPREHENSIVE UNDERSTANDING

▌ COMFORT

➤ Define *comfort,* as described by Yolcaba (1991): ____

_____

_____

_____

➤ A holistic view of comfort helps to identify four contexts. Explain each one.

Physical: _____

_____

_____

_____

Social: _____

_____

_____

_____

Psychospiritual: _____

_____

_____

_____

Environmental: _____

_____

_____

_____

▌ NATURE OF PAIN

➤ Define *pain* as described by Mahon (1994): _____

_____

_____

_____

➤ Identify the four defining attributes for the pain experience (Mahon):

a. _____

_____

b. _____

_____

c. _____

_____

d. _____

_____

Prejudices and Misconceptions

➤ The medical model of illness describes pain as ____

_____

_____

_____

➤ List the seven common biases and misconceptions about pain.

a. _____

b. _____

c. _____

d. _____

e. _____

f. _____

g. _____

■ PHYSIOLOGY OF PAIN

➤ Pain is a complex mixture of physical, emotional, and behavioral reactions.
➤ The three physiological components of pain are

_____, _____,

and _____.

Reception

➤ All cellular damage caused by _____,

_____, _____,

or _____ stimuli results in the release of painful substances.

➤ Define *nociceptor:* _____

_____

_____

➤ Define *pain threshold:* _____

_____

_____

_____

➤ Compare the two types of peripheral nerve fibers responsible for conducting painful stimuli by completing the grid below.
➤ Identify the neurophysiological function of the following neuroregulators:

Substance P _____

_____

_____

_____

Prostaglandins _____

_____

_____

_____

Serotonin _____

_____

_____

_____

Endorphins _____

_____

_____

Bradykinin _____

_____

_____

➤ Describe the basic concept underlying the gate-control theory of pain: _____

_____

_____

_____

_____

Type	A Fibers	C Fibers
Fiber type		
Myelination		
Transmission speed		
Nature of pain message		

Perception

➤ Perception is the point at which _____
_____.

➤ List the three interactional systems of pain perception described by Meinhart and McCaffery (1983).

a. _____

b. _____

c. _____

Reaction

➤ Stimulation of the autonomic nervous system results in physiological responses to pain. Give five examples of each and their effect:

Sympathetic stimulation

a. _____
b. _____
c. _____
d. _____
e. _____

Parasympathetic stimulation

a. _____
b. _____
c. _____
d. _____
e. _____

➤ Identify four behavioral changes that occur when the client experiences pain, and give two examples of each.

a. _____
_____
_____

b. _____
_____
_____

c. _____
_____
_____

d. _____
_____
_____

➤ Define *pain tolerance:* _____
_____
_____

➤ Describe the pain pattern for the following disorders:

Kidney disease _____

Angina pectoris _____

Ruptured intravertebral disk _____

Gastric ulcer _____

Trigeminal neuralgia _____

■ ACUTE AND CHRONIC PAIN

➤ List four characteristics of acute pain.

a. _____
b. _____
c. _____
d. _____

➤ List four symptoms associated with chronic pain.

a. _____
b. _____
c. _____
d. _____

➤ Define *intractable pain:* _____
_____

➤ Define *euphoria:* _____
_____

➤ Remission is _____,
and exacerbation is _____.

■ FACTORS INFLUENCING PAIN

Age

➤ Explain how the following types of clients react to pain:

Young children _____
_____
_____

Toddlers and preschoolers _____

_____

_____

Older adults _____

_____

_____

➤ Identify five reasons why older clients may not report pain.

a. _____

b. _____

c. _____

d. _____

e. _____

Gender

➤ Describe the cultural influences on gender in relation

to expressing pain: _____

_____

_____

Culture

➤ Explain the different meanings and attitudes associated with pain with regard to the following cultural
groups:

Americans _____

_____

_____

_____

Mexican-Americans _____

_____

_____

_____

Chinese _____

_____

_____

➤ Briefly explain the following factors that influence
pain:

Meaning of Pain _____

_____

_____

Attention _____

_____

_____

Anxiety _____

_____

_____

_____

Fatigue _____

_____

_____

_____

Previous experience _____

_____

_____

_____

Coping style

a. Internal loci of control _____

_____

_____

b. External loci of control _____

_____

_____

_____

Family and Social Support _____

_____

_____

_____

■ NURSING PROCESS AND PAIN

➤ Pain management extends beyond pain relief, encom-

passing the client's _____,

_____, and _____.

Assessment

➤ Complete the following grid describing the location,
characteristics, and examples of causes of pain.

Location	Characteristics	Causes
Superficial		
Deep visceral		
Referred		
Radiating		

➤ For clients with chronic pain, assessment should be

focused on _____,

_____, and _____
dimensions of the pain experience and on its history
and context.

➤ List four examples of nonverbal expressions of pain:

_____, _____,

_____, _____.

➤ Cognitively impaired clients require simple assessment approaches involving close observation of behavior changes.

➤ List and briefly describe the three phases of the pain
experience.

a. _____

_____

b. _____

_____

c. _____

_____

➤ Briefly explain the following common characteristics
of pain:

Onset and duration _____

_____

_____

_____

Location _____

_____

_____

_____

Severity _____

_____

_____

_____

Quality _____

_____

_____

_____

Pain pattern _____

_____

_____

_____

Concomitant symptoms _____

_____

_____

_____

➤ Describe the following descriptive scales for measuring the severity of pain:

Verbal descriptor scale (VDS) _____

_____

_____

_____

Numerical rating scale (NRS) _____

_____

_____

_____

Visual analog scale (VAS) _____

_____

_____

_____

Faces scale _____

_____

_____

_____

➤ When a client has pain. the nurse should assess

_____, _____,

and _____.

➤ Identify the behavioral effects the nurse should assess when a client has pain.

a. _____

b. _____

c. _____

d. _____

➤ Explain how pain can influence activities of daily living in regard to the following:

Sleep _____

_____

_____

_____

Hygiene _____

_____

_____

_____

Sexual relations _____

_____

_____

_____

Employment _____

_____

_____

_____

Social activities _____

_____

_____

➤ Any factor (neurological status) that interrupts or influences normal pain reception or perception affects the client's awareness and response to pain.

➤ List three therapies to influence pain perception and response.

a. _____

_____

b. _____

_____

c. _____

_____

Nursing Diagnosis

➤ List 10 potential or actual nursing diagnoses related to a client in pain.

a. _____

b. _____

c. _____

d. _____

e. _____

f. _____

g. _____

h. _____

i. _____

j. _____

Planning

➤ List five goals appropriate for the client experiencing pain.

a. _____

b. _____

c. _____

d. _____

e. _____

➤ To write an effective care plan, the nurse establishes the following for a client with pain. Explain each one:

Therapeutic relationship _____

_____

_____

_____

_____

Education _____

_____

_____

_____

_____

Implementation

➤ List the general guidelines for individualizing approaches to a client's pain relief:

_____

_____

_____

_____

_____

_____

_____

_____

_____

_____

➤ List three ways that a nurse can convey caring to a client in pain.

a. _____

b. _____

c. _____

➤ Explain the following two types of touching behaviors:

Task-oriented _____

_____

_____

Affective _____

_____

_____

➤ Define the holistic health approach to pain control:

_____

_____

_____

➤ Three holistic health approaches are _____,

_____, and _____.

➤ Define *therapeutic touch:* _____

_____

_____

_____

➤ The four basic steps to therapeutic touch are_____

_____, _____,

_____, and _____.

➤ Briefly explain how acupuncture is effective in pain control: _____

_____

_____

_____

➤ The five types of relaxation techniques for a client in pain are _____, _____,

_____, _____,

and _____.

➤ Relaxation techniques are taught only when the client is not in acute discomfort because _____

_____

_____.

➤ Briefly explain how the nurse would lead a client through guided imagery: _____

_____

_____

_____

_____

➤ Briefly explain how the nurse would guide a client through progressive relaxation exercises: _____

_____

_____

_____

_____

➤ Pain can impair the ability to perform self-care activities. Describe the nursing measures that are appropriate: _____

_____

_____

_____

_____

_____

_____

Nonpharmacological Pain-relief Measures

➤ Nonpharmacological pain-relief measures include the following. Explain the goal of each:

Cognitive-behavioral _____

_____

_____

_____

Physical agents _____

_____

_____

_____

➤ The AHCPR guidelines for acute pain management cite nonpharmacological interventions to be appropriate for clients who meet certain criteria. List those criteria.

a. _____

b. _____

c. _____

d. _____

e. _____

➤ List the information the nurse would give to the client to prevent misinterpretation of the painful event and promote understanding of what to expect.

a. _____

b. _____

c. _____

d. _____

e. _____

f. _____

➤ Define *distraction*, and list one disadvantage and advantage of using distraction: _____

_____

_____

_____

_____

_____

➤ Describe the effects of using music as a distraction to control pain: _____

_____

_____

_____

_____

➤ List five ways to use music effectively.

a. _____

b. _____

c. _____

d. _____

e. _____

➤ Define the following pain-relief measures and the rationale for their use:

Biofeedback _____

_____

_____

_____

Self-hypnosis _____

_____

_____

_____

Reducing pain perception _____

_____

_____

_____

Cutaneous stimulation _____

_____

_____

➤ What is *TENS*, and how is it believed to reduce pain?

_____

_____

_____

_____

Pharmacological Pain Therapy

➤ Analgesics are the most common method of pain relief.
➤ Identify the three types of analgesics, and explain what they are generally prescribed for.

a. _____

_____

b. _____

_____

c. _____

_____

➤ List the seven characteristics of an ideal analgesic.

a. _____

b. _____

c. _____

d. _____

e. _____

f. _____

g. _____

➤ Describe four major principles for analgesic administration.

a. _____

b. _____

c. _____

d. _____

➤ Define *PCA:* _____

_____

➤ Describe three benefits of PCA.

a. _____

b. _____

c. _____

➤ Describe what a local anesthetic is, and give its physiological properties: _____

_____

_____

_____

➤ Identify four types of local anesthesic.

a. _____

b. _____

c. _____

d. _____

➤ List the seven advantages of an epidural analgesia.

a. _____

b. _____

c. _____

d. _____

e. _____

f. _____

g. _____

➤ List four goals and one action for each goal related to the care of a client with epidural infusions.

a. _____

b. _____

c. _____

d. _____

➤ List five client teaching strategies for the safe and effective use of PCAs.

a. _____

b. _____

c. _____

d. _____

e. _____

➤ Explain the following surgical measures used to relieve pain:

Dorsal rhizotomy _____

_____

_____

Chordotomy _____

_____

_____

_____

➤ Define *intractable pain:* _____

_____

➤ Identify the three-step approach to cancer pain management recommended by the World Health Organization (1990).

a. _____

b. _____

c. _____

➤ Identify four conditions in which continuous infusion of morphine is recommended.

a. _____

b. _____

c. _____

d. _____

➤ List four guidelines for safe administration of morphine sulfate via ambulatory infusion pumps.

a. _____

b. _____

c. _____

d. _____

➤ Define the following types of pain clinics:

Syndrome-oriented _____

_____

_____

_____

Modality-oriented _____

_____

_____

_____

➤ Explain hospice programs: _____

_____

_____

_____

Evaluation

➤ Identify three evaluative criteria in determining the outcomes of pain-relief measures.

a. _____

b. _____

c. _____

REVIEW QUESTIONS

(The student should select the appropriate answer and cite the rationale for choosing that particular answer.)

1. Pain is a protective mechanism warning of tissue injury and is largely a (an):
   a. Symptom of a severe illness or disease
   b. Subjective experience
   c. Objective experience
   d. Acute symptom of short duration

Answer ( ) Rationale: _____

_____

_____

2. A substance that can cause analgesia when it attaches to opiate receptors in the brain is:
   a. Substance P
   b. Serotonin
   c. Prostaglandin
   d. Endorphin

Answer ( ) Rationale: _____

_____

_____

3. Which of the following is true of pain?
   a. Children are typically overmedicated for pain.
   b. African-Americans express pain more often than European-Americans.
   c. Emotionally healthy persons are usually able to tolerate moderate pain better than those less stable emotionally.
   d. Men and women differ significantly in their respective pain responses.

Answer ( ) Rationale: _____

_____

_____

4. To adequately assess the quality of a client's pain, which statement by the nurse would be appropriate?
   a. "Tell me what your pain feels like."
   b. "Is your pain a crushing sensation?"
   c. "How long have you had this pain?"
   d. "Is it a sharp pain or a dull pain?"

Answer ( ) Rationale: _____

_____

_____

5. Mr. Ricardo has an epidural catheter in place and is receiving morphine sulfate through it for postoperative pain. When the nurse enters the room, Mr. Ricardo is short of breath, and his respirations are 12 per minute (baseline is 18 per minute). What action should the nurse take first?
   a. Call the physician immediately.
   b. Speak to Mr. Ricardo in a quiet tone of voice, and reassure him that his anxiety will ease.
   c. Stop the morphine infusion.
   d. Reposition Mr. Ricardo and offer him a backrub.

Answer ( ) Rationale: _____

_____

_____

6. Which of the following descriptions of pain is the one given by the International Association for the Study of Pain (IASP)?
   a. Easily measured and described
   b. Rarely influenced by psychosocial and cultural factors
   c. A protective mechanism or warning of tissue damage
   d. Associated only with acute illness or disease states

Answer ( ) Rationale: _____

_____

_____

7. The use of client distraction in pain control is based on the principle that:
   a. Small C fibers transmit impulses via the spinothalamic tract.
   b. The reticular formation can send inhibitory signals to gating mechanisms.
   c. Large A fibers compete with pain impulses to close gates to painful stimuli.
   d. Transmission of pain impulses from the spinal cord to the cerebral cortex can be inhibited.

Answer ( ) Rationale: _____

_____

_____

8. Pain that has periods of remission and exacerbation would most appropriately be described as:
   a. Acute
   b. Intractable
   c. Chronic
   d. Psychosomatic

Answer ( ) Rationale: _____

_____

_____

9. Teaching a child about painful procedures is best achieved by:
   a. Early warnings of the anticipated pain
   b. Storytelling about the upcoming procedure
   c. Relevant play directed toward procedure activities
   d. Avoiding explanations until the pain is experienced

Answer ( ) Rationale: _____

_____

_____

10. Which action is appropriate when using music to control pain?
    a. Encourage the client to concentrate on the music's rhythm.
    b. When pain is acute, reduce the volume.
    c. When the client's mood is low, select music that is upbeat.
    d. Avoid selecting music based on client age and background.

Answer ( ) Rationale: _____

_____

_____

11. The nurse has taught a relaxation technique to a client with chronic tension headaches. The client subsequently develops a tension headache and finds that the technique is ineffective in reducing pain. The best action by the nurse would be to:
    a. Tell the client that the technique was probably done incorrectly.
    b. Teach the client a new technique because this one is ineffective.
    c. Inform the client that relaxation techniques are inappropriate for tension headaches.
    d. Assure the client that the technique may need to be practiced repeatedly to be effective.

Answer (   ) Rationale: _____
_____
_____

12. Which statement about analgesic administration is correct?
    a. Narcotic injections provide longer, more sustained relief for clients with chronic pain.
    b. The same dose of a drug, when administered by a different route, will produce the same level of analgesia.
    c. The best time to administer analgesics is after the client has been active.
    d. Severe pain requires a greater amount of analgesic for relief.

Answer (   ) Rationale: _____
_____
_____

CLINICAL SITUATIONS

1. Mr. Jasper and Mr. Stern are clients experiencing back pain. Mr. Jasper's pain resulted from falling off a ladder 48 hours ago. Mr. Stern's pain has been bothering him for more than eight months with no known cause.
    a. As the nurse caring for both clients, how might you anticipate differences in assessment and treatment.

    _____
    _____
    _____
    _____
    _____

    b. What might influence your approach to assessment if Mr. Stern were 39 rather than 80 years of age?

    _____
    _____
    _____

2. Mr. Lake is a 45-year-old man who experienced a traumatic injury to his left arm following an industrial accident 24 hours ago. His arm is in a very bulky dressing, and pain is aggravated when he lies on his left side. He has an intravenous line with a continuous infusion of IV fluids in his right arm. What non-pharmacologic pain-relief measures might be helpful for Mr. Lake?

    _____
    _____
    _____
    _____
    _____
    _____

Chapter 44

Oxygenation

The cardiac and respiratory systems function to supply the body's oxygen demands.

PRELIMINARY READING

Chapter 44, pp. 1191-1246

COMPREHENSIVE UNDERSTANDING

■ CARDIOVASCULAR PHYSIOLOGY

➤ The function of the cardiac system is to deliver

_____, _____,

and other _____ and to

remove the _____ through the

_____, _____,

and the _____.

Structure and Function

➤ The right ventricle pumps blood through the _____

_____ while the left ventricle

pumps blood to the _____,
supplying oxygen and nutrients to the tissues and removing wastes from the body.

➤ Identify three conditions that decrease myocardial
pump effectiveness, and explain the results of these
conditions.

a. _____

b. _____

c. _____

➤ The chambers of the heart fill during _____

_____ and empty during _____.

➤ Describe the Frank-Starling law of the heart: _____

_____

_____

_____

➤ Briefly describe the myocardial blood flow through the

heart: _____

_____

_____

_____

_____

_____

➤ Describe the following types of circulation:

Coronary artery _____

_____

_____

_____

_____

_____

Systemic _____

_____

_____

_____

_____

_____

➤ Give a description of the following cardiac terms:

Cardiac output _____

_____

_____

_____

Cardiac index _____

_____

_____

_____

Stroke volume _____

_____

_____

_____

Preload _____

_____

_____

_____

Afterload _____

_____

_____

_____

Myocardial contractility _____

_____

_____

_____

Conduction System

➤ The autonomic nervous system influences the rate of impulse generation as well as the speed of transmission through the conductive pathway and the strength of atrial and ventricular contractions.

➤ Describe how the following affect the conduction system of the heart:

Sympathetic nerve fibers _____

_____

_____

_____

Parasympathetic nerve fibers _____

_____

_____

_____

➤ Diagram and label the electrical conduction system of the heart:

➤ Diagram and label the components of the ECG waveform for normal sinus rhythm (NSR):

▌ RESPIRATORY PHYSIOLOGY

➤ The three steps in the process of oxygenation are

_____, _____,

and _____.

Structure and Function

➤ The _____, _____,

_____, and _____

are essential for ventilation, perfusion, and exchange
of respiratory gases.

Ventilation

➤ Define *ventilation:* _____

_____

_____

➤ Define the following terms related to the work of
breathing:

Compliance _____

_____

_____

_____

Surfactant _____

_____

_____

_____

Airway resistance _____

_____

_____

Expiration _____

_____

_____

Accessory muscles _____

_____

_____

_____

➤ List four conditions that may show variations in
lung volumes.

a. _____

b. _____

c. _____

d. _____

➤ Gases are moved into and out of the lungs through
pressure changes. Describe the changes that must occur

to facilitate air into the lungs: _____

_____

_____

_____

Perfusion

➤ Define *perfusion:* _____

_____

_____

_____

➤ Briefly describe pulmonary circulation: _____

_____

_____

_____

_____

_____

➤ Identify the normal distribution of pressures within

the pulmonary circulation: _____

_____

_____

_____

Exchange of Respiratory Gases

➤ Respiratory gases are exchanged in the _____

_____ and the _____
of the body tissues.

➤ Define *diffusion:* _____

_____

➤ The rate of diffusion can be affected by _____

_____.

➤ List four factors required for oxygen transport and
delivery.

a. _____

b. _____

c. _____

d. _____

➤ Describe the breakdown of carbon dioxide as it is diffused into the red blood cells: _____

_____

_____

_____

_____

Regulation of Respiration

➤ Describe the main purpose of respiratory regulation:

_____

_____

_____

_____

➤ List and briefly describe two regulatory mechanisms of respiration.

a. _____

_____

_____

b. _____

_____

_____

■ FACTORS AFFECTING OXYGENATION

➤ List the four factors that influence oxygenation.

a. _____

b. _____

c. _____

d. _____

Physiological Factors

➤ Describe the mechanism affecting oxygenation in the following physical conditions:

Fever _____

_____

Anemia _____

_____

Heart failure _____

_____

Stroke _____

_____

Rib fracture _____

_____

Hypovolemia _____

_____

Pregnancy _____

_____

Muscular dystrophy _____

_____

Cigarette smoking _____

_____

Kyphosis _____

_____

Obesity _____

_____

Myasthenia gravis _____

➤ List the basic mechanisms contributing to anemia.

a. _____

b. _____

c. _____

➤ The clinical findings of anemia are _____

_____

_____

_____.

➤ Identify three situations that would decrease the fraction of inspired oxygen concentration.

a. _____

b. _____

c. _____

➤ Damage to the spinal cord can affect respiration in two ways. Name and describe them:

a. _____

_____

_____

b. _____

_____

_____

Developmental Factors

➤ List at least one physiological factor influencing tissue oxygenation for each developmental level listed.

Premature infant: _____

_____

_____

_____

Infant and toddler: _____

_____

_____

_____

School-age child and adolescent: _____

_____

_____

_____

Young and middle-age adult: _____

_____

_____

_____

Older adult: _____

_____

_____

_____

Behavioral Factors

➤ Briefly describe how the following behavioral (lifestyle) factors influence respiratory function:

Nutrition _____

_____

_____

_____

Exercise _____

_____

_____

_____

Cigarette smoking _____

_____

_____

_____

Substance abuse _____

_____

_____

_____

Environmental Factors

➤ List four occupational pollutants.

a. _____

b. _____

c. _____

d. _____

➤ A continuous state of anxiety increases the body's metabolic rate and oxygen demand.

▌ ALTERATIONS IN CARDIAC FUNCTIONING

➤ Alterations in cardiac functioning are caused by illnesses and conditions that affect _____,

_____, _____,

_____, and _____.

Disturbances in Conduction

➤ Define *dysrhythmias:* _____

_____

_____

➤ Briefly describe the following dysrhythmias:

Sinus tachycardia _____

_____

_____

_____

Sinus bradycardia _____

_____

_____

Sinus dysrhythmia _____

_____

_____

_____

PSVT _____

_____

_____

_____

PVCs _____

_____

_____

_____

Ventricular tachycardia _____

_____

_____

Altered Cardiac Output

➤ Failure of the myocardium to eject sufficient volume to the systemic and pulmonary circulations can result in left-sided and right-sided failure. Complete the grid below.

Impaired Valvular Function

➤ Define *valvular heart disease:* _____

_____

_____

_____

➤ Define *stenosis:* _____

_____

➤ Define *regurgitation:* _____

_____

Myocardial Ischemia

➤ Define the following:

Myocardial ischemia _____

_____

_____

_____

Angina pectoris _____

_____

_____

_____

Myocardial infarction _____

_____

_____

_____

➤ Describe the chest pain associated with myocardial infarction: _____

_____

_____

_____

■ ALTERATIONS IN RESPIRATORY FUNCTIONING

➤ The three primary alterations in respiratory function are _____, _____, and _____.
Complete the grid on the next page.

➤ Define the following terms:

Cyanosis _____

_____

Central cyanosis _____

_____

Peripheral cyanosis _____

_____

Type of Failure	Clinical Findings
Left-sided	
Right-sided	

NURSING PROCESS AND OXYGENATION

Assessment

➤ The nursing assessment of a client's cardiopulmonary functioning should include data from the following areas. Briefly explain each.

Nursing history _____

_____

_____

Physical examination _____

_____

_____

_____

Laboratory and diagnostic tests _____

_____

_____

_____

NURSING HISTORY
➤ List eight areas to include in a nursing history for oxygenation.

a. _____

b. _____

c. _____

d. _____

e. _____

f. _____

g. _____

h. _____

➤ Define *dyspnea:* _____

_____

➤ Identify the differences between the two types of dyspnea:

Physiological _____

_____

Pathological _____

_____

➤ Define *orthopnea:* _____

_____

➤ Define *cough:* _____

_____

➤ Define *productive cough:* _____

_____

Alterations	Causes	Signs and Symptoms
Hyperventilation		
Hypoventilation		
Hypoxia		

➤ List the five major characteristics to be included in a description of sputum.

a. _____

b. _____

c. _____

d. _____

e. _____

➤ Wheezing is characterized by _____

_____

_____

_____

➤ Describe the following types of chest pain:

Cardiac _____

_____

Pleuritic _____

_____

Musculoskeletal _____

_____

➤ List the three most common types of environmental exposures in the home.

a. _____

b. _____

c. _____

➤ List three common drugs that may affect cardiopulmonary functioning.

a. _____

b. _____

c. _____

PHYSICAL EXAMINATION

➤ Briefly explain the following techniques used in assessing tissue oxygenation:

Inspection _____

_____

_____

_____

Palpation _____

_____

_____

_____

Percussion _____

_____

_____

_____

Auscultation _____

_____

_____

_____

DIAGNOSTIC TESTS

➤ Describe the following tests used to determine adequacy of the cardiac conduction system:

Electrocardiogram _____

_____

_____

_____

Holter monitor _____

_____

_____

_____

Exercise stress test _____

_____

_____

_____

Electrophysiological studies _____

_____

_____

_____

➤ Describe the following tests to determine myocardial contraction and blood flow:

Echocardiography _____

_____

_____

_____

Scintigraphy _____

_____

_____

_____

Cardiac catheterization and angiography _____
_____
_____
_____

➤ Describe the following tests used to measure the adequacy of ventilation and oxygenation:

Pulmonary function tests _____
_____
_____
_____

Peak expiratory flow rate _____
_____
_____
_____

Arterial blood gases _____
_____
_____
_____

Oximetry _____
_____
_____
_____

Complete blood count _____
_____
_____
_____

➤ Describe the following tests used to visualize structures of the respiratory system:

Chest x-ray _____
_____
_____
_____

Bronchoscopy _____
_____
_____
_____

Lung scan _____
_____
_____
_____

➤ Describe the following tests used to determine abnormal cells or infection in the respiratory tract:

Throat cultures _____
_____
_____
_____

Sputum specimens _____
_____
_____
_____

Skin testing _____
_____
_____
_____

Thoracentesis _____
_____
_____
_____

➤ Identify the most important information to present to a client before thoracentesis, and give the rationale:
_____
_____
_____
_____

Nursing Diagnosis

➤ List six potential or actual nursing diagnoses for a client with altered oxygenation.

a. _____
b. _____
c. _____
d. _____
e. _____
f. _____

Planning

➤ List six goals appropriate for a client with actual or potential oxygenation needs.

a. _____

b. _____

c. _____

d. _____

e. _____

f. _____

Implementation

➤ Briefly explain the following types of nursing interventions for promoting and maintaining adequate oxygenation:

Dependent nursing actions _____

_____

_____

_____

Interdependent-dependent nursing actions _____

_____

_____

_____

Health Promotion in a Primary Care Setting

➤ Describe the purpose of the influenza and pneumococcal vaccine, and explain for whom the vaccines are

recommended: _____

_____

_____

_____

_____

➤ Avoiding exposure to secondhand smoke is essential to maintaining optimal cardiopulmonary function.

Acute and Tertiary Care

➤ Nursing interventions for the client with acute pulmonary illnesses are directed toward _____

_____, _____,

and _____.

➤ List five treatment modalities appropriate for a client with dyspnea.

a. _____

b. _____

c. _____

d. _____

e. _____

MAINTENANCE OF A PATENT AIRWAY

➤ Describe selected nursing interventions used to promote and maintain adequate oxygenation by completing the grid on the next page. Include the purpose of the intervention.

MOBILIZATION OF PULMONARY SECRETIONS

➤ Nursing interventions that promote mobilization of pulmonary secretions include the following. Briefly explain each one:

Hydration _____

_____

_____

_____

Humidification _____

_____

_____

_____

Nebulization _____

_____

_____

_____

MAINTENANCE OR PROMOTION OF LUNG EXPANSION

➤ Nursing interventions to maintain or promote lung expansion include the following noninvasive techniques. Briefly explain each one:

Positioning _____

_____

_____

_____

Incentive spirometry _____

_____

_____

_____

Nursing Interventions	Purpose
Cascade cough	
Huff cough	
Quad cough	
Oropharyngeal and nasopharyngeal suctioning	
Orotracheal and nasotracheal suctioning	
Tracheal suctioning	
Oral airway	
Tracheal airway	

Chest physiotherapy (CPT) _____

_____

_____

➤ List and briefly describe the three activities involved in CPT.

a. _____

b. _____

c. _____

➤ Identify the three reasons for inserting chest tubes.

a. _____

b. _____

c. _____

➤ Define the following:

Hemothorax _____

_____

Pneumothorax _____

_____

➤ List the four types of drainage systems used with chest tubes.

a. _____

b. _____

c. _____

d. _____

➤ Identify five special considerations the nurse needs to address when dealing with chest tubes.

a. _____

b. _____

c. _____

d. _____

e. _____

MAINTENANCE AND PROMOTION OF OXYGENATION

➤ Identify the goals of oxygen therapy: _____

_____

_____

_____

_____

➤ List four safety measures to be instituted when a client receives oxygen administration.

a. _____

b. _____

c. _____

d. _____

➤ Describe the following methods of oxygen delivery and the usual flow rates:

Nasal cannula _____

_____

Nasal catheter _____

_____

Transtracheal oxygen _____

_____

Face mask _____

_____

Venturi mask _____

_____

➤ Identify the indications for a client to use home oxygen:

_____

_____

_____

➤ Identify the teaching required by the client for use of home oxygen therapy: _____

_____

_____

_____

_____

_____

RESTORATION OF CARDIOPULMONARY FUNCTIONING

➤ Define *cardiac arrest:* _____

_____

➤ List the three goals of cardiopulmonary resuscitation (CPR).

a. _____

b. _____

c. _____

Restorative Care

➤ Cardiopulmonary rehabilitation is _____

_____

_____

_____

_____

_____

➤ Respiratory muscle training improves muscle strength and endurance, resulting in improved activity tolerance. Briefly explain ISRBD (incentive spirometer resistive breathing device): _____

_____

_____

_____

_____

_____

➤ Briefly explain the following breathing exercises used to improve ventilation and oxygenation:

Pursed-lip breathing _____

_____

_____

_____

Diaphragmatic breathing _____

_____

_____

_____

_____

Evaluation

➤ List three evaluative criteria for a client with alterations in oxygenation.

a. _____

b. _____

c. _____

REVIEW QUESTIONS

(The student should select the appropriate answer and cite the rationale for choosing that particular answer.)

1. Ventilation, perfusion, and exchange of gases are the major purposes of:
   a. Respiration
   b. Circulation
   c. Aerobic metabolism
   d. Anaerobic metabolism

Answer ( ) Rationale: _____

_____

_____

2. Afterload refers to:
   a. The amount of blood ejected from the left ventricle each minute
   b. The amount of blood ejected from the left ventricle with each contraction
   c. The resistance to left ventricle ejection
   d. The amount of blood in the left ventricle at the end of diastole

Answer ( ) Rationale: _____

_____

_____

3. The movement of gases into and out of the lungs depends on the:
   a. 50% Oxygen content in the atmospheric air
   b. Pressure gradient between the atmosphere and the alveoli
   c. Use of accessory muscles of respiration during expiration
   d. Amount of carbon dioxide dissolved in the fluid of the alveoli

Answer ( ) Rationale: _____

_____

_____

4. The client's ECG shows an abnormal rhythm that slows during inspiration and increases with expiration. The rate is 70 to 80 beats per minute. The P-wave, PR interval, and QRS complex are normal. This is referred to as:
   a. Sinus tachycardia
   b. Sinus dysrhythmia
   c. Supraventricular tachycardia
   d. Premature ventricular contractions

Answer ( ) Rationale: _____

_____

_____

5. Which of the following is *not* a symptom of alveolar hyperventilation:
   a. Lethargy
   b. Dizziness
   c. Carpopedal spasm
   d. Tinnitus

Answer ( ) Rationale: _____

_____

_____

6. An effect of hypoxia that results from desaturated hemoglobin in the capillaries is:
   a. Pallor
   b. Cyanosis
   c. Erythema
   d. Polycythemia

Answer ( ) Rationale: _____

_____

_____

7. Mr. Issac comes to the ER complaining of difficulty breathing. An objective finding associated with his dyspnea might include:
   a. Statements about a sense of impending doom
   b. Complaints of shortness of breath
   c. Feelings of heaviness in the chest
   d. Use of accessory muscles of respiration

Answer ( ) Rationale: _____

_____

_____

8. For which client would the use of a finger oximeter be appropriate?
   a. Client W, who is in shock following an auto accident
   b. Client X, who has chronic obstructive pulmonary disease
   c. Client Y, who was brought to the emergency room following prolonged exposure to the cold
   d. Client Z, a diabetic, who has poor capillary refill

Answer ( ) Rationale: _____

_____

_____

9. The physician suspects that the client has tuberculosis and orders a sputum specimen to be obtained. The nurse will collect which type of specimen?
   a. Sputum for culture and sensitivity
   b. Sputum for cytology
   c. Sputum for acid-fast bacillus
   d. Sputum for blood

Answer ( ) Rationale: _____

_____

_____

10. A common cause for the nursing diagnosis of ineffective airway clearance is:
    a. Incisional pain
    b. Acid-base imbalances
    c. Elevated temperature
    d. Decreased cardiac output

Answer ( ) Rationale: _____

_____

_____

11. The use of chest physiotherapy to mobilize pulmonary secretions involves the use of:
    a. Hydration
    b. Percussion
    c. Nebulization
    d. Humidification

Answer ( ) Rationale: _____

_____

_____

12. What is the first step of the cardiopulmonary resuscitation process?
    a. Call for help.
    b. Open the victim's airway.
    c. Assess victim for unresponsiveness.
    d. Place victim supine on a firm, flat surface.

Answer ( ) Rationale: _____

_____

_____

CLINICAL SITUATIONS

1. You have just begun your morning rounds when one of your clients, Mr. Havens, complains of chest pain. State how you would assess his pain. What are three important interventions for this client?

_____

_____

_____

_____

_____

_____

_____

_____

2. You are caring for a client who had abdominal surgery 24 hours ago. This client has a 10-year history of chronic pulmonary disease. What assessments and interventions are necessary to maintain a patent airway?

_____

_____

_____

_____

_____

_____

_____

_____

_____

Fluid, electrolyte, and acid-base balances are
maintained by the intake, distribution, and
output of water and electrolytes, and their regulation by the renal and pulmonary systems.

PRELIMINARY READING

Chapter 45, pp. 1247-1292

COMPREHENSIVE UNDERSTANDING

■ FLUID AND ELECTROLYTE BALANCES

Distribution of Body Fluids

➤ Body fluids are distributed in two distinct compartments. Briefly explain each one.

Extracellular: _____

_____

_____

Intracellular: _____

_____

_____

Composition of Body Fluids

➤ Define *electrolyte:* _____

_____

_____

➤ Define the following terms related to the composition of body fluids:

Cations _____

_____

Anions _____

_____

mEq/L _____

_____

Minerals _____

_____

Cells _____

_____

Movement of Body Fluids

➤ Fluids and electrolytes shift from compartment to
compartment to facilitate body processes.

➤ List and briefly describe the four factors responsible
for movement of body fluids:

a. _____

_____

_____

b. _____

_____

_____

c. _____

_____

_____

d. _____

_____

_____

➤ Define the following terms related to osmosis:

Osmotic pressure _____

_____

_____

_____

Isotonic _____

_____

Hypotonic _____

_____

Hypertonic _____

_____

➤ Define the following terms related to filtration:

Hydrostatic pressure _____

_____

_____

_____

Regulation of Body Fluids

➤ Briefly describe the physiological stimuli triggering the

thirst mechanism: _____

_____

_____

_____

_____

_____

➤ List the four organs contributing to body fluid loss.

a. _____

b. _____

c. _____

d. _____

➤ Define:

Insensible water loss _____

_____

_____

_____

Sensible water loss _____

_____

_____

_____

➤ For each hormone, identify the stimuli for its release and its influence on fluid and electrolyte balance in the grid below.

Regulation of Electrolytes

➤ The major cations are _____,

_____, _____, and

_____. They are located in the

_____ and _____ fluid.

➤ The major anions are_____,

_____, and _____.

➤ Give the normal values, function, and regulatory mechanisms for the major body electrolytes in the grid on the next page.

■ ACID-BASE BALANCE

➤ Acid-base balance exists when the _____

_____

_____

_____.

➤ The concentration of hydrogen ions in a body fluid is

expressed as _____.

➤ A pH value of _____ is neutral.

Below _____ is acid, and

above _____ is alkaline.

➤ The types of acid-base regulators within the body are

_____, _____,

and _____ buffering systems.

➤ A buffer is a _____

_____.

Hormone	Stimuli	Action
ADH		
Aldosterone		
Glucocorticoids		

Electrolyte	Values	Function	Regulatory Mechanism
Sodium			
Potassium			
Calcium			
Magnesium			
Chloride			
Bicarbonate			
Phosphate			

➤ Identify and describe the acid-base regulatory mechanisms for each of the following buffering systems:

Chemical Regulation _____

_____

_____

_____

_____

Biological Regulation _____

_____

_____

_____

_____

_____

Physiological Regulation _____

_____

_____

_____

_____

➤ Describe the physiological mechanism in which the lungs regulate hydrogen ion concentration: _____

_____

_____

_____

_____

➤ List three ways in which the kidneys can regulate hydrogen concentration.

a. _____

b. _____

c. _____

■ DISTURBANCES IN FLUID, ELECTROLYTE, AND ACID-BASE BALANCES

Fluid Disturbances

➤ Define and briefly describe the two major classifications of fluid imbalance.

a. _____

_____

b. _____

_____

Fluid Disturbances	Causes	Signs and Symptoms
Fluid volume deficit (FVD)		
Fluid volume excess (FVE)		
Third-space syndrome		
Hyperosmolar imbalance		
Hypoosmolar imbalance		

➤ Complete the grid above giving the causes, signs, and symptoms of the listed fluid disturbances.

Electrolyte Imbalances

➤ For each electrolyte disturbance, identify the diagnostic laboratory finding, and list at least four characteristic signs and symptoms in the grid on p. 322.

Acid-Base Imbalances

➤ For each acid-base imbalance, identify the diagnostic laboratory finding, and list the characteristic signs and symptoms in the grid at the top of p. 323.

■ VARIABLES AFFECTING NORMAL FLUID, ELECTROLYTE, AND ACID-BASE BALANCES

➤ List the four major factors that can affect fluid and electrolyte imbalances.

a. _____

b. _____

c. _____

d. _____

➤ Briefly describe the fluid changes that are associated with aging and development.

Infants: _____

_____

_____

_____

Children: _____

_____

_____

_____

Adolescents: _____

_____

_____

_____

Older adults: _____

_____

_____

_____

➤ Briefly describe how the following affect total body water:

Body size _____

_____

_____

_____

Environmental temperature _____

_____

_____

_____

➤ Briefly describe the influence of each habit on fluid and electrolyte balance.

Diet: _____

_____

_____

_____

_____

Imbalance	Lab Finding	Signs and Symptoms
Hyponatremia		
Hypernatremia		
Hypokalemia		
Hyperkalemia		
Hypocalcemia		
Hypercalcemia		
Hypomagnesemia		
Hypermagnesemia		

Acid-Base Imbalance	Lab Findings	Signs and Symptoms
Respiratory acidosis		
Respiratory alkalosis		
Metabolic acidosis		
Metabolic alkalosis		

Stress: _____

_____

_____

_____

_____

_____

Exercise: _____

_____

_____

_____

_____

_____

■ NURSING PROCESS AND FLUID, ELECTROLYTE, AND ACID-BASE IMBALANCES

Assessment

➤ The eight major categories of risk factors for fluid, electrolyte, and acid-base imbalances are _____

_____, _____,

_____, _____,

_____, _____,

_____, and _____.

➤ Indicate the possible fluid, electrolyte, or acid-base imbalance associated with each assessment finding:

Weight loss of 6% to 9% _____

_____

Irritability _____

_____

Lethargy _____

_____

Bulging fontanels (infant) _____

_____

Periorbital edema _____

_____

Sticky, dry mucous membranes _____

_____

Chvostek's sign _____

_____

Distended neck veins _____

_____

Dysrhythmias _____

_____

Weak pulse _____

_____

Low blood pressure _____

_____

Third heart sound _____

_____

Increased respiratory rate _____

_____

Crackles _____

_____

Anorexia _____

_____

Abdominal cramps _____

_____

Poor skin turgor _____

_____

Oliguria or anuria _____

_____

Increased specific gravity _____

_____

Muscle cramps, tetany _____

_____

Hypertonicity of muscles on palpation _____

_____

Decreased or absent deep tendon reflexes _____

_____

Increased temperature _____

_____

Distended abdomen _____

_____

Cold, clammy skin _____

_____

2+ edema _____

_____

➤ Recording I & O is essential for obtaining an accurate data base. This information helps maintain an ongoing evaluation of hydration status to prevent severe imbalances.

➤ Indicate the normal values for each of the following lab tests:

Calcium _____

Carbon dioxide content _____

Chloride _____

Magnesium _____

Phosphate _____

Potassium _____

Sodium _____

Serum osmolality _____

Urine specific gravity _____

Arterial blood gas levels: pH _____

$PaCO_2$ _____ PaO_2 _____

SaO_2 _____ HCO_3 _____

Nursing Diagnosis

➤ List five potential or actual nursing diagnoses for a client with fluid, electrolyte, or acid-base imbalances.

a. _____

b. _____

c. _____

d. _____

e. _____

Planning

➤ List three goals appropriate for a client with altered fluid, electrolyte, or acid-base imbalances.

a. _____

b. _____

c. _____

Implementation

Correcting Fluid and Electrolyte Imbalances

➤ List and briefly describe the enteral replacements of fluids.

a. _____

_____

b. _____

_____

➤ Briefly explain the need for a restricted fluid intake and how the nurse would implement the restriction:

_____

_____

_____

_____

_____

➤ List the three methods of parenteral replacement.

a. _____

b. _____

c. _____

➤ State the primary goal of IV fluid replacement: _____
_____
_____

➤ Define the following types of electrolyte solutions:

Isotonic _____
_____

Hypotonic _____
_____

Hypertonic _____
_____

➤ List two major purposes of infusion pumps.

a. _____

b. _____

➤ List three groups of clients in whom venipunctures may be difficult.

a. _____

b. _____

c. _____

➤ List four factors that may affect IV flow rates.

a. _____

b. _____

c. _____

d. _____

➤ Indicate the sequence to be followed when changing a gown of a client with an IV line.

a. _____

b. _____

c. _____

d. _____

e. _____

f. _____

➤ List four interventions that can reduce the risk of infusion-related infections.

a. _____

b. _____

c. _____

d. _____

➤ Complete the grid below describing complications of IV therapy.

➤ List three objectives of blood transfusion.

a. _____

b. _____

c. _____

Complication	Assessment Finding	Nursing Action
Infiltration		
Phlebitis		
Fluid overload		
Bleeding		

➤ Complete the grid below describing the major blood groups.

➤ Define *autotransfusion:* _____

_____

_____

_____

➤ Identify the five nursing interventions associated with blood transfusions, and give the rationale for each.

a. _____

_____

b. _____

_____

c. _____

_____

d. _____

_____

e. _____

_____

➤ Define *transfusion reaction,* and give its cause: _____

_____

_____

_____

_____

_____

➤ List the five signs and symptoms most commonly associated with transfusion reactions.

a. _____

b. _____

c. _____

d. _____

e. _____

➤ Define the following risks associated with blood transfusions:

Hyperkalemia _____

_____

_____

_____

Hypocalcemia _____

_____

_____

_____

Iron overload (hemosiderosis) _____

_____

_____

_____

Circulatory overload _____

_____

_____

➤ List the nine steps the nurse should follow if a transfusion reaction is suspected.

a. _____

b. _____

c. _____

d. _____

e. _____

f. _____

g. _____

h. _____

i. _____

	A	B	O	AB
Antigens present				
Antibodies present				

Correcting Acid-Base Imbalances

➤ Identify three nursing interventions to correct acid-base imbalances, and give the rationale for each.

a. _____

_____

b. _____

_____

c. _____

_____

Evaluation

➤ List three expected outcomes for a client with an alteration in fluid, electrolyte, or acid-base imbalances.

a. _____

b. _____

c. _____

REVIEW QUESTIONS

(The student should select the appropriate answer and cite the rationale for choosing that particular answer.)

1. The body fluids comprising the interstitial fluid and blood plasma are:
   a. Intracellular
   b. Extracellular
   c. Hypotonic
   d. Hypertonic

Answer (   ) Rationale: _____

_____

_____

2. The movement of body fluids and electrolytes that requires metabolic function and energy expenditure is:
   a. Diffusion
   b. Osmosis
   c. Active transport
   d. Fluid pressure

Answer (   ) Rationale: _____

_____

_____

3. Which of the following statements is true with regard to the lungs' regulation of acid-base balance?
   a. They serve a minor role in the physiological buffering of H ions.
   b. It takes several days for the lungs to restore pH to a normal level.
   c. They correct imbalances by alternating the rate and depth of respiration.
   d. The lungs maintain normal pH by either retaining or excreting bicarbonate.

Answer (   ) Rationale: _____

_____

_____

4. Mr. Bernsen has a serum potassium level of 5.8. The nurse should assess for:
   a. Pitting edema
   b. Respiratory depression
   c. Decreased deep tendon reflexes
   d. Irregularity in heart rate or rhythm

Answer (   ) Rationale: _____

_____

_____

5. Mrs. Green's arterial blood gas results are as follows: pH 7.32, $Paco_2$ 52, Pao_2 78, HCO_3 24. Mrs. Green has:
   a. Respiratory acidoses
   b. Respiratory alkalosis
   c. Metabolic acidosis
   d. Metabolic alkalosis

Answer (   ) Rationale: _____

_____

_____

6. Mr. Frank is an 82-year-old client who has had a 3-day history of vomiting and diarrhea. Which symptom would you expect to find on a physical examination?
   a. Neck vein distention
   b. Crackles in the lungs
   c. Tachycardia
   d. Hypertension

Answer (   ) Rationale: _____

_____

_____

7. Mrs. Heithaus was admitted to your unit with a head injury in a motor vehicle accident. Her urine output during the last 24 hours has been 1000 ml, despite a 3000 ml IV fluid intake. Her sodium level is 124. The nurse knows that Mrs. Heithaus' symptoms may be indicative of:
   a. Diabetic insipidus
   b. Secretion of inappropriate ADH (SIADH)
   c. Hypernatremia
   d. Metabolic alkalosis

   Answer ( ) Rationale: _____
   _____
   _____

8. Which of the following is most likely to result in respiratory alkalosis?
   a. Fad dieting
   b. Hyperventilation
   c. Chronic alcoholism
   d. Steroid use

   Answer ( ) Rationale: _____
   _____
   _____

9. Which of the following is a correctly stated nursing diagnosis for the client with an alteration in fluid and electrolyte status?
   a. Fluid volume deficit related to NPO status
   b. Fluid volume excess related to congestive heart failure
   c. Fluid volume deficit related to difficulty swallowing
   d. Fluid volume excess related to physician ordering too many IV fluids

   Answer ( ) Rationale: _____
   _____
   _____

10. Mr. Kellogg is on a fluid restriction of 1500 ml per day. How much fluid should the nurse plan for Mr. Kellogg to receive on the day shift (7 AM to 3 PM)?
    a. 1500 ml
    b. 500 ml
    c. 1200 ml
    d. 750 ml

    Answer ( ) Rationale: _____
    _____
    _____

11. Ten minutes after her blood transfusion started, Ms. White began experiencing fever, chills, and difficulty breathing. The nurse should:
    a. Realize that this is a harmless reaction and continue to monitor the blood transfusion.
    b. Slow the transfusion rate.
    c. Turn off the blood, and turn on the normal saline on the Y-tubing infusion set.
    d. Turn off the blood and "piggyback" 0.9% saline into the IV line.

    Answer ( ) Rationale: _____
    _____
    _____

12. For which condition can having the client breathe into a paper bag be helpful?
    a. Respiratory alkalosis
    b. Respiratory acidosis
    c. Metabolic acidosis
    d. Metabolic alkalosis

    Answer ( ) Rationale: _____
    _____
    _____

CLINICAL SITUATIONS

1. Mrs. Calhoun has heart failure and is taking Lanoxin and Lasix to treat the heart failure. The nurse practitioner managing Mrs. Calhoun's care noted that her serum potassium in March was 3.6 mEq/L and, in consultation with the physician, ordered a potassium supplement to be given. In September of the same year, Mrs. Calhoun was admitted to the hospital because she fractured her right hip and has a total hip replacement. Three days after surgery, she began taking oral medications and the Lanoxin, Lasix, and potassium supplement are again ordered. At this time, the nurse notes that Mrs. Calhoun's heart rate is irregular, her previous 24-hour input and output showed intake of 2050 ml and output of 800 ml and that her urine now is very dark amber. What serum electrolyte level should the nurse immediately check? What other assessment data should the nurse gather? Which medication(s) should be held until the staff nurse consults with Mrs. Calhoun's health care provider?

2. Mr. Jones is receiving IV fluids because he is NPO after surgery earlier today. His fluid order is 1000 ml lactated Ringer's with 20 mEq/L KCl to run over six hours. What IV tubing should be used to administer these fluids in terms of drop size? The nurse hangs a new bag of IV fluids at 5 PM. At 8 PM, the nurse notes that 300 ml have infused from the bag. Are these fluids on time? If not, what assessments should be done to determine the reason?

Chapter 46 | Urinary Elimination

When the urinary system fails to function properly, virtually all organ systems will be eventually affected.

PRELIMINARY READING

Chapter 46, pp. 1293-1339

COMPREHENSIVE UNDERSTANDING

▮ PHYSIOLOGY OF URINE ELIMINATION

➤ Summarize the function of each of the following organs in the urinary system:

Kidneys _____

_____

_____

_____

Ureters _____

_____

_____

_____

Bladder _____

_____

_____

_____

Urethra _____

_____

_____

_____

➤ Define the following terms related to urine elimination:

Renal artery _____

_____

Nephron _____

_____

Glomerulus _____

_____

Proteinuria _____

_____

Erythropoietin _____

_____

Renin _____

_____

Meatus _____

_____

Act of Urination

➤ Number the steps describing the normal act of micturition in sequential order.

_____ Parasympathetic impulses from the micturition center cause the detrusor muscle to begin contracting.

_____ The external bladder sphincter relaxes.

_____ Impulses travel to the cerebral cortex, making the person conscious of the need to void.

_____ The detrusor muscle contracts.

_____ The internal urethral sphincter relaxes, allowing urine to enter the urethra.

_____ Urine passes through the urethral meatus.

_____ Urine volume stretches the bladder walls, sending impulses to the spinal cord.

▮ FACTORS INFLUENCING URINATION

➤ Disease processes that primarily affect renal function (changes in urine volume or quality) are generally categorized as the following. Briefly explain.

Prerenal: _____

_____

_____

Renal: _____
_____
_____
_____

Postrenal: _____
_____
_____
_____

➤ Define *oliguria:* _____
_____

➤ Define *anuria:* _____
_____

Growth and Development

➤ Briefly explain the normal micturition patterns that occur in the following developmental stages:

Infants _____
_____
_____
_____

Children _____
_____
_____
_____

Adult _____
_____
_____
_____

Older adult _____
_____
_____
_____

➤ Define the following terms related to urination:

Nocturia _____
_____

Urinary frequency _____
_____

Residual urine _____
_____

➤ Briefly explain the following factors that influence urination:

Sociocultural Factors: _____
_____
_____
_____

Psychological Factors: _____
_____
_____
_____

Personal Habits: _____
_____
_____
_____

Muscle Tone: _____
_____
_____
_____

Volume Status

➤ Explain how the following affect urine production:

Alcohol _____
_____

Caffeine drinks _____
_____

Fruits and vegetables _____
_____

Febrile conditions _____
_____

Disease Conditions

➤ Describe how the following conditions affect micturition:

Neuropathic conditions _____
_____
_____
_____

Degenerative joint disease _____
_____
_____

End-stage renal disease _____

_____

_____

➤ Define *uremic syndrome:* _____

_____

_____

_____

➤ Name the two types of renal replacement therapies.

   a. _____

   b. _____

➤ Briefly describe the two methods of dialysis.

   Peritoneal dialysis: _____

   _____

   _____

   _____

   Hemodialysis: _____

   _____

   _____

   _____

Surgical Procedures

➤ Briefly explain how the stress of surgery affects urine

   output: _____

   _____

   _____

   _____

➤ Briefly explain how anesthetics and narcotic analgesics

   affect urine output: _____

   _____

   _____

   _____

➤ Explain what a urinary diversion is: _____

   _____

   _____

   _____

Medications

➤ List five medications that affect urination.

   a. _____

   b. _____

   c. _____

   d. _____

   e. _____

➤ Explain what a cystoscopy is and how it may affect uri-

   nation: _____

   _____

   _____

   _____

❚ ALTERATIONS IN URINARY ELIMINATION

➤ Clients with urinary problems have disturbances in the act of micturition. List the three most common.

   a. _____

   b. _____

   c. _____

Urinary Retention

➤ Define *urinary retention:* _____

   _____

   _____

   _____

➤ Define *retention with overflow:* _____

   _____

   _____

   _____

Lower Urinary Tract Infections

➤ List six signs or symptoms of urinary tract infections (UTIs).

   a. _____

   b. _____

   c. _____

   d. _____

   e. _____

   f. _____

➤ Identify the most common cause of UTIs: _____

   _____

➤ Identify the three common causes of UTIs in women.

a. _____

b. _____

c. _____

➤ Define the following terms related to UTIs:

Bacteriuria _____

_____

Dysuria _____

_____

Hematuria _____

_____

Pyelonephritis _____

_____

Urinary Incontinence

➤ Define *urinary incontinence:* _____

_____

_____

➤ Briefly explain the five types of urinary incontinence.

Functional: _____

_____

_____

_____

Overflow: _____

_____

_____

_____

Stress: _____

_____

_____

_____

Urge: _____

_____

_____

_____

Total: _____

_____

_____

_____

Urinary Diversions

➤ Briefly explain the following urinary diversions:

Ileal loop or conduit _____

_____

_____

_____

Ureterostomy _____

_____

_____

_____

Nephrostomy _____

_____

_____

_____

▌NURSING PROCESS FOR URINARY PROBLEMS

Assessment

Nursing History

➤ List the three major factors to be explored during a nursing history concerning urinary elimination.

a. _____

b. _____

c. _____

Physical Assessment

➤ List and briefly explain the organs that the nurse would assess to determine the presence and severity of urinary problems.

a. _____

_____

b. _____

_____

c. _____

_____

d. _____

_____

Assessment of Urine

➤ Assessment of urine involves _____

and _____.

➤ Explain the following characteristics of urine:

Color _____
_____
_____
_____

Clarity _____
_____
_____
_____

Odor _____
_____
_____
_____

➤ Explain the following types of urine specimens collected for testing:

Random _____
_____
_____
_____

Clean-voided, or midstream _____
_____
_____
_____

Sterile _____
_____
_____
_____

Timed urine _____
_____
_____
_____

➤ Briefly explain on how to collect a urine specimen from a young child: _____
_____
_____
_____
_____

➤ Common urine tests include the following. Briefly explain each:

Urinalysis _____
_____
_____
_____

Specific gravity _____
_____
_____
_____

Urine culture _____
_____
_____
_____

➤ Briefly explain the following types of diagnostic examinations, and give the nursing implications for each:

Abdominal roentgenogram _____
_____
_____
_____
_____
_____

Intravenous pyelogram (IVP) _____
_____
_____
_____
_____

➤ Identify the specific nursing implications for a client receiving an IVP.

a. _____

b. _____

c. _____

➤ Identify the specific nursing implications for a client after an IVP test.

a. _____

b. _____

c. _____

d. _____

➤ List the nursing implications for a client before a renal scan.

a. _____

b. _____

c. _____

d. _____

e. _____

➤ Name the two nursing implications for a client during a renal scan.

a. _____

b. _____

➤ Briefly explain the following diagnostic tests, and give the nursing implications for each:

CT _____

_____

_____

_____

Renal ultrasound _____

_____

_____

_____

Cystometrogram (CMG) _____

_____

_____

_____

➤ List the three types of invasive procedures.

a. _____

b. _____

c. _____

➤ List the nursing implications for a cystoscopy.
Before the test:

a. _____

b. _____

c. _____

d. _____

e. _____

f. _____

g. _____

h. _____

During the test:

a. _____

b. _____

c. _____

d. _____

After the test:

a. _____

b. _____

c. _____

d. _____

e. _____

f. _____

➤ List the nursing implications related to a renal biopsy.
Before the test:

a. _____

b. _____

c. _____

d. _____

e. _____

f. _____

During the test:

a. _____

b. _____

c. _____

After the test:

a. _____

b. _____

c. _____

d. _____

e. _____

f. _____

g. _____

h. _____

➤ List the nursing implications related to an angiography (arteriogram).
Before the test:

a. _____

b. _____

c. _____

d. _____

e. _____

After the test:

a. _____

b. _____

c. _____

d. _____

e. _____

f. _____

g. _____

Nursing Diagnosis

➤ List 12 potential or actual nursing diagnoses related to urinary elimination.

a. _____

b. _____

c. _____

d. _____

e. _____

f. _____

g. _____

h. _____

i. _____

j. _____

k. _____

l. _____

Planning

➤ List the six goals appropriate for a client with a urinary elimination problem.

a. _____

b. _____

c. _____

d. _____

e. _____

f. _____

Implementation

Health Promotion

➤ List five teaching strategies aimed at eradicating or minimizing urinary elimination problems.

a. _____

b. _____

c. _____

d. _____

e. _____

➤ List five techniques that may be used to stimulate the micturition reflex.

a. _____

b. _____

c. _____

d. _____

e. _____

➤ Identify at least two types of treatment options to promote micturition in the following types of urinary incontinence:

Functional incontinence _____

_____

_____

_____

Overflow _____

_____

_____

_____

Stress incontinence _____

_____

_____

_____

Urge incontinence _____

_____

_____

_____

Total incontinence _____

_____

_____

_____

➤ Urine is normally acidic and tends to inhibit growth of microorganisms. List four types of foods that increase urine acidity.

a. _____

b. _____

c. _____

d. _____

Acute Care

➤ Briefly explain how the nurse could help the hospitalized client maintain normal elimination habits:

_____
_____
_____
_____

➤ List and explain three types of medications that can be used to treat incontinence or retention.

a. _____
_____

b. _____
_____

c. _____
_____

➤ Briefly explain the following types of catheters:

Straight single-use _____
_____
_____

Indwelling _____
_____
_____

Coude' _____
_____
_____

➤ List eight indications for catheterization and the method used.

a. _____

b. _____

c. _____

d. _____

e. _____

f. _____

g. _____

h. _____

➤ Explain the following in relation to preventing infection and maintaining an unobstructed flow of urine:

Fluid intake _____
_____
_____

Perineal hygiene _____
_____
_____

Catheter care _____
_____
_____

Ostomy care _____
_____
_____

➤ List six ways to minimize the risk of urinary tract infection in catheterized clients.

a. _____

b. _____

c. _____

d. _____

e. _____

f. _____

➤ Briefly describe catheter irrigations and instillations:

_____
_____
_____
_____

➤ Name two important principles to follow when removing an indwelling catheter.

a. _____

b. _____

➤ Briefly explain the two alternatives for urinary drainage, and give the nursing implications for each.

Suprapubic catheter _____

_____

_____

_____

_____

_____

Condom catheter _____

_____

_____

_____

_____

➤ Name two precautions that should be taken to ensure client safety and comfort when using a condom catheter.

a. _____

b. _____

Restorative Care

➤ Define *Kegel exercises:* _____

_____

_____

_____

➤ List and describe four pelvic floor exercises.

a. _____

_____

b. _____

_____

c. _____

_____

d. _____

_____

➤ State the goal of bladder retraining: _____

_____

_____

➤ List 12 measures the nurse can teach the client to gain control over urination.

a. _____

b. _____

c. _____

d. _____

e. _____

f. _____

g. _____

h. _____

i. _____

j. _____

k. _____

l. _____

➤ A client with functional incontinence may benefit from habit training, which helps clients improve voluntary control over urination.

➤ Explain prompted voiding: _____

_____

_____

_____

➤ List the nursing measures used to maintain skin integrity when urine comes in contact with the skin.

a. _____

b. _____

c. _____

d. _____

➤ List two comfort measures for a client with the following sources of discomfort:

Incontinence _____

_____

_____

_____

Dysuria _____

_____

_____

_____

Painful distention _____

_____

_____

_____

_____

Evaluation

➤ List three expected outcomes for a client with urinary problems.

a. _____

b. _____

c. _____

REVIEW QUESTIONS

(The student should select the appropriate answer and cite the rationale for choosing that particular answer.)

1. All of the following factors will influence the production of urine *except:*
   a. Anxiety
   b. Acute renal disease
   c. Febrile conditions
   d. Diuretic medications

Answer ( ) Rationale: _____

_____

_____

2. Mrs. Rantz complains of leaking urine when she coughs or laughs. This is known as:
   a. Functional incontinence
   b. Stress incontinence
   c. Urge incontinence
   d. Reflex incontinence

Answer ( ) Rationale: _____

_____

_____

3. Ms. Hathaway has a urinary tract infection. Which of the following symptoms would you expect her to exhibit?
   a. Proteinuria
   b. Dysuria
   c. Oliguria
   d. Polyuria

Answer ( ) Rationale: _____

_____

_____

4. Which of the following is an appropriate action for the nurse in collecting a midstream urine specimen for culture from a female client?
   a. Instruct client to cleanse the perineum from back to front.
   b. Instruct client to collect initial flow of urine into a sterile specimen jar.
   c. Make sure urine specimen reaches laboratory within 1 hour of collection.
   d. Use only clear water for cleansing the perineum.

Answer ( ) Rationale: _____

_____

_____

5. The nurse is working in the radiology department with a client who is having an intravenous pyelogram. Which of the following complaints by the client is an abnormal response?
   a. Shortness of breath and audible wheezing
   b. Feeling dizzy and warm with obvious facial flushing
   c. Thirst and feeling "worn out"
   d. Frequent, loose stools

Answer ( ) Rationale: _____

_____

_____

6. Mr. Singh has been scheduled for a cystoscopy tomorrow morning. Nursing interventions would include:
   a. Instructing the client to lie still during the testing
   b. Explaining that insertion of the cystoscope is painless
   c. Instructing him in how to assume the Sims' position
   d. Withholding all sedatives and analgesics

Answer ( ) Rationale: _____

_____

_____

7. Which of the following is a correctly stated nursing diagnosis for the client with an alteration in urinary elimination?
   a. Functional incontinence related to weakened detrusor muscle
   b. Urinary retention related to nursing staff not following intermittent catheterization schedule
   c. Toileting self-care deficit related to myocardial infarction
   d. High risk for altered maintenance related to lack of knowledge of proper technique for self-catheterization

Answer ( ) Rationale: _____

_____

_____

8. The urinalysis of Ms. Hathaway reveals a high bacteria count. Ampicillin is prescribed for her urinary tract infection. The teaching plan for a UTI should include all of the following *except:*
   a. Drink at least 2000 ml of fluid daily.
   b. Always wipe perineum from front to back.
   c. Explain the possible side effects of medication.
   d. Drink plenty of orange and grapefruit juices.

Answer ( ) Rationale: _____

_____

_____

9. The nurse helps the client with voiding by compressing downward with both hands below the umbilicus and above the symphysis pubis. This procedure is called:
   a. Credé's maneuver
   b. Kegel exercise
   c. Micturition
   d. Trigone stimulation

Answer ( ) Rationale: _____

_____

_____

10. Mr. Davidson, 87 years old, is scheduled for a chest x-ray examination this afternoon. He is ambulatory and has an indwelling Foley catheter. The technician will accompany him to radiology. What instructions or information should the nurse give the technician before he leaves?
    a. The drainage bag should be kept below bladder level while ambulating.
    b. The drainage bag should be disconnected before leaving his room.
    c. Abdominal pressure may be felt while ambulating.
    d. The drainage bag should be placed on the x-ray table beside him during the procedure.

Answer ( ) Rationale: _____

_____

_____

11. Which of the following is not a correctly stated projected outcome for the client with an alteration in urinary elimination?
    a. Client will have less than 150 ml of residual urine after voiding.
    b. Client will be able to state components of the lower urinary tract that assist to maintain continence.
    c. Client will empty the bladder using the procedural maneuvers taught.
    d. Client's bladder will not be palpable.

Answer ( ) Rationale: _____

_____

_____

CLINICAL SITUATIONS

1. Mrs. Jaynes is 8 hours postpartum and has not voided. The physician has written an order for catherization. What criteria do you use to determine if you will use a straight or an indwelling catheter?

_____

_____

_____

_____

_____

_____

2. You have just removed an external condom catheter for routine hygiene care. What assessments are needed to determine the skin integrity of the client's penis and scrotum?

_____

_____

_____

_____

_____

_____

Chapter 47

Bowel Elimination

To manage clients' elimination problems, the nurse must understand normal elimination and factors that promote or impede elimination.

PRELIMINARY READING

Chapter 47, pp. 1340-1378

COMPREHENSIVE UNDERSTANDING

■ NORMAL DIGESTION AND ELIMINATION

➤ List the three major purposes of the gastrointestinal tract.

a. _____

b. _____

c. _____

➤ The volume of fluids absorbed by the GI tract is high, making fluid balance a key function of the GI system.

➤ Summarize the functions of each of the following:

Mouth _____

_____

_____

_____

Esophagus _____

_____

_____

_____

Stomach _____

_____

_____

_____

Small Intestine _____

_____

_____

_____

_____

Large Intestine _____

_____

_____

_____

➤ Define the following terms, and state what they are related to in the GI tract:

Bolus _____

_____

Refluxing _____

_____

Peristalsis _____

_____

Chyme _____

_____

Haustral contractions _____

_____

Flatus _____

_____

Feces _____

_____

Valsalva maneuver _____

_____

➤ List and briefly describe the four functions of the colon.

a. _____

_____

b. _____

_____

c. _____

_____

d. _____

_____

➤ Indicate the correct sequence of mechanisms involved in normal defecation.

_____ Increased intraabdominal pressure or the Valsalva maneuver occurs.

_____ The external sphincter relaxes.

_____ The internal sphincter relaxes, and awareness of the need to defecate occurs.

_____ The levator ani muscles relax.

_____ Sensory nerves are stimulated via rectal distention.

■ FACTORS AFFECTING ELIMINATION

Age

➤ Briefly describe the normal elimination pattern of an infant: _____

_____

_____

_____

➤ List six changes occurring in the GI system of the older adult that impair normal digestion and elimination.

a. _____

b. _____

c. _____

d. _____

e. _____

f. _____

Diet

➤ Identify the mechanisms that cause high-fiber diets to promote elimination: _____

_____

_____

_____

➤ List five types of foods that are considered high in fiber (bulk).

a. _____

b. _____

c. _____

d. _____

e. _____

➤ Define *lactose intolerance:* _____

_____

_____

_____

_____

Fluid Intake

➤ Summarize how an inadequate intake of fluids affects the character of feces: _____

_____

_____

_____

Physical Activity

➤ Physical activity _____ peristalsis; immobilization _____ colonic motility.

➤ Weakened abdominal and pelvic floor muscles impair the ability to _____

and to _____.

Psychological Factors

➤ List three diseases of the GI tract that may be associated with stress.

a. _____

b. _____

c. _____

➤ Summarize how the stress response affects elimination:

_____

_____

_____

_____

Personal Habits

➤ List four personal elimination habits that influence bowel function.

a. _____

b. _____

c. _____

d. _____

Position during Defecation

➤ Describe how the position of squatting facilitates defecation: _____

_____

_____

_____

Pain

➤ List five conditions that may result in painful defecation.

a. _____

b. _____

c. _____

d. _____

e. _____

Pregnancy

➤ Identify the common problems that occur during pregnancy, and explain why they occur: _____

_____

_____

_____

Surgery and Anesthesia

➤ Summarize the effects of anesthetic agents and peristalsis: _____

_____

_____

_____

Medications

➤ Describe the effect of each medication on elimination.

Mineral oil: _____

_____

Dicyclomine HCl (Bentyl): _____

_____

Narcotics: _____

_____

Anticholinergics: _____

_____

Antibiotics: _____

_____

Diagnostic Tests

➤ List three types of diagnostic tests for visualization of GI structures.

a. _____

b. _____

c. _____

▌ COMMON BOWEL ELIMINATION PROBLEMS

➤ List four factors that place a client at risk for elimination problems.

a. _____

b. _____

c. _____

d. _____

Constipation

➤ Define constipation: _____

_____

_____

➤ List and briefly describe four causes of constipation.

a. _____

_____

b. _____

_____

c. _____

_____

d. _____

_____

➤ List three groups of clients in whom constipation could pose a significant health hazard.

a. _____

b. _____

c. _____

➤ Describe how the Valsalva maneuver can be avoided:

_____

_____

_____

Impaction

➤ Define *fecal impaction:* _____

_____

➤ List four signs and symptoms of fecal impaction.

a. _____

b. _____

c. _____

d. _____

Diarrhea

➤ Define *diarrhea:* _____

_____

➤ Name the two major complications associated with diarrhea.

a. _____

b. _____

➤ List five conditions and the physiological effects that cause diarrhea.

a. _____

b. _____

c. _____

d. _____

e. _____

➤ List the six nursing responsibilities in the management of diarrhea.

a. _____

b. _____

c. _____

d. _____

e. _____

f. _____

Incontinence

➤ Define *fecal incontinence:* _____

_____

_____

_____

Flatulence

➤ Flatulence is _____. It is a common cause of _____,

_____, and _____.

Hemorrhoids

➤ Define *hemorrhoids:* _____

_____

➤ List four conditions that cause hemorrhoids.

a. _____

b. _____

c. _____

d. _____

▐ BOWEL DIVERSIONS

➤ Define the following:

Stoma _____

_____

Ostomies _____

_____

Ileostomy _____

_____

Colostomy _____

_____

Incontinent ostomy _____

_____

Continent ostomy _____

_____

Incontinent Ostomies

➤ The location of the ostomy determines the consistency of the stool.

➤ Describe the normal consistency and appearance of feces the nurse would expect from:

An ileostomy _____

_____

A sigmoid colostomy _____

_____

A transverse colostomy _____

_____

An ascending colostomy _____

_____

➤ List and briefly describe the three types of colostomy construction.

a. _____

_____

_____

b. _____

_____

_____

c. _____

_____

_____

Continent Ostomies

➤ Briefly describe the following surgical procedures that provide continence:

Ileoanal pull-through _____

_____

_____

_____

Restorative proctocolectomy _____

_____

_____

_____

Kock continent ileostomy _____

_____

_____

_____

Psychological Considerations

➤ Identify a major concern of a client with an ostomy:

_____

_____

_____

▌ NURSING PROCESS AND BOWEL ELIMINATION

Assessment

➤ List 14 factors to be included in a nursing history for clients with altered elimination status.

a. _____

b. _____

c. _____

d. _____

e. _____

f. _____

g. _____

h. _____

i. _____

j. _____

k. _____

l. _____

m. _____

n. _____

➤ Describe the assessment strategies for the following parameters in the physical assessment.

Mobility _____

_____

Dexterity _____

_____

Anorectal sensation _____

_____

Anal sphincter function _____

_____

Abdominal muscle contractility _____

_____

➤ Summarize the following steps for assessing the abdomen:

Inspection _____

_____

_____

_____

Auscultation _____

_____

_____

_____

Palpation _____

_____

_____

_____

Percussion _____

_____

_____

_____

➤ Explain the normal fecal characteristics.

Color: _____

_____

Odor: _____

_____

Consistency: _____

_____

Frequency: _____

_____

Amount: _____

_____

Shape: _____

_____

Constituents: _____

_____

➤ For each of the following fecal characteristics, indicate the possible cause:

White or clay color _____

_____

Black or tarry _____

_____

Melena _____

_____

Liquid consistency _____

_____

Narrow, pencil shaped _____

_____

➤ Briefly describe the appropriate technique for collecting a stool specimen: _____

_____

_____

_____

➤ Define *guaiac test:* _____

_____

_____

➤ Define *endoscopy,* or *gastroscopy:* _____

_____

_____

_____

➤ List the nursing implications for a client having an endoscopy.
Before the test:

a. _____

b. _____

c. _____

d. _____

e. _____

f. _____

g. _____
During the test:

a. _____

b. _____

c. _____
After the test:

a. _____

b. _____

c. _____

➤ List the nursing implications related to a client receiving a sigmoidoscopy, or proctoscopy.
Before the test:

a. _____

b. _____

c. _____

d. _____

e. _____

f. _____

g. _____
During the test:

a. _____

b. _____

c. _____

d. _____
After the test:

a. _____

b. _____

➤ Define *UGI:* _____

➤ List the nursing implications appropriate for a client receiving a UGI.
Before the test:

a. _____

b. _____

c. _____

d. _____

During the test:

a. _____

After the test:

a. _____

b. _____

➤ Define *small bowel follow-through:* _____

_____

_____

_____

➤ List the appropriate nursing implications for a client receiving a barium enema.
Before the test:

a. _____

b. _____

c. _____

d. _____

e. _____

f. _____

g. _____

h. _____

During the test:

a. _____

After the test:

a. _____

b. _____

c. _____

Nursing Diagnosis

➤ List nine potential or actual nursing diagnoses for a client with alteration in bowel elimination.

a. _____

b. _____

c. _____

d. _____

e. _____

f. _____

g. _____

h. _____

i. _____

Planning

➤ List the seven goals appropriate for clients with elimination problems.

a. _____

b. _____

c. _____

d. _____

e. _____

f. _____

g. _____

Implementation

➤ List three ways to promote regular bowel habits in the hospitalized client.

a. _____

b. _____

c. _____

➤ Explain the proper technique for positioning a client on a bedpan: _____

_____

_____

_____

_____

➤ Identify the primary action of the following laxatives and cathartics:

Bulk forming _____

_____

_____

Emollient (wetting) _____

_____

_____

Saline _____

_____

_____

Stimulant cathartics _____

_____

_____

_____

Lubricants _____

_____

_____

_____

➤ Identify the most effective antidiarrheal agent, and give its primary action: _____

_____

_____

_____

➤ The primary reason for an enema is _____.

➤ Briefly describe the following types of enemas:

Tap water _____

_____

_____

_____

Normal saline _____

_____

_____

_____

Soapsuds solution _____

_____

_____

_____

Low-volume hypertonic saline _____

_____

_____

_____

Oil-retention _____

_____

_____

_____

Carminative _____

_____

_____

_____

Harris flush _____

_____

_____

_____

Medicated _____

_____

_____

_____

➤ Explain the physician's order, "Give enemas till clear:"

_____

_____

➤ List the three complications of digital removal of stool.

a. _____

b. _____

c. _____

➤ Summarize the goal of a bowel training program:

_____

_____

_____

_____

_____

➤ List five factors to consider when selecting a pouching system for an ostomate.

a. _____

b. _____

c. _____

d. _____

e. _____

➤ List six contraindications to colostomy irrigation.

a. _____

b. _____

c. _____

d. _____

e. _____

f. _____

➤ Summarize the diet restrictions for ostomy clients:

_____

_____

_____

_____

_____

➤ Describe two exercises for prevention of constipation in the bedridden client.

a. _____

_____

b. _____

_____

➤ Describe two nursing interventions that promote comfort for clients who experience the following:
Hemorrhoids

a. _____

b. _____

Flatulence

a. _____

b. _____

Skin breakdown

a. _____

b. _____

➤ List and describe six interventions that may assist in restoring self-concept in a client with bowel elimination problems.

a. _____

_____

b. _____

_____

c. _____

_____

d. _____

_____

e. _____

_____

f. _____

_____

Evaluation

➤ List four expected outcomes for a client with an alteration in bowel elimination.

a. _____

b. _____

c. _____

d. _____

REVIEW QUESTIONS

(The student should select the appropriate answer and cite the rationale for choosing that particular answer.)

1. Most nutrients and electrolytes are absorbed in the:
   a. Esophagus
   b. Small intestine
   c. Colon
   d. Stomach

Answer ( ) Rationale: _____

_____

_____

2. Which of the following factors will most likely result in regular bowel elimination?
   a. Sedentary life-style
   b. Vegetarian diet
   c. Use of narcotic analgesics
   d. Emotional depression

Answer ( ) Rationale: _____

_____

_____

3. Which of the following should be included in the teaching plan for the client who is scheduled for a gastroscopy?
   a. Avoid eating and drinking for 2 to 4 hours after the test.
   b. A cleansing enema will be given the evening before the procedure.
   c. General anesthetic is usually used for the procedure.
   d. Moderate abdominal pain is common after the procedure.

Answer ( ) Rationale: _____

_____

_____

4. A correctly stated nursing diagnosis for the client with an alteration in bowel function would be:
   a. Toileting self-care deficit related to history of colon cancer
   b. Diarrhea related to infection with an intestinal parasite
   c. Constipation related to decreased mobility
   d. Bowel incontinence related to high-fiber diet

Answer ( ) Rationale: _____

_____

_____

5. Mrs. Deutch is 8 months pregnant with her first child and complaining of constipation. Your nutritional teaching plan for her should include all of the following *except:*
   a. Whole-grain breads
   b. Pastas
   c. Fruit and fruit juices
   d. Hot beverages

Answer ( ) Rationale: _____

_____

_____

6. Mrs. Anthony is concerned about her breast-fed infant's stool, stating it is yellow instead of brown. The nurse explains to Mrs. Anthony that:
   a. A change to formula may be necessary.
   b. Her infant is dehydrated, and she should increase his fluid intake.
   c. The stool is normal for an infant.
   d. It will be necessary to send a stool specimen to the lab.

Answer ( ) Rationale: _____

_____

_____

7. After positioning a client on the bedpan, the nurse should:
   a. Leave the head of the bed flat.
   b. Raise the head of the bed 30 degrees.
   c. Raise the head of the bed to a 90-degree angle.
   d. Raise the bed to the highest working level.

Answer ( ) Rationale: _____

_____

_____

8. An example of a bulk-forming, cathartic drug would be:
   a. Colace
   b. Lomotil
   c. Metamucil
   d. Milk of magnesia

Answer ( ) Rationale: _____

_____

_____

9. The physician has ordered a cleansing enema for 7-year-old Michael. The nurse realizes the maximum volume to be given would be:
   a. 100 to 150 ml
   b. 150 to 250 ml
   c. 300 to 500 ml
   d. 600 to 700 ml

Answer ( ) Rationale: _____

_____

_____

10. The nurse has an order to give enemas until clear. After administering the second enema, the nurse observes that the client is passing brown liquid stool. The nurse should:
    a. Give a third enema.
    b. Notify the physician.
    c. Administer an oil retention enema.
    d. Stop the procedure since the client is no longer passing formed stool.

Answer ( ) Rationale: _____

_____

_____

CLINICAL SITUATIONS

1. A 25-year-old man with a history of good health is admitted to your unit following a motor vehicle accident. His injuries and treatments are such that he has been prescribed bed rest for the next 2 weeks. What type of plan would you design to prevent him from becoming constipated during this period of immobility?

_____

_____

_____

_____

_____

_____

_____

_____

_____

_____

2. An elderly woman with a new, permanent colostomy is about to be discharged from your unit to her daughter's home. The skin around her stoma has no breakdown. Both she and her daughter realize the importance of maintaining this skin integrity. How would you go about advising them?

_____

_____

_____

_____

_____

_____

_____

_____

Chapter
48 | Surgical Client

Perioperative nursing care includes nursing care given before (preoperative), during (intra-operative), and after surgery (postoperative).

PRELIMINARY READING

Chapter 48, pp. 1380-1427

COMPREHENSIVE UNDERSTANDING

▌HISTORY OF SURGICAL NURSING

➤ List the benefits for the client who has ambulatory surgery.

a. _____

b. _____

c. _____

d. _____

▌CLASSIFICATION OF SURGERY

➤ Define the following surgical procedure classifications:

Palliative _____

_____

Ablative _____

_____

Emergency _____

_____

Minor _____

_____

Urgent _____

_____

Major _____

_____

Reconstructive _____

_____

Constructive _____

_____

Elective _____

_____

Transplant _____

_____

Diagnostic _____

_____

▌PREOPERATIVE SURGICAL PHASE

➤ The ability to establish rapport and maintain a professional relationship is an essential component of the perioperative phase.

▌NURSING PROCESS AND THE SURGICAL CLIENT

➤ List and describe the six nursing responsibilities during the preoperative phase.

a. _____

_____

b. _____

_____

c. _____

_____

d. _____

_____

e. _____

_____

f. _____

_____

◗ Assessment

➤ Assessment of the surgical client involves collecting a nursing history, performing a physical examination, reviewing the client's and family members' emotional health, and analyzing risk factors and diagnostic data.

Nursing History

➤ List the data the nurse would collect from the client's

medical history: _____

_____

➤ Describe how each condition increases the risk associated with surgery.

Bleeding disorders: _____

_____

Diabetes mellitus: _____

_____

Heart disease: _____

_____

Respiratory infections: _____

_____

Liver disease: _____

_____

Fever: _____

_____

Chronic respiratory disease: _____

_____

Immunological disorders: _____

_____

➤ A client's past experience with surgery can influence physical and psychological responses to a procedure. List four factors to assess.

a. _____

b. _____

c. _____

d. _____

➤ Briefly explain how the nurse can prepare clients and their family members for the surgical experience:

_____

_____

_____

_____

➤ Describe how each of the following drugs have special implications for the surgical client:

Antibiotics _____

_____

Antidysrhythmics _____

_____

Anticoagulants _____

_____

Anticonvulsants _____

_____

Antihypertensives _____

_____

Corticosteroids _____

_____

Insulin _____

_____

Diuretics _____

_____

➤ Briefly describe how the following factors may place the client at risk for a surgical procedure:

Allergies _____

_____

_____

Smoking habits _____

_____

_____

Alcohol ingestion and substance abuse _____

_____

_____

Family support _____

_____

_____

Occupation _____

_____

_____

Previous pain experience _____

_____

_____

➤ To understand the impact of surgery on a client's and family's emotional health, the following factors are assessed. Briefly explain each:

Feelings _____

_____

_____

_____

Self-concept _____

_____

_____

_____

Body image _____

_____

_____

_____

Coping resources _____

_____

_____

_____

➤ Briefly describe the findings on which the nurse would focus related to the physical examination of the following body systems:

General survey _____

_____

_____

_____

Head and neck _____

_____

_____

_____

Integument _____

_____

_____

_____

Thorax and lungs _____

_____

_____

_____

Heart and vascular system _____

_____

_____

_____

_____

Abdomen _____

_____

_____

_____

Neurological status _____

_____

_____

_____

➤ Briefly describe how the following conditions and factors increase a person's risk in surgery:
Age

Infants _____

_____

_____

_____

Older adults _____

_____

_____

_____

Nutrition

Malnourished client _____

_____

_____

_____

Obesity _____

_____

_____

_____

Other

Radiotherapy _____

_____

_____

_____

Fluid and electrolyte balance _____

_____

_____

_____

➤ Describe the following routine screening tests for surgical clients:

CBC _____

_____

Serum electrolytes _____

_____

Coagulation studies _____

_____

Serum creatinine _____

_____

Urinalysis _____

_____

Nursing Diagnosis

➤ List 10 potential or actual nursing diagnoses appropriate for the preoperative client.

a. _____

b. _____

c. _____

d. _____

e. _____

f. _____

g. _____

h. _____

i. _____

j. _____

Planning

➤ List the eight goals of care for the perioperative client.

a. _____

b. _____

c. _____

d. _____

e. _____

f. _____

g. _____

h. _____

Implementation

Informed Consent

➤ Surgery cannot be performed until a client understands the _____ ,

_____ , _____ ,

_____ , and _____ .

➤ The primary responsibility for informing the client rests with the _____ .

➤ A client's signature on a consent form implies _____

_____ .

Preoperative Teaching

➤ Describe the five ways in which structured preoperative teaching may influence a client's postoperative recovery.

a. _____

b. _____

c. _____

d. _____

e. _____

➤ Describe the criteria developed by the Association of Operating Room Nurses (AORN) that may be used in determining the client's understanding of the surgical procedure.

a. _____

b. _____

c. _____

d. _____

e. _____

f. _____

g. _____

h. _____

➤ Every preoperative teaching program includes explanation and demonstration of the following five postoperative exercises. Briefly explain the rationale for each:

Diaphragmatic breathing _____

_____

_____

Incentive spirometry _____

_____

_____

Controlled coughing _____

_____

_____

Turning _____

_____

_____

_____

Leg exercises _____

_____

_____

Physical Preparation

➤ Briefly describe the purpose of each of the following orders:

NPO after midnight _____

_____

_____

Shower with antimicrobial soap the evening before the surgery _____

_____

_____

Enemas till clear _____

_____

_____

Dalmane, 15 mg PO, at bedtime (night before surgery)

_____

_____

_____

Day of Surgery

➤ List the 11 responsibilities of a nurse caring for a client the morning of surgery.

a. _____

b. _____

c. _____

d. _____

e. _____

f. _____

g. _____

h. _____

i. _____

j. _____

k. _____

➤ Explain the purpose for the following types of nasogastric (NG) intubation:

Lavage _____

_____

Decompression _____

_____

Gavage _____

_____

Compression _____

_____

Evaluation

➤ List three expected outcomes for a preoperative client.

a. _____

b. _____

c. _____

Transport to the Operating Room

➤ List the 10 pieces of equipment that should be present in the postoperative bedside unit.

a. _____

b. _____

c. _____

d. _____

e. _____

f. _____

g. _____

h. _____

i. _____

j. _____

■ INTRAOPERATIVE SURGICAL PHASE

Holding Area

➤ Describe the nursing responsibilities to the client in

the holding area: _____

_____

_____

_____

Admission to the Operating Room

➤ Describe the responsibilities of the nurse in the operating room: _____

_____

_____

_____

Introduction of Anesthetic

➤ Briefly explain the four stages of general anesthesia:

Stage 1 _____

Stage 2 _____

Stage 3 _____

Stage 4 _____

➤ List the risks of general anesthesia: _____

_____

_____

_____

_____

➤ Regional anesthesia is _____

_____

_____

_____.

➤ Briefly list and explain the four types of regional induction methods:

a. _____

_____

b. _____

_____

c. _____

_____

d. _____

_____

➤ Local anesthesia involves _____

_____

_____

_____.

Positioning the Client for Surgery

➤ Explain the principles of positioning the client for

surgery: _____

_____

_____

Nurse's Role during Surgery

➤ Describe the responsibilities of the nurse during the surgical procedure in the following roles:

Scrub nurse _____

_____

_____

_____

Circulating nurse _____

_____

_____

_____

Documentation of Intraoperative Care

➤ During the intraoperative phase, the nursing staff continues the preoperative plan. Documentation of intraoperative care provides useful data for the nurse who cares for the client postoperatively.

▌POSTOPERATIVE SURGICAL PHASE

➤ Identify the two phases of the postoperative period and the usual time frame for ambulatory and hospitalized clients.

a. _____

_____

_____

_____

b. _____

_____

_____

_____

Immediate Postoperative Recovery

➤ Describe the responsibilities of the nurse in the PACU:

_____

_____

_____

_____

_____

RESPIRATION

➤ List three major causes of airway obstruction in the postoperative client.

a. _____

b. _____

c. _____

➤ List six areas of assessment used to determine the respiratory status of a postoperative client.

a. _____

b. _____

c. _____

d. _____

e. _____

f. _____

➤ List the four measures that will maintain airway patency.

a. _____

b. _____

c. _____

d. _____

CIRCULATION

➤ List four areas for assessment to determine a postoperative client's circulatory status.

a. _____

b. _____

c. _____

d. _____

➤ Describe the characteristic findings associated with postoperative hemorrhage in the grid on the next page.

TEMPERATURE CONTROL

➤ Define the following terms related to temperature:

Shivering _____

_____

Malignant hyperthermia _____

_____

NEUROLOGICAL FUNCTIONS

➤ List the areas of assessment to determine a postoperative client's neurological status.

a. _____

b. _____

c. _____

d. _____

➤ Briefly describe a dermatome assessment: _____

_____

_____

_____

SKIN INTEGRITY AND CONDITION OF THE WOUND

➤ The nurse assesses the condition of the skin for

_____, _____,

_____, and _____.

➤ Describe how the nurse would assess the amount of

drainage from a wound: _____

_____

_____

_____

GENITOURINARY FUNCTION

➤ The client may regain voluntary control over urinary

function in _____ hours after anesthesia.

Area of Assessment	Characteristic Findings
Blood pressure	
Heart rate	
Respiratory rate	
Pulse volume	
Skin	
Client behavior	

GASTROINTESTINAL FUNCTION

➤ Normally during the immediate recovery phase,

_____ bowel sounds are auscultated in all four quadrants.

➤ Distention may occur in the client who develops a

_____.

➤ List three nursing measures used to minimize nausea in the immediate postoperative period.

a. _____

b. _____

c. _____

FLUID AND ELECTROLYTE BALANCE

➤ List three areas the nurse assesses to determine fluid and electrolyte alterations.

a. _____

b. _____

c. _____

COMFORT

➤ Postoperative pain can be perceived when _____

_____ is regained.

➤ Assessment of the client's discomfort and evaluation of pain relief therapies are essential nursing functions.

➤ Identify three types of pain relief measures the client may receive in the PACU.

a. _____

b. _____

c. _____

Recovery in Ambulatory Surgery

➤ Briefly describe the two types of recovery phases for the ambulatory surgical client:

Phase 1 _____

_____

Phase 2 _____

_____

➤ List the teaching instructions that would be given to a client in Phase 2 recovery.

a. _____

b. _____

c. _____

d. _____

Postoperative Convalescence

➤ List the criteria that must be present to discharge ambulatory surgical clients: _____

_____

_____

_____

_____

➤ List nine criteria for evaluating recovery room discharge readiness.

a. _____

b. _____

c. _____

d. _____

e. _____

f. _____

g. _____

h. _____

i. _____

▮ THE NURSING PROCESS IN POSTOPERATIVE CARE

Assessment

➤ List the items that the nurse's assessment includes after the client returns to the nursing division.

a. _____

b. _____

c. _____

d. _____

e. _____

f. _____

Nursing Diagnosis

➤ List six potential or actual nursing diagnoses that are appropriate for a postoperative client.

a. _____

b. _____

c. _____

d. _____

e. _____

f. _____

Planning

➤ List the typical surgeon's postoperative orders.

a. _____

b. _____

c. _____

d. _____

e. _____

f. _____

g. _____

h. _____

i. _____

➤ State five typical goals of care for the postoperative client.

a. _____

b. _____

c. _____

d. _____

e. _____

Implementation

➤ Complete the grid on the next page, identifying three nursing interventions for each of the following areas of need in the postoperative client:

Area of Need	Nursing Intervention
Maintaining respiratory function	
Preventing circulatory status	
Promoting normal bowel elimination	
Promoting adequate nutrition	
Promoting urinary elimination	
Promoting wound healing	
Promoting rest and comfort	
Maintaining self-concept	

Evaluation

➤ State three expected outcomes appropriate for the postoperative client.

a. _____

b. _____

c. _____

REVIEW QUESTIONS

(The student should select the appropriate answer and cite the rationale for choosing that particular answer.)

1. Palliative surgery:
   a. Involves surgical exploration that allows the surgeon to make a diagnosis
   b. Relieves or reduces the intensity of disease symptoms
   c. Must be done immediately to save the client's life
   d. Is necessary for the client's physical health

Answer ( ) Rationale: _____
_____
_____

2. Mrs. Young, a 45-year-old diabetic client, is having a hysterectomy in the morning. Because of her history, the nurse would expect:
   a. An increased risk of hemorrhaging
   b. Fluid and electrolyte imbalances
   c. Altered elimination of anesthetic agents
   d. Impaired wound healing

Answer ( ) Rationale: _____
_____
_____

3. The purposes of the nursing history for the client who is to have surgery include all of the following except:
   a. Identifying the client's perception and expectations about surgery
   b. Obtaining information about the client's past experience with surgery
   c. Deciding whether or not surgery is indicated
   d. Understanding the impact surgery has on the client's and family's emotional health

Answer ( ) Rationale: _____
_____
_____

4. During her admission history, the nurse inquires about Mrs. Young's alcohol consumption. It is important to assess a client's history of alcohol ingestion before surgery because:
   a. Higher than normal amounts of anesthetic agents will be needed
   b. Postoperative narcotic agents should not be administered
   c. Surgery time will be lengthened
   d. The type of surgical procedure may be altered

Answer ( ) Rationale: _____
_____
_____

5. All of the following clients are at risk for developing serious fluid and electrolyte imbalances during and after surgery except:
   a. Client E, who is 81 years old and is having emergency surgery for a bowel obstruction following four days of vomiting and diarrhea
   b. Client F, who is 1 year old and having a cleft palate repair
   c. Client G, who is 55 years old and has a history of chronic respiratory disease
   d. Client H, who is 79 years old and has a history of congestive heart failure

Answer ( ) Rationale: _____
_____
_____

6. Mr. McNail, a 39-year-old police officer, is scheduled for an exploratory laparotomy this morning. By witnessing the signing of an informed consent form, the nurse affirms that:
   a. Mr. McNail was properly informed of the procedure.
   b. The signature on the form is Mr. McNail's.
   c. The surgical procedure will be performed as stated on the form.
   d. The surgeon's explanation to Mr. McNail was witnessed by the nurse.

Answer ( ) Rationale: _____
_____
_____

7. The purpose of leg exercises postoperatively is to:
   a. Promote venous return
   b. Maintain muscle tone
   c. Assess range of motion
   d. Exercise fatigued muscles

Answer ( ) Rationale: _____
_____
_____

8. Guidelines for ensuring that all nursing interventions are completed on the day of surgery are located on which document?
   a. Nurse's notes
   b. Anesthesia record
   c. Preoperative checklist
   d. Physician's order sheet

Answer (   ) Rationale: _____
_____
_____

9. To prevent airway obstruction, the nurse in the PACU positions the client:
   a. With arms over or across the chest
   b. On one side with the face down and the neck slightly extended
   c. In the Trendelenburg position
   d. Prone with the neck extended

Answer (   ) Rationale: _____
_____
_____

10. Mr. Smith has been admitted to the PACU following abdominal surgery. The nurse notes that his blood pressure is decreasing; his pulse rate is increasing, his skin is cool and clammy; and his abdominal dressing has a large area of bright red drainage. The nurse should:
    a. Notify the physician immediately.
    b. Understand that this is normal and continue to monitor.
    c. Apply a specially warmed blanket to increase the client's metabolic rate.
    d. Realize that these are symptoms of acute pain and treat accordingly.

Answer (   ) Rationale: _____
_____
_____

11. The PACU nurse notices that the client is shivering. This is most commonly caused by:
    a. The use of a reflective blanket on the operating room table
    b. Side effects of certain anesthetic agents
    c. Cold irrigations used during surgery
    d. Malignant hypothermia, a serious condition

Answer (   ) Rationale: _____
_____
_____

CLINICAL SITUATIONS

1. Mrs. Tice is a 40-year-old mother of two entering the outpatient surgery clinic for a breast biopsy. She has not had surgery before. She is a smoker and takes medication for high blood pressure. What factors will the nurse assess preoperatively in developing a plan for surgical care?

_____
_____
_____
_____
_____
_____
_____
_____
_____

2. Ms. Lyons is recovering from surgery on the first postoperative day. The nurse finds that the client's abdomen is distended. What might this indicate?

_____
_____
_____
_____
_____
_____
_____
_____
_____

Chapter 49 — Clients With Wounds

The integument is a protective barrier against disease-causing organisms; is a sensory organ for pain, temperature, and touch; and can synthesize vitamin D. Injury to the integument poses risks to safety and triggers a complex healing response.

PRELIMINARY READING

Chapter 49, pp. 1428-1464

COMPREHENSIVE UNDERSTANDING

∎ NORMAL INTEGUMENT

➤ Define the following terms related to the integument:

Epidermis _____

_____

Dermis _____

_____

Desquamation _____

_____

Collagen _____

_____

➤ Briefly describe the functions of the epidermis and the dermis: _____

_____

_____

_____

➤ Describe the normal changes that occur in aging skin:

a. _____

_____

b. _____

_____

c. _____

_____

d. _____

_____

e. _____

_____

f. _____

_____

∎ WOUND CLASSIFICATIONS

➤ A wound is _____.

➤ Wound classification systems describe the _____

_____, _____,

_____, _____,

or _____.

➤ Define the following wound classifications:

Clean-contaminated _____

_____

Unintentional _____

_____

Open _____

_____

Perforating _____

_____

Infected _____

_____

Closed _____

_____

Laceration _____

_____

Contusion _____

_____

Intentional _____

_____

Clean _____

_____

Colonized _____

_____

Contaminated _____

_____

Superficial _____

_____

Abrasion _____

_____

Penetrating _____

_____

▌WOUND HEALING PROCESS

➤ The nature of healing is the same for all wounds, with variations depending on the location, severity, and extent of injury.

➤ Describe the two types of healing processes.

Primary intention: _____

_____

Secondary intention: _____

_____

Healing by Primary Intention

➤ List in sequence and briefly describe the three stages of healing by primary intention.

a. _____

_____

_____

b. _____

_____

_____

c. _____

_____

_____

Healing by Secondary Intention

➤ Briefly describe the healing process that occurs with

secondary intention: _____

_____

_____

_____

➤ Granulation tissue is _____.

▌COMPLICATIONS OF WOUND HEALING

Hemorrhage

➤ Briefly describe how the nurse can detect the following:

External hemorrhage _____

_____

_____

_____

Internal hemorrhage _____

_____

_____

_____

➤ A hematoma is _____

_____.

Infection

➤ Wound infection is the second most common nosocomial infection.

➤ List and describe four signs and symptoms of wound infection.

a. _____

_____

b. _____

_____

c. _____

_____

d. _____

_____

Dehiscence

➤ Define *dehiscence:* _____

_____

_____

_____

➤ List three causes of wound dehiscence.

a. _____

_____

b. _____

_____

c. _____

_____

Evisceration

➤ Define *evisceration:* _____

_____

_____

➤ Explain the action the nurse should take when a client's
wound eviscerates: _____

_____

_____

_____

Fistulas

➤ Define *fistula:* _____

_____

➤ List four causes of a fistula.

a. _____

_____

b. _____

_____

c. _____

_____

d. _____

_____

Delayed Wound Healing

➤ Define *third-intention wound healing:* _____

_____

_____

■ FACTORS INFLUENCING WOUND HEALING

Nutrition

➤ List the five nutrients needed for wound healing and
describe their contribution to the healing process.

a. _____

_____

b. _____

_____

c. _____

_____

d. _____

_____

e. _____

_____

➤ Describe how each factor impairs wound healing.

Age: _____

_____

_____

_____

Malnutrition: _____

_____

_____

_____

Obesity: _____

_____

_____

_____

Impaired oxygenation: _____

_____

_____

_____

Smoking: _____

_____

_____

_____

_____

Steroids: _____

_____

_____

_____

Antibiotics: _____

_____

_____

_____

Chemotherapeutic drugs: _____

_____

_____

_____

Diabetes: _____

_____

_____

_____

Radiation: _____

_____

_____

_____

Wound stress: _____

_____

_____

_____

■ PSYCHOSOCIAL IMPACT OF WOUNDS

➤ Body image changes can impose a great stress on the client's adaptive mechanisms.
➤ List three factors that may affect the client's perception of the wound.

a. _____

b. _____

c. _____

■ NURSING PROCESS AND WOUND HEALING

Assessment

➤ List four areas for assessment of a wound in an emergency setting.

a. _____

b. _____

c. _____

d. _____

➤ List six areas for assessment of a wound in a stable setting (for example, after surgery or treatment).

a. _____

b. _____

c. _____

d. _____

e. _____

f. _____

➤ Describe the normal appearance of a wound: _____

_____

_____

➤ Describe the characteristics of the following types of wound drainage:

Serous _____

_____

Purulent _____

_____

Serosanguineous _____

_____

Sanguineous _____

_____

➤ Explain the purposes for the use of drains and the nursing implications: _____

_____

_____

_____

_____

_____

➤ Surgical wounds are closed with _____,

_____, or _____.

➤ Explain the technique of inspecting and palpating a wound: _____

_____

_____

_____

➤ If the client experiences serious discomfort while the nurse inspects or palpates the wound, the nurse should look for underlying problems.
➤ Compare the techniques used to obtain the following wound cultures:

Aerobic _____

_____

_____

_____

_____

Anaerobic _____

_____

_____

_____

Nursing Diagnosis

➤ List nine potential or actual nursing diagnoses for wound healing.

a. _____

b. _____

c. _____

d. _____

e. _____

f. _____

g. _____

h. _____

i. _____

Planning

➤ List seven goals appropriate for the client with a wound.

a. _____

b. _____

c. _____

d. _____

e. _____

f. _____

g. _____

Implementation

First Aid for Wounds

➤ List and explain, in order of priority, the four first aid interventions for clients with a traumatic wound.

a. _____

_____

_____

_____

b. _____

_____

_____

_____

_____

c. _____

_____

_____

_____

d. _____

_____

_____

➤ List the topical agents used for cleansing wounds.

a. _____

b. _____

c. _____

d. _____

e. _____

Dressings

➤ The choice of dressings and the method of dressing a wound influence the progress of wound healing.

➤ Ideally, a dressing leaves a wound slightly _____

_____to promote _____.

➤ List the seven purposes of dressings.

a. _____

b. _____

c. _____

d. _____

e. _____

f. _____

g. _____

➤ Explain the purpose of pressure dressings: _____

_____

_____

➤ List and briefly explain the purpose of each of the three layers of a surgical dressing.

a. _____

_____

b. _____
_____

c. _____
_____

➤ List the seven AHCPR clinical guidelines for selection of dressings.

a. _____

b. _____

c. _____

d. _____

e. _____

f. _____

g. _____

➤ Describe the following types of dressings, and give the purpose of each:

Woven gauze _____

_____

_____

_____

Wet-to-dry _____

_____

_____

_____

Self-adhesive _____

_____

_____

_____

Hydrocolloid _____

_____

_____

_____

Hydrogel _____

_____

_____

_____

➤ List the four guidelines for the dressing change procedure recommended by the CDC.

a. _____

b. _____

c. _____

d. _____

➤ List four nursing actions appropriate in preparing a client for a dressing change.

a. _____

b. _____

c. _____

d. _____

➤ List the eight principles for packing a wound.

a. _____

b. _____

c. _____

d. _____

e. _____

f. _____

g. _____

h. _____

➤ The choice of securing dressings depends on the

_____, _____,

_____, _____,

and _____.

➤ Briefly describe the method the nurse uses to remove tape safely: _____

_____

_____

_____

➤ List five nursing interventions used to minimize discomfort during wound care:

a. _____

b. _____

c. _____

d. _____

e. _____

Cleansing Skin and Drain Sites

➤ Cleansing a wound or drain site may be required if a dressing does not properly absorb drainage or if an open drain deposits drainage onto the skin.

➤ List the three principles that are important when cleansing an incision or the area around the drain.

a. _____

b. _____

c. _____

➤ List the three purposes of wound irrigation.

a. _____

b. _____

c. _____

Suture Care

➤ Sutures are _____,

_____, and _____,

and _____ determine the suture
material to be used.

➤ A Steri-strip is _____.

➤ Describe the procedure for removing staples: _____

_____

_____

Drainage Evacuation

➤ Describe a drainage evacuator: _____

_____

_____

_____

Bandages and Binders

➤ List six purposes for the use of a binder or bandage.

a. _____

b. _____

c. _____

d. _____

e. _____

f. _____

➤ Describe four nursing responsibilities that must be
performed before applying a bandage or binder.

a. _____

b. _____

c. _____

d. _____

➤ Briefly describe the following types of binder applications:

Abdominal binder _____

_____

_____

_____

T-binders _____

_____

_____

_____

➤ Sling supports are used for _____.

➤ Describe the following types of bandage applications:

Circular _____

_____

Spiral _____

_____

Spiral-reverse _____

_____

Figure eight _____

_____

Recurrent _____

_____

Heat and Cold Therapy

➤ List four factors the nurse must consider before using heat or cold therapy.

a. _____

b. _____

c. _____

d. _____

➤ List five conditions that increase the risk of injury
from heat and cold applications.

a. _____

b. _____

c. _____

d. _____

e. _____

➤ List five physiological responses of heat application,
and give their therapeutic benefit.

a. _____

_____

b. _____

_____

c. _____

_____

d. _____

_____

e. _____

➤ List five physiological responses of cold application, and give their therapeutic benefit.

a. _____

_____

b. _____

_____

c. _____

_____

d. _____

_____

e. _____

_____

➤ The body's response to heat and cold therapies depends on six factors. List them, and explain each one.

a. _____

_____

b. _____

_____

c. _____

_____

d. _____

_____

e. _____

_____

f. _____

_____

➤ List the four areas to assess before applying heat or cold therapies.

a. _____

b. _____

c. _____

d. _____

➤ Complete the safety chart below describing the *do's* and *dont's* for application of heat or cold therapy.
➤ Complete the grid on the next page describing the advantages and disadvantages of moist and dry applications.
➤ Explain the following types of heat or cold applications, and give the nursing implications for each:

Warm soaks _____

_____

_____

_____

Sitz baths _____

_____

_____

_____

_____

	Do's	Dont's
Heat therapy		
Cold therapy		

Applications	Advantages	Disadvantages
Moist applications		
Dry applications		

Aquathermia pads _____

_____

_____

_____

_____

Warm air blower _____

_____

_____

_____

_____

Commercial hot packs _____

_____

_____

_____

Electric heating pads _____

_____

_____

_____

_____

Cold, moist, and dry compresses _____

_____

_____

_____

Cold soaks _____

_____

_____

_____

Ice bags or collars _____

_____

_____

_____

Evaluation

➤ List three expected outcomes for the client with impaired skin integrity.

a. _____

b. _____

c. _____

REVIEW QUESTIONS

(The student should select the appropriate answer and cite the rationale for choosing that particular answer.)

1. An example of an injury that heals by secondary intention is a/an:
   a. Burn
   b. Appendectomy incision
   c. Fracture
   d. Sprained ankle

   Answer ( ) Rationale: _____

   _____

   _____

2. Obesity can influence wound healing because:
   a. Adipose tissue is fragile.
   b. There is a decrease in functional hemoglobin levels in fatty tissue.
   c. There are fewer blood vessels in adipose tissue.
   d. Cell growth and differentiation in structure are slower in the obese client.

   Answer ( ) Rationale: _____

   _____

   _____

3. Which of the following complications of wound healing is considered a medical emergency?
   a. Hematoma
   b. Dehiscence
   c. Fistula
   d. Evisceration

   Answer ( ) Rationale: _____

   _____

   _____

4. While assessing the client's dressing, the nurse finds pale watery red drainage. This is documented as:
   a. Serous
   b. Sanguineous
   c. Serosanguineous
   d. Purulent

   Answer ( ) Rationale: _____

   _____

   _____

5. When cleansing Mr. Pearson's wound, the nurse cleans from the least contaminated to the most contaminated area. The rationale for this is to:
   a. Prevent contaminating previously cleaned areas
   b. Promote proper absorption of drainage
   c. Reduce excess moisture that may harbor microorganisms
   d. Prevent introduction of organisms into the wound

   Answer ( ) Rationale: _____

   _____

   _____

6. Mrs. Palmer's wound is healing by secondary intention. Which of the following cleansing agents should *not* be used?
   a. Hibiclens
   b. Betadine
   c. Hydrogen peroxide
   d. Normal saline

   Answer ( ) Rationale: _____

   _____

   _____

7. Which of the following techniques is performed when removing sutures?
   a. The visible portion is pulled through first.
   b. Each suture is clipped as far away from the skin as possible.
   c. Tweezers are necessary only for removal of continuous sutures.
   d. The suture is clipped close to the skin and pulled through from the other side.

   Answer ( ) Rationale: _____

   _____

   _____

8. Dr. Smith orders a heat application for Mrs. Hyde, age 75. When carrying out this order the nurse bases his or her actions on the fact that the elderly have:
   a. Alterations in nerve pathways
   b. Thickened skin areas
   c. Reduced sensitivity to pain
   d. Increased sensitivity to temperature stimuli

   Answer ( ) Rationale: _____

   _____

   _____

9. In which situation is the application of heat appropriate?
   a. Client A, admitted with possible appendicitis, would like a heating pad applied to his abdomen.
   b. Client B, who had knee surgery this morning and has large areas of serous drainage on his dressing, would like a hot water bottle over his bandage.
   c. Client C has peripheral vascular problems and likes to apply a heating pad to her feet at night.
   d. Client D has swelling in his left ankle, which he sprained 3 days ago, and would like to apply warm compresses.

Answer ( ) Rationale: _____

_____

10. An advantage of a moist application over a dry one is that the moist application:
    a. Has less risk of burns to the skin
    b. Does not cause skin maceration
    c. Retains temperature longer
    d. Penetrates deeply into tissue layers

Answer ( ) Rationale: _____

_____

11. Ms. Sampson is to apply an ice bag to her jaw following dental surgery. All of the following instructions are appropriate *except:*
    a. Apply the ice bag to the jaw for 1 hour; bag may be reapplied in 30 minutes.
    b. Fill the bag two-thirds full with crushed ice.
    c. Remove air from the bag by squeezing its sides before securing the cap.
    d. Cover the bag with a towel before applying.

Answer ( ) Rationale: _____

_____

_____

CLINICAL SITUATIONS

1. Your client is admitted for abdominal pain. Upon visual inspection, you identify a red, blistering area over the lower abdomen. The client reports having used a hot water bottle at home. Please list additional assessment parameters needed, and identify a treatment and teaching plan.

_____

_____

_____

_____

_____

_____

_____

_____

_____

_____

2. There is an order to cleanse a lower abdominal wound with normal saline with each dressing change. Upon inspection, you identify a 1-cm diameter wound with a depth of 4.5 cm. You are unable to visualize the base. What steps should you take in caring for this client?

_____

_____

_____

_____

_____

_____

_____

_____

ANSWERS TO REVIEW QUESTIONS AND CLINICAL SITUATIONS

Chapter 1
REVIEW QUESTIONS

1. c (p. 10)
2. d (p. 11)
3. b (p. 13)
4. b (p. 14)
5. d (p. 6)
6. b (p. 6-7)
7. d (p. 5)
8. c (p. 13)

Chapter 2
REVIEW QUESTIONS

1. d (p. 22)
2. a (p. 23)
3. d (p. 27)
4. a (p. 27)
5. a (p. 28)
6. d (p. 30)
7. a (p. 31)
8. c (p. 32)
9. a (p. 34)
10. a (p. 36-37)
11. a (p. 39, 42)

Chapter 3
REVIEW QUESTIONS

1. c (p. 48)
2. a (p. 54)
3. b (p. 48)
4. a (p. 52)
5. b (p. 52)
6. c (p. 55)

Chapter 4
REVIEW QUESTIONS

1. d (p. 65)
2. a (p. 67)
3. d (p. 68)
4. b (p. 73)
5. d (p. 76)
6. c (p. 71)

Chapter 5
REVIEW QUESTIONS

1. c (p. 81)
2. d (p. 82)
3. d (p. 83)
4. c (p. 84)
5. a (p. 92)
6. c (p. 92)
7. b (p. 84)

Chapter 6
REVIEW QUESTIONS

1. b (p. 100)
2. c (p. 103)
3. c (p. 105)
4. b (p. 105)
5. a (p. 105)
6. c (p. 105)
7. e (p. 105)
8. d (p. 105)

Chapter 7
REVIEW QUESTIONS

1. c (p. 112)
2. a (p. 114)
3. a (p. 114)
4. b (p. 114)
5. b (p. 120)
6. d (p. 111)
7. c (p. 111)
8. c (p. 115)
9. b (p. 121)
10. a (p. 121)
11. d (p. 121)

Chapter 8
REVIEW QUESTIONS

1. a (p. 125)
2. c (p. 128)
3. a (p. 129)
4. b (p. 129)
5. d (p. 132)
6. c (p. 129)
7. d (p. 129)
8. a (p. 131-132)
9. b (p. 128, 132)

Chapter 9
REVIEW QUESTIONS

1. c (p. 138)
2. d (p. 138)
3. b (p. 138)
4. d (p. 139)
5. c (p. 141)
6. c (p. 137-138)
7. d (p. 137)
8. b (p. 152-153)
9. a (p. 144)

Chapter 10
REVIEW QUESTIONS

1. b (p. 156)
2. d (p. 157)
3. b (p. 157-158)
4. d (p. 158)
5. a (p. 159)
6. c (p. 160)
7. a (p. 156)
8. c (p. 160-161)
9. a (p. 161)
10. b (p. 159)

Chapter 11
REVIEW QUESTIONS

1. c (p. 166)
2. c (p. 166)
3. b (p. 166-167)
4. b (p. 168)
5. a (p. 168)
6. c (p. 168-169)
7. d (p. 172-173)
8. b (p. 173)
9. c (p. 175)
10. c (p. 175)

Chapter 12
REVIEW QUESTIONS

1. b (p. 180)
2. c (p. 183)
3. a (p. 184)
4. c (p. 200)
5. c (p. 202-204)
6. d (Table 12-3)
7. a (p. 187)
8. a (p. 186)
9. d (p. 186)
10. d (p. 193, 197)
11. b (p. 197)

Chapter 13
REVIEW QUESTIONS

1. a (p. 208)
2. a (p. 211)
3. c (p. 216)
4. d (p. 217)
5. c (p. 217)
6. c (p. 218)
7. c (p. 222)
8. a (p. 222-223)
9. d (p. 223)
10. a (p. 225)

Chapter 14
REVIEW QUESTIONS

1. b (p. 234)
2. b (p. 236)
3. b (p. 236)
4. b (p. 241)
5. a (p. 244)
6. d (p. 255)
7. a (p. 233)
8. b (p. 240)
9. c (p. 240)
10. b (p. 250)
11. c (p. 252)

Chapter 15
REVIEW QUESTIONS

1. a (p. 262)
2. c (p. 262)
3. b (p. 265)
4. c (p. 264)
5. d (p. 266)
6. c (p. 267)
7. c (p. 271)
8. b (p. 272)
9. a (p. 276)
10. c (p. 281)

Chapter 16
REVIEW QUESTIONS

1. b (p. 291)
2. b (p. 292)
3. d (p. 292)
4. c (p. 292-293)
5. b (p. 293)
6. d (p. 293)
7. c (p. 293)
8. b (p. 287)
9. d (p. 294)

Chapter 17
REVIEW QUESTIONS

1. a (p. 299)
2. d (p. 299)
3. d (p. 299-300)
4. d (p. 299)
5. c (p. 303-304)
6. c (p. 301)
7. d (p. 301)
8. b (p. 300)
9. a (p. 300)

Chapter 18
REVIEW QUESTIONS

1. d (p. 307)
2. b (Table 18-1)
3. a (p. 312-314)
4. c (p. 314)
5. b (p. 308)
6. a (Table 18-1)
7. b (p. 313)
8. d (p. 313)
9. d (p. 312-313)

Chapter 19
REVIEW QUESTIONS

1. d (p. 323)
2. c (p. 320)
3. c (p. 323)
4. d (p. 327)
5. a (p. 329)
6. b (p. 328)
7. c (p. 326)
8. d (p. 322)

Chapter 20
REVIEW QUESTIONS

1. a (p. 333)
2. c (p. 334)
3. d (p. 335)
4. b (p. 336)
5. b (p. 340)
6. a (p. 341)
7. d (p. 342)
8. d (p. 341)
9. b (p. 346)
10. b (p. 344)

Chapter 21
REVIEW QUESTIONS

1. a (p. 353-354)
2. c (p. 357)
3. b (p. 360-361)
4. b (p. 358)
5. b (p. 360)
6. a (p. 352)
7. a (p. 357)
8. b (p. 366)

Chapter 22
REVIEW QUESTIONS

1. d (p. 371)
2. a (p. 371)
3. b (p. 372)
4. d (p. 377)
5. a (p. 371)
6. d (p. 374)
7. c (p. 375)
8. b (p. 376)
9. c (p. 378)
10. d (p. 380-381)
11. d (p. 382-383)

Chapter 23
REVIEW QUESTIONS

1. c (p. 390)
2. c (p. 390-391)
3. b (p. 391)
4. d (p. 397)
5. a (p. 390)
6. c (p. 390-391)
7. b (p. 391)
8. d (p. 398)
9. b (p. 395)

Chapter 24
REVIEW QUESTIONS

1. c (p. 412)
2. c (p. 415-416)
3. d (p. 416)
4. b (p. 418)
5. d (p. 418)
6. c (p. 419-420)
7. b (p. 420-421)
8. a (p. 422)
9. d (p. 422)
10. c (p. 424)
11. d (p. 427)
12. c (p. 429)

Chapter 25
REVIEW QUESTIONS

1. a (p. 477)
2. d (Table 25-3)
3. a (p. 452)
4. a (Table 25-3)
5. a (p. 449)
6. c (p. 451)

Chapter 26
REVIEW QUESTIONS

1. c (p. 458)
2. c (p. 459)
3. c (p. 462)
4. c (p. 464)
5. b (p. 472)
6. d (p. 460)
7. c (Table 26-2)
8. c (p. 466)
9. d (p. 467)
10. a (p. 468)
11. a (p. 472-473)

Chapter 27
REVIEW QUESTIONS

1. a (p. 478)
2. a (p. 478)
3. b (p. 480)
4. c (p. 480)
5. a (p. 485)
6. c (p. 485)
7. c (p. 482)
8. c (p. 487)
9. c (p. 489)
10. a (p. 485)

CLINICAL SITUATIONS

1. Although the focus of the family as client is the family, itself, the focus of the family as context is the health and development of an individual member within his or her family environment. Although distinctions can be made between the two approaches, they are not necessarily mutually exclusive, and it is important that the nurse recognize that a nursing intervention for one member impacts all family members. For example, a newly diagnosed diabetic client will need to learn to care for all aspects of his or her disease, and the family will also have adjustments to make and new information to understand. When other family members are not available or refuse to be involved, an individual approach is the only possibility. However, the nurse recognizes that the client's family background influences behavior.
2. Suggestions to the parents would include specific instructions on how to meet the physical and emotional needs of the ill child, while remembering that the other members of the family continue to have needs; how to avoid contagion to other members of the family, and how to share the added tasks and responsibilities of caring for an ill family member. In addition, suggestions for a single-parent family must also consider that the added tasks and responsibilities are likely to be more overwhelming since there is only one adult available. The nurse may need to help the single parent identify and use outside resources and suggest ways to allocate time.

Chapter 28
REVIEW QUESTIONS

1. c (p. 497)
2. d (p. 497)
3. a (p. 504)
4. c (p. 505)
5. c (p. 505-506)
6. d (p. 506-507)
7. b (p. 510-511)
8. c (p. 513)
9. d (p. 514-515)
10. a (p. 515-516)

CLINICAL SITUATIONS

1. The development of attachment is essential for optimal infant growth and development. Close physical contact and interaction facilitates attachment. Parents and family members should be provided with opportunities to touch, feed, comfort, care for, and play with the newborn. Nursing interventions should reduce attachment-inhibiting factors such as parental fatigue, hunger, pain, and stress, as well as limitations on the newborn's ability to respond. Nurses should assess the progress of attachment and facilitate interaction by demonstrating care measures, pointing out newborn's reciprocal responses, and providing explanations regarding newborn health status and behaviors. Sibling visitation is another helpful measure that nurses can recommend and arrange.
2. Preschoolers demonstrate an increased ability to cooperate, share thoughts, and interact and communicate. When teaching about health, nurses should consider that cognitive development is at the preoperational level and is characterized by egocentricity, concrete and causal thinking, and the mixing of fantasy and reality. Preschoolers continue to rely on caregivers for support and security, especially in times of stress or illness. Nursing measures are required that maintain close family contact and foster trust in health care providers. Play facilitates expression in concerns and emotions and can be used to teach. Participating in their own care and learning about their health enhances the preschooler's health concept, reduces fear, and preserves a sense of control.

Chapter 29
REVIEW QUESTIONS

1. c (p. 534)
2. c (p. 529)
3. b (p. 532)
4. a (p. 536)
5. d (p. 537)
6. c (p. 539)
7. d (p. 540)
8. a (p. 541-542)
9. b (p. 533)
10. b (p. 540)
11. c (p. 542)

CLINICAL SITUATIONS

1. Sexual maturation and interest in sexual matters requires the education of the adolescent. Formal operations and abstract thinking characterize adolescent cognition, allowing them to acquire decision-making skills, understand complex information, define appropriate sex role behaviors, and consider the impact of their actions on themselves and others. They may respond more positively to instruction from adults other than their parents. Peers are major influences on behavior. One-on-one discussions, peer-group work, role playing, and decision-making practice are effective modalities to help adolescents see the consequences of sexual activity (including transmission of AIDS) and make decisions that are right for them. Safe sex practices must be addressed.
2. a. The rate of growth during adolescence is slower. The average increase in height is 2 inches per year, and weight increases by 4 to 7 lb per year. Also during adolescence cardiovascular functioning is refined and stabilized. Heart rate averages 70 to 90 beats/min, B/P 110/70 mm Hg, respiration rate 19 to 21 breaths per minute. Assess fine and gross motor skills (refer to Table 29-3), and note any deficiencies in iron, vitamin A, or calcium.
   b. According to Freud the developmental stage is called *latency*. This is a tranquil period when Freud believed sexual drives were dominant; however, child may engage in erogenous activities with same-sex peers. Child's use of coping and defense mechanisms emerge at this time. Any sexual interest may be sublimated through vigorous play and skill acquisition.
   c. According to Erickson, this stage is called *industry versus inferiority*. Feelings of inferiority may occur when adults perceive child's attempt to learn how things work through manipulation by being silly or troublesome. Lack of success in school, development of physical skills, and making friends also contribute to inferiority.

Chapter 30
REVIEW QUESTIONS

1. a (p. 551)
2. b (p. 554)
3. b (Table 30-3)
4. c (Table 30-4)
5. d (p. 564)
6. d (p. 550)
7. d (p. 552-554)
8. b (Table 30-4)
9. a (p. 559)

CLINICAL SITUATIONS

1. Changes during pregnancy are complex, requiring health guidance and counseling, discussion of feelings and stressors, stress reduction techniques, and physical care. Research has demonstrated that early, ongoing prenatal care reduces the rate of low birth weight as well as maternal-newborn morbidity and mortality. The nurse must emphasize how prenatal care influences the outcome of pregnancy. A connection should be made between the changes that occur during pregnancy and the need for health care to promote effective adaptation to these changes and to prevent problems from occurring. The client must learn that pregnancy is a dynamic state and that risk status can change as pregnancy progresses and other stressors (e.g., job, building a home) occur.
2. a. According to Erickson's theory, the primary developmental task of the middle years is to achieve generativity, the willingness to care for and guide others. The effects of treating cervical cancer may affect the roles and responsibilities assumed by the middle adult. Strained family relationships, modifications in family activities, increased health care tasks, increased financial stress, the need for housing adaptation, social isolation, medical concerns, and grieving.
   b. In the middle years, as children depart from the household, the family enters the postparental family stage. Time and financial demands on the parents decrease, and the couple faces the task of redefining their own relationship. The departure of the last child from the home may be a stressor. Many parents welcome freedom from child-rearing responsibilities, whereas others feel lonely or without direction because of the change. Eventually parents must reassess their marriage, resolve conflicts, and plan for the future.
   c. Potential for ineffective family or individual coping; Altered family processes; Potential for altered sexuality patterns; Altered health maintenance.
   d. Improved knowledge about the impact of risk factors on level of health; improved health-promotion activities; improved communication within their family structures; fewer experiences of illnesses and inability to problem-solve.

Chapter 31
REVIEW QUESTIONS

1. b (p. 571)
2. a (p. 577)
3. c (p. 577)
4. d (p. 577)
5. b (p. 583)
6. b (p. 589)
7. c (p. 579)
8. d (p. 587)
9. c (Table 31-1)
10. b (p. 578)

CLINICAL SITUATIONS

1. The client's concept of a meaningful retirement, current type and degree of socialization, adequacy of income to meet needs and desired leisure pursuits, and coping and adaptation skills.
2. Decreased peristalsis, hemorrhoids, anal fissures, and decreased mobility secondary to age-related musculoskeletal disorders.

Chapter 32
REVIEW QUESTIONS

1. d (p. 596-597)
2. b (p. 601, 608)
3. d (p. 597-598)
4. b (p. 601)
5. d (p. 614)
6. c (p. 614)
7. c (p. 614)
8. c (p. 633, Table 31-11)
9. b (p. 621)
10. c (p. 633)

CLINICAL SITUATIONS

1. The nurse would assess core body temperature, followed by heart rate and blood pressure. Body temperature would most easily and accurately be measured with a tympanic device. A rectal temperature would be acceptable if a tympanic monitor were not available. Risk factors for this client include age and homeless status.
2. Provide fluids to prevent dehydration. Consult with a physician about whether antibiotics are to be ordered. If so, give on time. Keep client comfortable with minimal covering but prevent shivering. Exposure of body parts increases radiation. Shivering can increase body temperature. Bathe in tepid water to increase convection.

Chapter 33
REVIEW QUESTIONS

1. d (p. 649)
2. d (p. 649)
3. a (p. 659)
4. b (p. 651-653)
5. c (p. 659)
6. c (p. 669)
7. a (p. 677-678)
8. c (p. 683-687)
9. b (Table 33-21)
10. a (p. 690-691)
11. d (p. 691-692)
12. c (p. 696)
13. a (p. 704)
14. b (p. 710)
15. c (p. 730)

CLINICAL SITUATIONS

1. When the client exhibits weight loss and fatigue, the nurse might assess further for involvement of the immune, gastrointestinal, and cardiac systems. Immune system alterations may be assessed through examination of lymph nodes coupled with a more detailed client history (e.g., exposure to a communicable disease, history of febrile episodes).
   Weight loss may be linked to both upper and lower GI problems. Thus the nurse would assess the oral cavity and the abdomen for evidence of alterations. Fatigue may be linked to cardiac disease and should not be discounted, although there may be a direct correlation to weight loss and cardiac disease.
2. Abdominal pain: abdominal palpation; inspection of patient's position and posture.
   Oral hygiene: inspection of gums, teeth, and mucosa.
   Cast application: assessment of circulation to involved extremity, including pulses, color and temperature of skin, and presence of edema.

Chapter 34
REVIEW QUESTIONS

1. d (p. 4)
2. b (p. 4)
3. b (p. 6)
4. d (p. 4)
5. a (p. 6)
6. a (p. 8)
7. c (p. 11)
8. b (p. 17)
9. b (p. 18)
10. d (p. 19)
11. d (p. 15)
12. a (p. 16-17)

CLINICAL SITUATIONS

1. The first tier contains precautions designed to care for all clients in health care facilities regardless of their diagnosis or presumed infectiousness. Standard precautions apply to blood, all body fluids regardless of whether or not they contain blood, nonintact skin, and mucous membranes. These precautions promote handwashing and use of gloves, masks, eye protection, or gowns when appropriate for client contact.

   Second tier precautions are designed for highly transmissible or epidemiologically important pathogens.

2. The nurse should include measures in the care plan emphasizing prevention of food-borne illness: careful handwashing before food preparation, adequate cooking of food, and prompt refrigeration of unused portions.

Chapter 35
REVIEW QUESTIONS

1. b (p. 794)
2. a (p. 794)
3. d (p. 795)
4. d (p. 795)
5. c (p. 796)
6. a (p. 797)
7. a (p. 799)
8. a (p. 801)
9. c (p. 802)
10. b (p. 803)
11. b (p. 809)
12. b (p. 822, 826)
13. a (p. 827)
14. d (p. 847)
15. b (p. 852)

CLINICAL SITUATIONS

1. The nurse should implement the following actions:
   - Determine the specific needs of the client regarding self-administration of medication.
   - Instruct the client and available support persons about the medications and their administration using enlarged print materials, pictures, or both.
   - Provide or recommend medication vials or packages with enlarged print labels, and cups or syringes with easy to read scales. Braille materials and labels may be obtained, if indicated, for clients who are blind.
   - Use color-coding to reinforce identification and scheduling of medications.
   - Refer the client to a community health resource, as appropriate.
2. Administration of medications to infants and children requires the following special considerations:
   - Calculating carefully with generally smaller dosage
   - Providing explanations that the child will understand (e.g., using pictures or puppets)
   - Offering simple choices for taking the medication (e.g., asking the child if fruit juice or water is preferred when taking the medication)
   - Giving injections only into the sites where the muscles are fully developed
   - Using spoons, plastic cups, and syringes for giving liquid medications
   - Restraining to prevent injury
   - Participation of parents or guardians in the administration of the medication
   - Praising positive medication experiences

Chapter 36
REVIEW QUESTIONS

1. d (p. 871)
2. d (p. 872)
3. c (p. 882-884)
4. c (p. 884-885)
5. b (p. 885)
6. d (p. 878)
7. d (p. 883)
8. c (p. 889)
9. b (Table 36-2)
10. a (p. 885)

CLINICAL SITUATIONS

1. Some alternatives to using restraints include the following: Make the environment as safe as possible and as homelike as possible. Determine client's behavior patterns. Meet physical needs such as providing pain relief and assisting with toileting needs. Modify the environment by keeping noise level low or playing soft music. Use night lights, and keep the bed in a low position. Identify the door of the client's room with a picture, sign, or some other device that the client will recognize. Spend time with the client. Allow the client to walk in the halls as much as possible, using a barrier to limit wandering from the designated area. Allow the client to assist the staff with simple tasks, and provide activities for client participation. Use pillows, wedges, and other devices to keep the client positioned safely. Involve the family in care as much as possible.
2. In deciding how to approach Mrs. Lopez the nurse must consider her cultural orientation and her socioeconomic status. Is this practice socially acceptable among her friends and family? Is she aware of the dangers? Why are all of them sitting in the front seat? Is the back seat occupied by clothing, furniture, or personal belongings? Can she afford a car seat? In this situation the nurse must be careful to teach about the hazards of this practice without being judgmental, accusatory, or condescending. If possible, it may be helpful to teach this and other safety practices to a group of young mothers at the clinic. Most communities have agencies that provide free car seats to families who cannot afford them, and the nurse could make appropriate referrals. Since most states have laws regarding mandatory use of car seats, referral to a social worker may be appropriate. (Depending on the results of the assessment the nurse may identify other problems and needs for teaching, such as family planning.)

Chapter 37
Chapter 37
REVIEW QUESTIONS

1. c (p. 894)
2. b (p. 896)
3. a (Table 37-2)
4. a (p. 910)
5. d (p. 915)
6. d (p. 919)
7. b (p. 927, 932)
8. d (p. 933)
9. d (p. 900-903)
10. a (p. 913)
11. d (p. 940)

CLINICAL SITUATIONS

1. The following basic guidelines should be discussed with Mr. Kauffman's daughter:
   a. Start with correct posture: muscles and joints do not function optimally when posture is faulty. Injury to bones, muscles, and joints can result.
   b. Maintain a wide base of support. Her feet should be positioned 6 to 8 inches apart. Keeping feet at shoulder width with one foot slightly in front of the other provides the greatest possible range of movement without straining to maintain balance.
   c. Use large muscle. Reaching and bending or twisting the spine while lifting or moving is likely to cause injury. The working surface should be at or slightly above the waist and directly in front of the body. This will allow maximum efficiency of the large muscles of the lower extremities.
   d. Use your body as a counterweight. When lifting or moving Mr. Kauffman, her body weight should be used to counteract the weight of her father. This technique is useful for both pushing and pulling.
   e. Minimize friction. Friction is the resistance created by a moving object on a surface. Friction can be diminished when the surface is smooth and well-lubricated, when the area of contact between surface and object is decreased, or when an object is rolled.
   f. Incorporate leverage when possible. Use elbows, hips, and knees as levers when lifting.
2. Priorities for this client include preventing skin and musculoskeletal changes. Because the client has been independent the nurse will want to promote independence and prevent complication so that the client can maintain her independence. Since the client has been healthy and independent, the most common potential problems will be with the integumentary and musculoskeletal system. Changes associated with aging and the usual treatment for fractured hips make the client particularly vulnerable to problems such as skin breakdown, muscle weakness and atrophy, bone demineralization, and decreased joint flexibility. These latter musculoskeletal problems put the elderly client at risk for falls, which are a major concern for the elderly client, especially one who has already broken a hip. Therefore pushing activity within therapeutic guidelines will be of major concern. Turning, positioning, ROM, and personal care will be important in preventing musculoskeletal and integumentary problems.

Chapter 38
REVIEW QUESTIONS

1. b (p. 953-954)
2. b (p. 956)
3. a (Table 38-3)
4. c (p. 957)
5. b (p. 955)
6. c (p. 959)
7. b (p. 967)
8. a (p. 968)
9. d (p. 983)
10. c (p. 976)

CLINICAL SITUATIONS

1. Interventions to reduce pressure ulcer formations
   a. Skin assessment, paying particular attention to pressure points
   b. Use a predictive assessment on this high risk patient
   c. Reduce shear and friction
   d. Use turning schedule based on client assessment findings
   e. Provide pressure-relief surfaces as needed
2. Know the location of the wound. Assess the wound to determine if it is clean, the type of drainage present, and the size of wound. Determine the presence of fluids; assess the client's mobility and activity status. Know what previous treatments were and if they were successful.

Chapter 39
REVIEW QUESTIONS

1. c (Table 39-1)
2. a (p. 997)
3. a (p. 998)
4. b (p. 1000)
5. c (p. 1007)
6. c (p. 1004)
7. b (p. 1007)
8. b (p. 1007-1008)
9. a (p. 1001)
10. c (p. 1009-1010)

CLINICAL SITUATIONS

1. Precautions should be taken when the two children are involved in activities associated with loud noise. Fireworks are dangerous and should only be used under adult supervision. If the children are exposed to loud noises, ear plugs are useful. Parents should also learn to inspect children's ears. Often children place objects in their ears.

2. Encourage the client to eliminate throw rugs to reduce the risk of falls from tripping. Ask a family
member if it is possible to install a new set of lights
to illuminate the stairwell. Bright paint along the
edge of each stair would also help the client see better. Handrails should be installed along the stairwell.

Chapter 40
REVIEW QUESTIONS

1. b (p. 1018-1019)
2. b (p. 1024)
3. a (p. 1021-1022)
4. c (p. 1025)
5. b (Table 40-3)
6. b (p. 1042-1043)
7. c (Table 40-4)
8. a (p. 1050)
9. c (Table 40-6)
10. d (p. 1062)
11. d (p. 1073)

CLINICAL SITUATIONS

1. Mrs. Jones requires attentive skin care. Lotion should
be applied to the skin regularly. Unless the client has
a source of drainage on the skin, reducing the frequency of bathing will help. The client should be
placed on a turning schedule to minimize pressure
on the skin. An appropriate pressure-relieving mat-
tress will reduce risk of pressure ulcer formation. The
patient may also require instruction on proper hygiene.
   Additional assessment measures should include mobility (ability to change position in bed), nutritional
habits, and hygiene habits at home.
2. First inspect the condition of the nails and surrounding skin. This is done to determine the condition of surrounding skin and the risk for infection.
Palpate peripheral pulses. This assesses the condition
of peripheral circulation to tissues. Obtain a physician's order before cutting the nails. This is usually
required in most institutions because of the potential risk to the client. Soak the feet well before performing nail care. If the client has not had regular
foot care, nails and surrounding tissues will be very
hard and brittle. Instruct client on the importance of
routine nail care. Clients must keep nails well
groomed to prevent tissue injury.

Chapter 41
REVIEW QUESTIONS

1. c (p. 1090)
2. d (p. 1092)
3. c (p. 1097)
4. c (p. 1103)
5. c (p. 1103)
6. d (p. 1107)
7. c (p. 1107-1108)
8. c (p. 1113)
9. b (p. 1118)
10. d (p. 1123)
11. a (p. 1112)

CLINICAL SITUATIONS

1. Additional assessment data include frequency of eating, types of foods offered, who "feeds" John Henry
most often, child's motor skills, actual height and
weight, birth weight, and gestational history, including maternal weight gain.
2. Additional assessments include an actual order for
tube feeding, tolerance to previous feedings, amount
of residual volume in the client's stomach, the presence or absence of bowel sounds, abdominal assessment (e.g., rigid, tender), and the actual location of
feeding tube.

Chapter 42
REVIEW QUESTIONS

1. a (p. 1130)
2. c (p. 1131)
3. d (p. 1134)
4. d (p. 1133)
5. a (p. 1135)
6. c (p. 1139)
7. d (p. 1143)
8. b (p. 1147)
9. b (p. 1141)
10. b (p. 1150)

CLINICAL SITUATIONS

1. The nurse's assessment should include a sleep history
so as to understand how the client's pain is influencing his ability to fall asleep and stay asleep. Is the pain
aggravated at night? Is the client using therapies for
pain relief that disrupt sleep? How are the client's
sleep habits affecting his wife's ability to sleep? It is
likely that they are experiencing insomnia.
2. The factors that suggest a sleep problem include an
excessive caffeine intake, inconsistent sleep schedule,
and a high level of physical activity just before bedtime. It would be helpful to assess how her daytime
activities might be affected when sleep is inadequate.
Also, the nurse can assess if she has tried any measures (e.g., sleeping pills) to fall asleep. A nursing care
plan should include introducing noncaffeinated beverages. A recommendation to try certain relaxing activities such as reading before attempting to fall

asleep might be helpful. The client should also be asked if it is possible to control the scheduling of meetings so that at least a few evenings allow for an earlier bedtime.

Chapter 43
REVIEW QUESTIONS

1. b (p. 1154)
2. d (p. 1158)
3. c (p. 1162)
4. a (p. 1168)
5. c (p. 1185)
6. c (p. 1154)
7. b (p. 1176)
8. c (p. 1160)
9. c (p. 1172)
10. a (p. 1176)
11. d (p. 1174)
12. d (p. 1178-1179)

CLINICAL SITUATIONS

1. a. Mr. Jasper's pain is acute. The nurse's assessment will be focused on quickly determining the character of the pain, its location, and any factors that may aggravate or alleviate it. The client will anticipate a quick response on the part of the caregiver to provide pain relief. The nurse will likely administer an appropriate analgesic and use any therapies known to provide relief, such as positioning.

   Mr. Stern's pain is chronic. With no known cause, it will be particularly important for the nurse to trust the client's perceptions of how the pain is affecting him. The nurse should be alert for symptoms of chronic pain such as fatigue, sleepiness, insomnia, anorexia, or depression. In addition the nurse needs to know if the client has any periods of remission or exacerbation. Chronic pain can influence a client's life-style. Has Mr. Stern had problems at work or with family life? Treatment may include activities such as relaxation and guided imagery, exercises prescribed by a physician or physical therapist, and heat applications. Analgesics may be more effective before bedtime or when the client participates in certain physical activities.

   b. An older client with chronic pain may suffer more loss in functional status than a younger client. If the client has cognitive impairment, he may be unable to provide the nurse with a complete history of the pain. It therefore might be helpful to include a family member in assessing how the pain affects the client. The nurse should also assess if the older client has other medical conditions that also cause back pain. Finally, it will be important to watch the client's posture and behaviors because older clients often do not report pain.

2. Position the client on his right side or supine, as determined by his tolerance to those positions. Be sure the dressing is not constricting the client's arm. A back massage may facilitate his ability to relax and lessen pain perception. Distraction and relaxation may be useful during time when the pain is less severe.

Chapter 44
REVIEW QUESTIONS

1. a (p. 1195)
2. c (p. 1194)
3. b (p. 1197)
4. b (p. 1203)
5. a (p. 1206)
6. b (p. 1207)
7. d (p. 1207)
8. b (p. 1211-1212)
9. c (p. 1214)
10. a (p. 1215)
11. b (p. 1227)
12. c (p. 1243)

CLINICAL SITUATIONS

1. Consider precipitating factors associated with chest pain, location, radiation, and duration of pain, presence of other symptoms associated with pain, and measures that relieve pain. Interventions are directed at reducing the pain (analgesics and vasodilators), maintaining or improving oxygenation (oxygen therapy), and reducing further injury (rest and interventional therapies).

2. Perform a complete pulmonary assessment, including chest wall motion; lung expansion and sounds; sputum; ability to cough and clear airway; mobility status; length and location of incision; type of pain control ordered; evaluation of preoperative learning regarding turn, cough, and deep breathing.

   Interventions: frequent turning and coughing to mobilize secretions. The actual schedule depends on client assessment. Suction if necessary. Assist the client to walk and sit up in a chair.

Chapter 45
REVIEW QUESTIONS

1. b (p. 1248)
2. c (p. 1249)
3. c (p. 1253)
4. d (Table 45-4)
5. a (Table 45-4)
6. c (Table 45-3)
7. b (p. 1250)
8. b (Table 45-5)
9. c (p. 1265)
10. d (p. 1267)
11. d (p. 1285)
12. a (p. 1290)

CLINICAL SITUATIONS

1. Because Mrs. Calhoun's urine output is markedly less than her intake, the ability of her kidneys to excrete serum potassium may be impaired, and here serum potassium may be elevated. Especially in light of her dysrhythmia, Mrs. Calhoun's serum potassium should be tested immediately. The nurse should ask Mrs. Calhoun if she is experiencing weakness, fatigue, or numbness and tingling (paresthesia). The nurse should test muscle tone, palpate for intestinal distention, and auscultate for decreased bowel sounds. The nurse should obtain an order for an ECG to determine the type of dysrhythmia present and the presence of U waves. The potassium supplement should be held at this time until the results of the serum potassium level are known.

2. The nurse should choose macrodrop tubing because Mr. Jones needs fairly rapid infusion of the IV fluids over 6 hours. At a rate of 176 ml/hr (1000 ml divided by 6 hr), 500 ml of IV solution should have been infused by 8 PM so that the IV fluids are behind. The nurse should check the rate of the IV solution and attempt to establish the ordered rate of 167 ml/hr by using the clamp on the tubing to verify the correct settings on the IV pump. If the fluids will not run that fast, the nurse should ensure that there are no kinks in the tubing. If the fluids still do not infuse correctly, the nurse should verify that the client's arm is positioned so that there is no impairment of venous return and that no dressing, clothing, or other item is so tight on the arm that it impairs venous return. If these measures do not restore the IV rate, the nurse should inspect the IV site for infiltration. If an infiltration is not evident, the nurse may manipulate the IV catheter to ensure that it is not adhering to the side of the vein, which can slow the rate.

Chapter 46
REVIEW QUESTIONS

1. a (p. 1296-1297)
2. b (Table 46-1)
3. b (p. 1300-1301)
4. c (p. 1308)
5. a (p. 1310)
6. a (p. 1311-1312)
7. d (p. 1313)
8. d (p. 1317)
9. a (Table 46-4)
10. a (p. 1326)
11. a (p. 1336-1337)

CLINICAL SITUATIONS

1. If the client has other children, assess for previous need for catherization. Examine perineum for extensive swelling from vaginal birth. It is most likely that the client's inability to void is due to perineal swelling. Using a straight catheter to relieve bladder distention and providing the client with perineal ice pack will reduce swelling as well as the need for additional catheterization. In most cases a straight catheter is used with the postpartum client because this is usually a one time need.

2. Assess both the scrotum and penile shaft for signs of swelling, edema, abrasions, or skin breakdown. Assess for excessive moisture and know if the client is circumcised.

Chapter 47
REVIEW QUESTIONS

1. b (p. 1342)
2. b (p. 1344)
3. a (p. 1357)
4. c (p. 1359)
5. b (p. 1372)
6. c (Table 47-6)
7. b (p. 1361-1362)
8. c (Table 47-7)
9. c (p. 1364)
10. a (p. 1364)

CLINICAL SITUATIONS

1. A comprehensive plan would consist of the following:
   a. Ascertaining the frequency with which he usually defecates
   b. Keeping an accurate daily record of his bowel movements to detect early evidence of constipation
   c. Ensuring a dietary intake high in fiber
   d. Ensuring a 24-hour fluid intake of 300 ml. Since he is young and otherwise in good health, he can tolerate a large intake of fluid but should be on accurate intake and output.

2. Advise both your client and the daughter to keep the area clean and dry. The skin can be cleaned with a mild soap and water or a commercial preparation such as PeriWash. Do not use hydrogen peroxide or alcohol around the area because both are irritating to the skin. If bleeding, swelling, redness, itching, or unusual tenderness occur, be sure to contact the physician, the enterostomal therapy nurse, or both.

Chapter 48

REVIEW QUESTIONS

1. b (Table 48-1)
2. d (Table 48-2)
3. c (p. 1382)
4. a (p. 1384)
5. c (p. 1389)
6. b (p. 1393)
7. a (p. 1398)
8. c (p. 1402)
9. b (p. 1415)
10. a (p. 1415)
11. b (p. 1416)

CLINICAL SITUATIONS

1. The nurse should determine to what extent Mrs. Tice is fearful of being diagnosed with cancer. Her anxiety regarding her diagnosis should be addressed in the nurse's plan of care. In addition, her unfamiliarity with surgery may further increase her anxiety and fears. The nurse will assess fully the client's level of understanding regarding surgery and her expectations for the procedure. It would also be useful to assess the physician's expectations.

   Mrs. Tice's history of smoking will require an assessment of pulmonary status as well as the ability of the client to perform coughing and deep breathing exercises. Since the client takes antihypertensive medications, the nurse will assess preoperative vital signs to monitor for any alterations preoperatively.

2. The first factor to consider is reduced peristalsis. Does the client have a return of bowel sounds? If not, and if the client is becoming nauseated, a physician may have a nasogastric tube inserted.

   If the client had abdominal surgery, the nurse might also assess for possible internal bleeding. If this is the case, the client also will show signs of falling blood pressure and a rising pulse.

Chapter 49

REVIEW QUESTIONS

1. a (p. 1431)
2. c (Table 49-2)
3. d (p. 1433)
4. c (Table 49-3)
5. d (p. 1447)
6. c (p. 1439)
7. d (p. 1450)
8. c (Table 49-5)
9. d (Table 49-6)
10. c (Table 49-7)
11. a (p. 1462)

CLINICAL SITUATIONS

1. Location and presentation are consistent with a burn. Further assessment should include the temperature of the water used to fill the hot water bottle, the material used to insulate the hot water bottle, whether the client distinguishes hot and cold, and the size and depth of the injury incurred. Treatment may include cold compresses to the area, if not contraindicated as the source of the abdominal pain is determined. Local care should be to cover the injured area with a nonadherent dressing. The physician may prescribe an antimicrobial ointment.

   Teaching should focus on the use of hot water bottles for hot/cold therapy. Temperature of the solution used, the insulating material used, and the length of time the modality is used should be reviewed with the client.

2. Installation of hydrogen peroxide into a tract is not recommended because of the risk of air embolism. In this client, where the base of the wound is not visible, cleansing in this manner is not recommended. Discuss alternative methods of cleansing this wound with the prescribing physician. Other methods may include using normal saline, water via syringe or handheld shower, or a manufactured wound cleanser.